Alcohol, psychiatry and society

Manchester University Press

SOCIAL HISTORIES OF MEDICINE

Series editors: David Cantor, Elaine Leong and Keir Waddington

Social Histories of Medicine is concerned with all aspects of health, illness and medicine, from prehistory to the present, in every part of the world. The series covers the circumstances that promote health or illness, the ways in which people experience and explain such conditions, and what, practically, they do about them. Practitioners of all approaches to health and healing come within its scope, as do their ideas, beliefs, and practices, and the social, economic and cultural contexts in which they operate. Methodologically, the series welcomes relevant studies in social, economic, cultural, and intellectual history, as well as approaches derived from other disciplines in the arts, sciences, social sciences and humanities. The series is a collaboration between Manchester University Press and the Society for the Social History of Medicine.

Previously published

Migrant architects of the NHS *Julian M. Simpson*

Mediterranean quarantines, 1750–1914 *Edited by John Chircop and Francisco Javier Martínez*

Sickness, medical welfare and the English poor, 1750–1834 *Steven King*

Medical societies and scientific culture in nineteenth-century Belgium *Joris Vandendriessche*

Vaccinating Britain *Gareth Millward*

Madness on trial *James E. Moran*

Early Modern Ireland and the world of medicine *Edited by John Cunningham*

Feeling the strain *Jill Kirby*

Rhinoplasty and the nose in early modern British medicine and culture *Emily Cock*

Communicating the history of medicine *Edited by Solveig Jülich and Sven Widmalm*

Progress and pathology *Edited by Melissa Dickson, Emilie Taylor-Brown and Sally Shuttleworth*

Balancing the self *Edited by Mark Jackson and Martin D. Moore*

Global health and the new world order *Edited by Jean-Paul Gaudillière, Claire Beaudevin, Christoph Gradmann, Anne M. Lovell and Laurent Pordié*

Accounting for health: Calculation, paperwork and medicine, 1500–2000 *Edited by Axel C. Hüntelmann and Oliver Falk*

Women's medicine *Caroline Rusterholz*

Germs and governance: The past, present and future of hospital infection, prevention and control *Edited by Anne Marie Rafferty, Marguerite Dupree and Fay Bound Alberti*

Leprosy and identity in the Middle Ages: From England to the Mediterranean *Edited by Elma Brenner and François-Olivier Touati*

Patient voices in Britain, 1840–1948 *Edited by Anne Hanley and Jessica Meyer*

Medical histories of Belgium: New narratives on health, care and citizenship in the nineteenth and twentieth centuries *Edited by Joris Vandendriessche and Benoît Majerus*

Alcohol, psychiatry and society

Comparative and transnational perspectives, *c.* 1700–1990s

Edited by

Waltraud Ernst and Thomas Müller

Manchester University Press

Published by Manchester University Press
Oxford Road, Manchester M13 9PL

www.manchesteruniversitypress.co.uk

British Library Cataloguing-in-Publication Data
A catalogue record for this book is available from the British Library

Published with support from the Centre for Psychiatry Suedwürttemberg / Clinic for Psychiatry and Psychotherapy I, The University of Ulm, FRG.

zfp
Südwürttemberg

ISBN 978 1 5261 5940 3 hardback

First published 2022

Typeset
by Cheshire Typesetting Ltd, Cuddington, Cheshire

Contents

Figures

Tables

Contributors

Jasmin Brötz obtained her PhD in history at the University of Koblenz, where she also studied for an MA in philosophy and history. She is a fellow in the research project 'Semantic transformations in the twentieth century' of the German Research Foundation (DFG). Her specialist field of enquiry concerns 'rationalisation, knowledge and scientification around 1900'. Previously she worked for the German Federal Archives for a critical edition entitled *Die Kabinettsprotokolle der Bundesregierung* (Cabinet Minutes of the Federal Government). Currently, she belongs to the staff of the Federal Archives' picture section and teaches at the Department for Cultural Studies at the University of Koblenz. Her general research interests include German history (nineteenth and twentieth centuries), history of science and historical semantics.

Ricardo Campos is a research scientist at the History Institute of the CSIC (Madrid). He has been secretary (2006–14) and editor-in-chief (2015–19) of *Asclepio. Revista de de historia de la medicina y de la ciencia* (Asclepio: Journal of History of Medicine and Science). Between 2017 and 2021 he was president of the Sociedad Española de Historia de la Medicina (Spanish Society for the History of Medicine). He is a founding member of the Red Iberoamericana de Historia de la Psiquiatría (Ibero-American Network of History of Psychiatry). He has worked on various topics in the fields of history of public health, social regulation of illness and history of psychiatry (especially care models and the concept of mental illness), as well as the relationship between insanity and crime. He is the author of, among other works, *Alcoholismo, medicina* *y sociedad en España (1876–1923)* (Alcoholism, Medicine and Society in Spain (1876–1923) (1997), *El caso Morillo: crimen, locura y subjetividad en la España de la Restauración* (The Morillo Trial: Crime, Madness and Subjectivity in Spain's Restoration) (2012) and *La sombra de la sospecha. Peligrosidad, psiquiatría y derecho en España (siglos XIX y XX)* (The Shadow of Suspicion: Dangerousness, Psychiatry and Law in Spain (Nineteenth and Twentieth Centuries) (2021).

Waltraud Ernst is Emerita Professor in the Department of History, Philosophy and Culture at Oxford Brookes University, UK. Her research focuses on the history of mental illness and alcohol in South Asia, and her publications include *Mad Tales from the Raj* (1991; 2010), *Colonialism and Transnational Psychiatry* (2013) and *Health and Medicine in the Indian Princely States* (2018; with B. Pati and T. V. Sekher). She has edited a number of books: *Alcohol Flows across Cultures* (2020), *Work, Psychiatry and Society* (2016), *Transnational Psychiatries* (2010/2015; with T. Müller), *Crossing Colonial Historiographies* (2010; with A. Digby and P.B. Mukharji), *India's Princely States* (2007; with B. Pati), *The Normal and the Abnormal* (2006), *Plural Medicine, Tradition and Modernity* (2002) and *Race, Science and Medicine* (1999; with B.J. Harris).

Adéla Gjuričová is Senior Researcher at the Institute of Contemporary History of the Czech Academy of Sciences in Prague. She focuses on politics and society during the late socialist era, the 1989 revolutions and post-communist transformations in Central Europe. She has worked on a number of projects dealing with parliamentary history and the history of expert cultures. Currently she leads the Czech team within the JPICH CADEAH project on 'European history reloaded: curation and appropriation of digital audio-visual heritage'. She is co-author of *Rozděleni minulostí: vytváření politických identit v České republice po roce 1989* (Divided by the Past: Political Identities in the Czech Republic after 1989) (2011), *Lebenswelten von Abgeordneten in Europa 1860–1990* (The Life-Worlds of Members of Parliament, 1860–1990) (2014), *Návrat parlamentu: Češi a Slováci ve Federálním shromáždění 1989–1992* (The Return of Parliament: The Czechs and Slovaks in the Federal Assembly 1989–1992) (2018) and *Architekti dlouhé změny. Expertní kořeny postsocialismu v Československu* (The Architects of Long Change: Expert Roots of Post-Socialism, 2019).

Kostis Gkotsinas studied history and archaeology at the National and Kapodistrian University of Athens. He completed his PhD dissertation on drugs in Greek inter-war society at the École des Hautes Études en Sciences Sociales in Paris. His research interests include the history of psychoactive substances, cultural and social history, deviance and state formation, gender and sexuality, the social aspects of armed conflicts and the urban setting of cultural practices. He is currently a scientific fellow at the École Française d'Athènes, working on the project '"Entre global et local". L'histoire civile d'une armée oubliée: l'Armée d'Orient, 1915–1919' (Left behind? The global and civilian history of a forgotten army: the Armée d'Orient, 1915–1919), with a particular interest in the leisure time of soldiers and civilians in the city of Salonika and in Macedonia during World War I. His monograph on the history of drugs in Greece (1875–1950) was published in French in 2022 and in Greek in 2020. He is currently working on an edited volume on alcohol in nineteenth- and twentieth-century Greece.

Akira Hashimoto is Professor of Social Welfare at Aichi Prefectural University, Japan. He received his PhD from the University of Tokyo in 1992 and studied on a German Academic Exchange Service scholarship at the University of Düsseldorf, Germany (1992–94). He has studied the history of psychiatry in Europe and Asia from a comparative point of view, specialising on the Belgian colony of Gheel and its international relevance in the nineteenth and twentieth centuries, as well as the history of institutionalised patients and their communities under the Mental Patients' Custody Act (1900–50) in Japan. He is currently researching the history of psychiatry in Japanese remote islands and other Far East countries in the nineteenth and twentieth centuries, from a colonial/post-colonial perspective. His publications include *Places of Treatment and the History of Psychiatry* (in Japanese; 2010) and *Mental Patients and Private Confinement at Home* (in Japanese; 2011).

Simon Heap is the long-standing editor of the African Studies Association of the UK (ASAUK) newsletter. With degrees from the University of Cambridge and the School of Oriental and African Studies, London, Simon was awarded a doctorate from the University of Ibadan on 'The liquor trade and the Nigerian economy, 1880–1939', funded by a Leverhulme Trust Study Abroad Studentship. He then held the Antony Kirk-Greene Junior Research Fellowship at St Antony's College, University of Oxford. After working in the international non-governmental organisation sector for fifteen years, Simon was the first holder of the Britain-Nigeria Educational Trust Commonwealth Fellowship in 2011 at his alma mater, the University of Ibadan. He is now in the Academic Office of Oxford Brookes University. Simon's published work and presentations can be found at https://oxfordbrookes.academia.edu/DrSimonHeap/. His latest work includes 'Processing delinquents at the Salvation Army's Boys' Industrial Home in Lagos, 1925–1944', in Saheed Aderinto (ed.), *Children and Childhoods in Colonial Nigerian Histories* (2015), and 'The postal service of Calabar, 1890–1960: historical cultural artefacts for contemporary tourism', in Paul Lovejoy et al. (eds), *Calabar on the Cross River* (2017).

David Korostyshevsky obtained his PhD at the University of Minnesota. He is a faculty member in the Department of History at Colorado State University. Focusing on the British Atlantic world and nineteenth-century America, he studies how changing chemical, medical and physiological understandings of alcohol were used to construct temperance arguments, discipline habitual drunkards in civil courts and exclude drinkers from life insurance.

Jacqueline Leckie is an adjunct research fellow with the Stout Centre for New Zealand Studies at Victoria University of Wellington and a conjoint associate professor in the School of Humanities and Social Sciences at the University of Newcastle, Australia. Her interdisciplinary research and publications are on the history and anthropology of Asia-Pacific. Jacqui taught for several years in the Department of Anthropology and Archaeology at Otago University, and earlier at the University of the South Pacific and Kenyatta University. In 2018 she was the J.D. Stout Research Fellow at the Stout Research Centre at Victoria University of Wellington. Her books include *Colonizing Madness: Asylum and Community in Fiji* (2020), *Indian Settlers: The Story of a New Zealand South Asian Community* (2007) and *To Labour with the State* (1997). She has edited *Development in an Insecure and Gendered World* (2009), *Migrant Cross-Cultural Encounters in Asia and the Pacific* (2016; with A. McCarthy and A. Wanhalla), *Asians and the New Multiculturalism in Aotearoa New Zealand* (2015; with G. Ghosh), *Localizing Asia in Aotearoa* (2011; with P. Voci), *Recentring Asia* (2011; with J. Edmond and H. Johnson) and *Labour in the South Pacific* (1990; with C. Moore and D. Munro).

Thomas Müller is Professor of the History and Ethics of Medicine at Ulm University, Germany. He is both a medical doctor (Charité Berlin) and a historian (MA, Free University, Berlin). He researched and lectured in the history of medicine at Free University and Humboldt University in Berlin from 1998 to 2006, and inaugurated a research unit for the history of medicine at Ulm University's Clinic for Psychiatry and Psychotherapy I / Centre of Psychiatry Südwürttemberg, Ravensburg, in 2006. He is head of the Württemberg Museum of Psychiatry. His topics of research include the history of psychotherapies and psychiatry, comparative history of medicine, medicine and Jewry, memorial culture (with a focus on National Socialist war crimes) and the integration of history of medicine into current concepts and reformed models of medical education. He is the author of *Von Charlottenburg zum Central Park West. Henry Lowenfeld und die Psychoanalyse in Berlin, Prag und New York* (From Charlottenburg to Central Park West: Henry Lowenfeld and Psychoanalysis in Berlin, Prague and New York) (2000) and has edited a number of volumes on the history of psychiatry and psychotherapy such as *Psychotherapie und Körperarbeit in Berlin. Geschichte und Praktiken der Etablierung* (Psychotherapy and Body Therapy in Berlin: Histories and Practices of Implementation) (2004); *Transnational Psychiatries: Social and Cultural Histories of Psychiatry in Comparative Perspective, c. 1800–2000* (2010, 2nd edn 2015; co-edited with Waltraud Ernst); and *Zentrum und Peripherie in der Geschichte der Psychiatrie. Regionale, nationale und internationale*

Perspektiven (Centre and Periphery in the History of Psychiatry) (2017).

Mauricio Becerra Rebolledo did his MA in the history of health sciences at COC-FIOCRUZ, Rio de Janeiro, and obtained his PhD in the history of science at CEHIC-UAB, Barcelona. He studied science in social communication in Pontificia Universidad Católica de Valparaíso (PUCV). He worked as a journalist and editor of the newspaper *El Ciudadano* (Chile) between 2009 and 2012. His research topics are the history of psychiatry and psychiatric therapy in Latin America. In his recent research he focuses on the figure of the 'drug addict' in medical discourse. Results of these investigations have been published in 'De psicosis tóxica a predisposición mórbida: emergencia de la figura del toxicómano en Chile, 1872–1954' (2009, http://repositorio.ucv.cl/handle/10.4151/52584); 'Ruina, degeneración y contagio: toxicomanía y peligrosidad social en Chile' (2013, www.redalyc.org/toc.oa?id=902&numero=39866); and the chapter 'Ensayos farmacológicos y medicina experimental: trayectorias de los discursos biomédicos sobre las drogas en Chile (1875–1929)' (Pharmacological trials and experimental medicine: trajectories of biomedical discourses on drugs in Chile (1875–1929)), in Claudia Araya et al. (eds), *República de la salud, fundación y ruinas de un país sanitario. Chile siglos XIX y XX* (2016). Mauricio is a member of the Red Iberoamericana de Historia de la Psiquiatría (Ibero-American Network of History of Psychiatry). His current research is on the development of experimental psychiatry in Peru and the trials conducted on psychotomimetic substances in mental hospitals in Latin America during the mid-twentieth century.

Mat Savelli is an assistant professor in the Department of Health, Aging and Society at McMaster University. After completing his DPhil at the University of Oxford in the history of medicine, he was a Haas postdoctoral fellow at the Science History Institute (Philadelphia, USA) and a Mellon postdoctoral fellow at the University of Pittsburgh. He has published widely on topics ranging from the history of Yugoslav psychiatry to the global advertising of psychiatric medications. He is the co-editor of *Psychiatry in Communist Europe* (with Sarah Marks; 2015) and *Global*

Transformations in the Life Sciences, 1945–1980 (with Patrick Manning; 2018).

Nina S. Studer is a historian and Arabist with a strong focus on gender and the history of psychiatry in colonial contexts. Her PhD, which she wrote at the Universities of Zürich and Oxford on descriptions of Muslim North African women by French colonial psychiatrists, was published as *The Hidden Patients: North African Women in French Colonial Psychiatry* in 2016. Since then, she has conducted research into medical and psychiatric descriptions of drinking habits in the colonial Maghreb – with a special focus on absinthe, coffee, tea, wine, champagne and Orangina – and written a series of articles and chapters on these different drinks. Among other things, she has written an article on the history of teaism in Tunisia ('"Was trinkt der zivilisierte Mensch?" Teekonsum und morbide Normalität im kolonialen Maghreb') for the *Schweizerische Zeitschrift für Geschichte* (2014) and on absinthe in the colonial Maghreb ('The green fairy in the Maghreb: absinthe, guilt and cultural assimilation in French colonial medicine') for *The Maghreb Review* (2015). In addition to research on the medicalisaton of consumption habits in the colonial Maghreb, she is also in the process of writing her professorial thesis on the participation of women in various protest movements in Syria and Lebanon during the French mandate period.

Christian Werkmeister is a research associate at the Ettersberg Foundation in Weimar, focusing on comparative research on European dictatorships. He studied Eastern European history, political science and law at Friedrich Schiller University, Jena, and wrote his doctorate thesis on late Soviet youth culture. He taught history and Polish studies at Martin Luther University, Halle/Wittenberg and Jena, Germany. His main fields of interest include popular culture, Soviet history and the history of genocide. His publications include *Jugendszenen und Kulturpolitik in der späten Sowjetunion, 1975–1991* (2020); 'Wahnsinn mit System. Psychiatrische Anstalten in der späten UdSSR' in *Osteuropa* (2014); 'Die Geschichte des GULag im RuNet: Möglichkeiten und Grenzen virtueller Erinnerungskulturen' (with Martin Müller-Butz), in Jörg

Ganzenmüller and Raphael Utz (eds), *Sowjetische Verbrechen und russische Erinnerung: Orte Akteure Deutungen* (2014); and 'Johannes Lepsius und die Verbrechen an den Armeniern. Die Vorgeschichte der UN-Genozidkonvention', in Sybille Steinbacher (ed.), *Holocaust und Völkermorde: Die Reichweite des Vergleichs* (2012).

Acknowledgements

The volume's development benefited from a research workshop held at St Anne's College, Oxford, from 29 to 30 June 2017. We acknowledge the financial support received from the Research Unit for the History of Medicine at the Centre for Psychiatry Südwürttemberg, Clinic for Psychiatry and Psychotherapy I, the University of Ulm at Ravensburg (Germany) and the Faculty of Humanities and Social Sciences at Oxford Brookes University (UK), which helped make the event enjoyable and productive. We also greatly appreciate the valuable contributions to the research workshop and discussions by Aude Fauvel, Tudor Georgescu, James Moran, Iain Smith, Len Smith, Oonagh Walsh and Melissa Stepney. We thank Jane Freebody for getting us organised so efficiently, the series editor, David Cantor, for his guidance and support and the reviewer of the final manuscript for their helpful comments.

Introduction: comparative and transnational perspectives on alcohol, psychiatry and society, *c.* 1500–1991

Waltraud Ernst and Thomas Müller

> I mix three kraters [large jars] only for those who are wise.
> One is for good health, which they drink first.
> The second is for love and pleasure.
> …
> The ninth to bile.
> The tenth to madness, in that it makes people throw things[1]
>
> (Eubulus, fourth century BCE)

Alcohol and madness in social historical context

In his humorously insightful list, the Athenian comedy poet Eubulus juxtaposed the amount of alcohol consumed and its effects on the drinker's physical and mental health. After one or two measures, love and pleasure were followed by sleep, conceit, shouting, carousal, black eyes and court proceedings, finally culminating, after all too many drinks, in the two aspects of the ancient Greek concept of melancholy: depression and mania or madness. LAs nowadays, commonplace emotions and conditions, morally flawed states and mental ailments were portrayed as being implicated in the consumption of varied volumes of alcoholic drink. This apparently enduring continuity shows that alcohol has a long history, both as a substance which could bring joy and conviviality or dejection and irascibility to those who imbibe it, and as a factor in disturbed mental health.

Many cultures understood the link between over-consumption of intoxicating beverages and the deterioration of physical and mental health. The idea that alcohol works as either medicine or poison for the body as well as for the mind, depending on the quantity consumed, is therefore neither new nor specific to the modern period. Nor is this idea restricted to particular geo-cultural locations. Beyond the Western, classical world of Greece and Rome, intoxicating substances and their quotidian, moral, physical and mental consequences were described at length in the Sanskrit medical compendia in South Asia, for example. Although the concept of 'alcohol' as a substance did not exist in the Vedas (*c.* 1500–1200 BCE), the oldest scriptures of Hinduism, the intoxicating (*madya)* effects of the many, widely imbibed beverages or *sura* (brewed from malted grains, sugar cane and a number of fruits and flower saps) as well as criteria for their beneficial use were listed in later Sanskrit medical collections such as the *Carakasamhita* (400–200 BCE).[2] There is indeed, as William Bynum put it, 'a long medical literature variously extolling the virtues and condemning the bad effects of alcohol'.[3]

For the modern period in Europe, historians of medicine such as Bynum, Roy Porter, Jonathan Reinarz and Rebecca Wynter have charted how doctors in Europe and North America warned and even preached against over-consumption of alcohol, while they also prescribed various alcoholic beverages in order to ameliorate a range of physical and mental conditions.[4] Even the American politician and physician Benjamin Rush (1746–1813), who favoured abstinence and was one of the first to define 'habitual drunkenness' as a disease,[5] reiterated blithely permissive, popular beliefs earlier in his life:

> Why all this noise about wine and strong drink? ... have we not seen hundreds who have made it a constant practice to get drunk almost everyday for 30 or 40 years, who notwithstanding, arrived to a great age, and enjoyed the same good health as those who have followed the strictest rules of temperance?[6]

Merrily light-hearted and sombre popular and medical ideas were intertwined in the minds of doctors. This was true also for the wider population, as the abundance of self-help compendia and nostrums that recommended and made use of alcohol attests.[7] In contrast to Rush's earlier contentions, the tenor of his famous 'Scale of the Progress of Temperance and Intemperance' of 1790 is more prescriptive and negative in its message about liquors' progressively harmful effects, which are evocatively rendered in their 'usual Order' (see Figure 0.1).

This measuring scheme of happiness, harm and doom has some heuristic resonance with Eubulus's outline, except for the wider range of beverages specified by the American. Both refer to common human qualities and experiences, moral and legal categories and medical conditions of both the purely physical and mental variety, and, in Rush's Judaeo-Christian version, the listing includes bad habits helpfully labelled 'vice', as well as obligingly instructive pointers to penances to be endured that enunciate their religiously informed provenance. While Eubulus's lyrical inventory aims to entertain and instruct, Rush's is based on a medley of medical categories and moral concepts, and serves as both religio-moral warning and medical spreadsheet of causes, diseases, symptoms, prognoses and consequences.

An investigation into the historical origin of beverages, and the ideas and practices connected with them, reveals an association between alcohol and madness as far back as ancient history and to medical frameworks in non-Graeco-Roman cultures. However, attempts at identifying similarities and apparent links across time and space tend to neglect the importance of the specific medical cosmologies within which ideas about alcohol were embedded, and the very different explanatory socio-economic reference points to which they were anchored. This gives grounds for analytical caution. First, on account of the historical and cultural specificity of medical ideas and practices, it is difficult to postulate a clear, universal continuity of the terms, concepts and experiences of drunkenness and of what was seen to constitute harmful over-consumption over time. Second, as drinking is not merely a medical concern or an act of individual preference for certain beverages but is also dependent on the availability of products, as well as the wider social, political and religious settings within which it occurs, historisation and contextualisation of alcohol in relation to mental health are at least as important as the identification of any similarities over time. A temporal limitation and hence an analytical focus on a shorter time span is therefore sensible and called for, especially when spatial

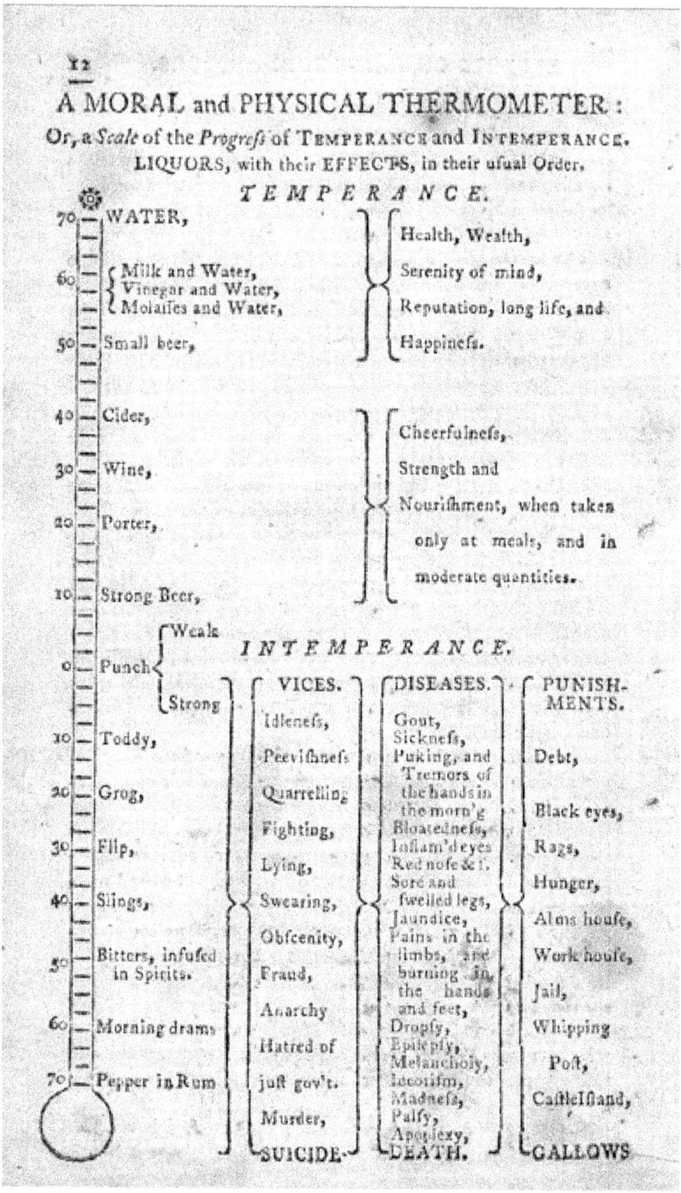

Figure 0.1 The moral thermometer from Benjamin Rush's *An Inquiry into the Effects of Spirituous Liquors on the Human Body and the Mind*, 1790

comparisons across different geo-cultural regions are intended, as is the case in this edited volume.

Admittedly, cultural attitudes to and medical prescriptions of alcohol may not be completely incommensurable over the *longue durée*, but there are certain limitations. Take the example of the South Asian tradition of medical writing as revealed in the *Carakasamhita*, which devoted a lengthy section (chapter 24) to alcohol: its properties, effects and uses. Notwithstanding structural affinities with modern Western compendia, the crucial point in this sophisticated medical system is that the actual effect of a substance depends on a person's physical and mental constitution. According to the Ayurvedic framework of the humours, intoxicating drinks are ascribed ten qualities (ranging from light and hot to sedative and rough). These are juxtaposed with the ten qualities of the vital fluids or *ojas* (heavy, cold, etc.) in the human body. According to this framework, when particular kinds of drinks or *suras* are imbibed, they create an imbalance in the person's heart, where the *ojas* reside, and affect her or his body and mind in either harmful or beneficial ways that are specific to the individual. The Ayurvedic schema therefore holds that any medical intervention dealing with alcohol-related problems or employing alcohol as a remedy needs to be applied in accordance with a person's singular bodily and mental makeup. Despite apparent resemblances between Ayurvedic and modern medical ideas – in terms of their recognition of the variously beneficial and damaging effects of alcohol, the stages of inebriety and even the role of moderation – the ways in which substances are seen to interact with the internal vital fluids and a person's physiological and mental constitution cannot easily be mapped on to each other. In other words, while the identification of the clear stages of intoxication in the *Carakasamhita* may reverberate with Eubulus's and Rush's schemas, the medical framework that guides the Ayurvedic doctor's diagnostic and therapeutic practice is distinctly different. In Ayurveda, drink is not universally and inherently good or bad; its effects and the treatment of over-consumption depend on a person's individual constitution. This principle applies to all beverages, not just intoxicating brews. As medicine is not a closed system, nor aloof from wider society, popular ideas and experiences of drinking too are bound to be shot through with principles and features that may be different from those espoused in modern medical and social contexts.

To avoid anachronistic and sweeping culture-centric accounts, historical contextualisation and 'thick description' need to be components of critical and nuanced writing on alcohol. This is important not only in regard to the medical system within which drinking was embedded but also in relation to the wider contexts that framed drinking behaviours and medical and popular responses to them. The Ayurveda extolled in the *Carakasamhita*, for example, was no 'folk medicine', but practised by highly trained physicians and not easily accessible to all strata of society. It was part of a socio-religious cosmology that considered intoxicating liquors as the drink of common people and of demons, and hence as impure and forbidden to the social elite.[8] The Hindu socio-economic and ritual hierarchy, which was seen to be adorned by the Brahmin caste at its apex, had a pivotal role in how different groups in society were supposed to relate to the consumption of substances, both intoxicating and otherwise. In theory, if not in practice, alcohol and religion were here the opium of the masses. Or, as Dietler puts it, the consumption of embodied material culture, like alcohol, 'constitutes a prime arena for the negotiation, projection, and contestation of power'.[9] The freedom to drink or the obligation to abstain from certain beverages simultaneously reifies social differences and enables stratified social cohesion, represented in either ritualised commensal consumption or refusal of consumption.[10] The chapters in this book pursue approaches that firmly locate drinking and mental health within their varied social contexts and in relation to the societal powers that govern them, and set out to avoid undue generalisations over time and place.[11]

The medicalisation of drunkenness and drinking in the Anglo-European world

A main trope in histories of alcohol has been the 'medicalisation' of drunkenness – if not of drinking *per se* – over the course of the modern period.[12] The suggestion is that something like a 'paradigm shift' began in Western countries around the late nineteenth century: a shift that replaced earlier perceptions of drunkenness as a moral problem or 'vice' with a conception – by the period between the two world wars – of alcoholism as a disease requiring medical therapeutic intervention. At the heart of this conceptual and representational trajectory was, it is argued, the transformation of 'intemperance' into 'alcoholism', and hence the move in debates on alcohol from the moral sphere to the realm of science-based medicine. As discussed above, during many periods and in many places both medicine and morals, as well as a range of other factors to boot, were implicated in the management of drinking and in the treatment of the physical and mental conditions arising from it. Moral and medical concerns have in fact been close drinking fellows for a long time. The question arises: what, if anything, is different in the professed new process of the medicalisation of alcohol consumption?

First, 'intemperance' and the emphasis on 'vice' and 'immoral' habits were connected with nineteenth-century reformers' ambition to exorcise the demon drink – through appeals to people's moral sense or religious duty – while 'alcoholism' emerged as a concomitant to the gradual consolidation of the medical profession as an interest group of state-accredited medical experts in Western countries. It is of course important to trace how new psychiatric categories such as alcohol insanity, dipsomania and, eventually, addiction and alcoholism came to subsume intemperate habits under the banner of a disease concept developed by a particular brand of newly professionalised medical experts: alienists, asylum doctors and psychiatrists.

However, an exclusive focus on the medical in relation to alcohol lacks nuance, as the medicalisation of drinking was set within and framed by responses to drinking and drunkenness that remained multiply determined, with ethical, mundane, religious, commercial, medical, superstitious, political, economic and other concerns intertwining to varying extents at any one time and place.[13] Even when a person is diagnosed as or is self-identifying with the medical category of 'alcoholic', they may still see themselves, or be considered by others, as morally culpable, politically irresponsible, psychologically weak or simply repulsive. Medical interventions and the prevalence of a medicalised discourse on alcohol do not preclude positive or negative social ascriptions or moral stigmatisation, and the medical is always also imbued with the morals of the time. Therefore, while the observed shift towards medicalisation – and the appearance of new medical concepts and of novel physiological understandings of alcohol consumption – may be historically distinct and clinically relevant, it does not provide us with a complete picture of the many and varied functions, meanings and popular representations of drinking and drunkenness. The aim in this book is therefore to identify how modern psychiatry's discourse on alcohol sat within and alongside, was fuelled by and drove other issues, such as those of empire, social class, religion, race, gender, population control, nationalism, oppression, medical power and politics.

Second, the postulated trend from 'moralisation' to 'medicalisation' occurred over the course of the long nineteenth and twentieth centuries, when science and medical power became consolidated as two important – and intrinsically linked – signifiers of Western modernity. This shift was predicated also on the marginalisation of heterodox medical discourses on alcohol that had prevailed during the presumed heyday of the moral, such as humoral medicine, naturopathy, homeopathy, mesmerism, balneology and a number of folk practices, to name but a few in relation to Western countries. Medical interventions had sat more or less comfortably alongside moral precepts. The perceived shift from moral to medical therefore owes much to the persistent and persuasive rhetoric and power of modern medicine and its historians, as well as to a certain historical amnesia about the prevalence of medical approaches before and during the age of reform. An exclusive historical focus on either the moral or the modern medical narrative of alcohol, in relation to mental health, neglects not only the social functions of alcohol but also drinkers' and over-drinkers' actual, mixed experiences, which cannot be reduced to just one dimension.

The role of culture

More recently, the important role of culture and community in alcohol consumption has been acknowledged among public health and policy officials, and a tendency towards the 'social-isation' and 'culturalisation' of drinking and drunkenness that draws on sociological and anthropological insights into the socio-cultural embeddedness of alcohol in both Western and non-Western countries has become more prominent.[14] Alcohol and drinking are beginning to be historicised and understood through the lenses of practice, politics, gender, race, age and communal bonding.[15] This kind of work owes much to anthropologists such as Mary Douglas and her classic *Constructive Drinking* of 1987, which paved the way for research on the social role of drinking, its ideological function and its economic significance.[16] A new focus on diverse and differentiated 'drinking cultures' and on their multiple, shifting and multifaceted nature – rather than on 'alcoholics, and their families' – has facilitated more nuanced research initiatives and therapeutic approaches.[17]

However, homogenising characterisations that are isolated from their historical context (such as 'dry' versus 'wet' cultures or 'Mediterranean drinking') and do not admit for fluidity of behaviours and changes over time, which have hitherto been prominent in some historical and sociological writing, have been challenged.[18] So has the prioritisation of the 'problem-focused' dimension that accentuates alcoholism and over-consumption and neglects the role of pleasure, social connection, intimacy, cultural belonging and cultural capital in drinking behaviours.[19] The need to develop historically grounded and context-specific multiple ethnographies of drinking and drunkenness is being seen as pressing at a time when alcoholism's financial burden to societies in high-income countries was estimated at 2.5 per cent of gross domestic product in 2009.[20] This need is not merely an academic issue. As alcohol constitutes a problem on a global scale, effective and sensible intervention would do well to focus on the factors that drive over-consumption, including those that are not narrowly pathologically and medically identifiable, such as pleasure, deprivation, social cohesion and historical factors.

Beyond the Anglo-European world of alcohol and drinking

An analysis of alcohol and drinking in colonial and post-colonial countries puts the multiple functions and meanings of alcohol consumption, as well as the global entanglements and local modifications of medical approaches to drinking, into sharp relief. The different socio-cultural and economic values and roles assigned to drinking and drunkenness, by colonisers and colonised and in regions outside Europe and North America, raise the question of whether the medical approaches forged in the minority world, or 'global north', were the sole and universally germane architypes of mental health interventions in regard to alcohol, rather than constituting but one, albeit an increasingly influential, trajectory among many others. Despite the importance of this issue, the regional scope remains sadly Euro- and Anglo-centric in the existing literature on alcohol and mental health. There are some notable exceptions, most of which focus on alcohol in relation to medicine more generally, such as Gretchen Pierce and Áurea Toxqui's and Deborah Toner's work on South and Central America respectively, Erica Wald's, Nandini Bhattacharya's and H. Fischer-Tine and J. Tschurenev's on South Asia, Gerard Sasges' on Indochina and Eric Engstrom and Ivan Crozier's on Indonesia.[21] Even within Europe, northern and Western countries have received far more attention than those in the east and the south of the continent, although Italy has been focused on more recently.[22] In North America, Australia and New Zealand, the history of drinking and alcohol abuse among First Nation people has been explored to a certain extent, while the African continent remains poorly covered.[23] The chapters in this book therefore offer insights into areas of analysis and geographical locations that have not hitherto figured prominently in histories of alcohol, let alone in regard to the nexus between drunkenness and mental health: southern Europe (Greece, Spain) and Eastern Europe (former Czechoslovakia, Yugoslavia, Soviet Union) as well as colonial and post-colonial countries (Brazil, Chile, Fiji, Nigeria, Algeria) and Japan.

In any historical analysis focused on colonial contexts, issues of economic power and political subjugation, military control and cultural hegemony, as well as race and religion, are central. This is no less so in regard to medical matters. The role of medicine and psychiatry in the justification of colonial rule and in the politics of the civilising mission has been well established in historical writing since the early 1990s.[24] Ideas on drinking and drunkenness among colonised people, and restrictive measures imposed despite the commercial value of alcohol imports and exports, therefore need to be set within these wider parameters. Medical concerns were, to a certain extent, a thorn in the side of commercial interest groups and colonial administrators alike, as both European alcohol and locally brewed 'country liquor' constituted good business for traders and manufacturers, as well as revenue for colonial tax departments. Restrictive alcohol policies therefore remained contested by many interest groups in the metropoles and colonies.

However, there were exceptions. First, on account of the importance of the military and navy in the process of colonisation, drunkenness among soldiers and sailors drew particular attention not only from medical officers, but also on the part of colonial authorities tasked with maintaining fighting power among the troops. Alcohol had traditionally been part of the same system of placatory disciplinary measures as, in the case of the British, generous rations of beef to ensure that men would willingly march or sail into battle on a full stomach. Excessive drinking did however take its toll on discipline, body and mind, especially in the tropics. In the case of colonial India, for example, the royal commission on the sanitary state of the army in India found in 1863 that each soldier consumed 18.5 gallons of raw spirit per annum, which is in stark contrast to the estimated 2.5 gallons consumed by adults in the United Kingdom in 2017.[25] In this situation, doctors and alcohol restrictions played an important role because, as the royal commission report put it: 'The value of a man who, with all his arms, costs the country £100 a year is considerable, and either the loss of his life, of his health, or of his efficiency, is not to be lightly regarded.'[26] Although medical interventions and restrictions on when and how alcohol was to be distributed had the potential to save colonial office resources, drunkenness continued to constitute a problem endemic among troops.[27]

Second, in regard to the wider colonial populations, both European alcohol and what was referred to as 'Country liquor' became increasingly, over the course of the nineteenth century, a fervently debated topic that paralleled concerns in the metropolises on the detrimental effect on people's bodies and minds of particular beverages, such as absinthe and other hard liquors. The impact of moral reformers' initiatives – and the flow of medical ideas and popular sentiments about alcohol and drinking from metropolitan centres to the colonial peripheries – was substantial, leading to colonial interventions that aimed at the emulation of measures taken in the colonial motherlands.[28] Yet, as several chapters in this book show, the starkly different socio-demographic, cultural and political circumstances prevalent in the colonies led to certain modifications of metropolitan blueprints. Such adaptations were rooted in the colonial prerequisite of racial exclusion as well as a multitude of essentialising tropes bound up with colonisers' perceptions of indigenous communities' assumed characteristics. One of them was the conjecture that traditional religious sentiment caused certain colonial communities such as 'the Muslims' to be abstinent and hence particularly susceptible to exposure to, and the harmful effects of, European alcohol. This assumption coexisted alongside the conviction that these groups lacked moral fibre and were hence prone to consume alcohol to excess. In regard to Africans in Nigeria, Europeans suggested that Africans could drink more alcohol without ill effects than they themselves could because they were physically stronger, while others contended that they were more susceptible to the effects of spirits.

Such varied and incommensurable, yet equally homogenising, narratives of assumed 'native' predispositions and propensities in contrast to the similarly sweeping, if sepia-toned, regard for the 'civilised European', fuelled the race-specific ascription of different 'vices' and medical conditions. In British India, for example, 'alcohol insanity' was seen to be mainly a European condition, while Indians were considered more prone to suffer from 'cannabis insanity'. However, the Indian psychiatrist and director at the Ranchi mental hospital, J.E. Dhunjibhoy, suggested in a 1930 article in the *Journal of Mental Science*, still cited by drugs and addiction researchers, that alcohol was 'largely consumed in those parts of India where the hemp drug is difficult to obtain or is unknown'.[29] His European colleague at the institution at Agra, in contrast, focused not so much on the availability of particular drugs as on Indians' cultural habits:

> Alcohol is not so frequent a cause of mental and nervous disorders in India as in countries where European races constitute the bulk of

> the population, mainly because of caste and religious customs, which prevent the Indian on the whole from indulging in it.[30]

Not surprisingly, in regard to types of 'alcoholic psychosis', Indian and British doctors disagreed about the role of racial factors, with the former arguing that they were 'the same as one sees in the West'[31] and the latter that 'The effects of alcohol vary greatly, not only between individuals, but between races.'[32]

However ill conceived, factually inaccurate and racially prejudiced such epidemiological assessments and diagnostic categories may have been – especially in view of the multitude of indigenous brews and liquors consumed by Indian communities – the exertion of medico-cultural power and the right to typify Indians' assumed racial habits became, alongside military force and economic profiteering, well-established core tenets of colonial rule. Sentiments of civilisationary superiority and racial difference were at their heart, and medical views on drinking and drunkenness among colonised populations both fuelled and mirrored these.

On the other hand, concerns about the 'diseases of civilisation' in European countries were rife from the eighteenth century onwards. This was demonstrated in George Cheyne's *The English Malady* of 1733. The 'Malady' was seen to be endemic in particular among the English upper classes and characteristic of the first postulated 'Age of Melancholy'.[33] As a French observer exclaimed: 'Surely, the people of England are the most unhappy people on the face of the earth – with liberty, property and three meals a day.'[34] Notwithstanding their laudable political, economic and social advancements, Cheyne saw his upper-class compatriots' excessive eating and drinking habits as the second most prominent cause of disease and madness.[35] Progress and civilisation came at a cost. By the late nineteenth century, the figure of Mr Hyde in Robert Louis Stevenson's novella *Dr Jekyll and Mr Hyde* of 1886 embodied well the destructive forces assumed to lurk beneath the veneer of Western civilisation.[36] In their Western incarnation, alcohol and civilisation were bound up almost intrinsically, and the consumption of beers, wines and spirits, preferably European-manufactured, became an idealised signature habit of polite socialising at home and in the colonies, while 'other races' were seen as requiring this habit in order to qualify – if they were even deemed capable of qualifying at all – as members of the league of civilised drinking nations. On the other hand, there were also those at home and abroad who proselytised from their wagons against the fearsome evils of alcohol. As O'Brien has shown, alcohol had a central role both in the unfolding of Western civilisations and as a social pathology that fed ambivalent attitudes to drinking.[37]

As science and Western fledgling psychiatry were projected as signifiers of modernity and rationality, ideas on alcohol and madness became closely enmeshed with debates on tradition and irrationality, on the one hand, and the progress of civilisation and the health of nations on the other – in both metropolitan and colonial countries.[38] In fact, the prominence of modern medicine and the upsurge of racial science coincided with the nineteenth-century heydays of British and French colonial expansion and the Scramble for Africa, bestowing a key role on medicine and psychiatry also in the management of drinking in the metropoles and colonies.[39] During this period, the discourses of civilisation, national decline and degeneration were fuelled by the twin concerns of diseases of civilisation and the degeneration or decline of the nation. Within this context, Cesare Lombroso's enduringly popular theories of 'criminal types' and of degenerationism, with its handmaiden eugenics, were arguably among the most disturbing scientific developments in which psychiatry became implicated.[40] Medical ideas and popular views on 'drunkards' and 'alcoholics' became embedded in and entrenched within these theories.[41]

After World War II, biologically focused psychiatric frameworks of alcohol abuse were increasingly complemented if not replaced by socio-psychological approaches, with institution-based treatments being supplemented with or replaced by community and self-help group initiatives – even, under certain circumstances, in totalitarian Eastern European countries. Nonetheless, as Western societal concerns and medical ideas about alcohol – especially those developed in France, Germany, Britain and the USA – percolated across national boundaries, they led to a diversity of medical and policy interventions in individual countries. Again, this was also the case in some of the party-controlled repressive states in Eastern Europe. Notwithstanding the diversity of national styles of alcohol interventions, certain issues remained consistently at the centre of medical debates in most regions. These included concerns such as whether alcohol over-consumption was bound to weaken the moral, physical and mental fabric of nation states, and identifying the adverse effects of diverse kinds of alcohol on the minds of different races or communities. The public kudos, official recognition and medical approval of imported as opposed to indigenous drinks and home brews were similarly dependent on their wider national and cultural provenance. From the late nineteenth century, the question emerged as to whether alcohol abuse would best be dealt with inside psychiatric or specialist institutions for inebriates, while the institutional response was challenged from the post-World War II period onwards, when medical expertise was seen to be not necessarily required, and families and self-help peer groups for alcoholics began to play an important role in the management of alcohol-related problems.

Popular representations of drinkers as 'jolly drunks' or as sad/bad 'drunkards' or 'alcoholics' remained ubiquitous, not least in relation to the long-enduring arguments on moderation and abstinence, when the issue of how much constituted too much drunkenness was at stake. This fuelled national stereotypes (such as 'the drunk Irish'), on the one hand, and boasting and national pride about who the biggest drinkers were, on the other, leading in turn to tension between popular conceptions and medical experts' views. Despite the rise of psychiatric expertise, religious concerns continued to inform popular attitudes and alcohol-related behaviours, as well as some medical practices and government policies. Gendered views on drinking and on 'the drunkard' prevailed in many cultural settings, with the latter being considered an overwhelmingly male problem, especially when admission statistics of medical and specialised institutions were focused on.[42] The entanglement of gender, social class and age complicated the public and medical visibility of women's drinking, the mental destructiveness of drink and the social and psychological cost of family violence. Overall, during the period covered in this book, popular discourses on drinking remained ambivalent and heterogeneous, and medical views were characterised by plurality despite progressive attempts towards the ossification of alcoholism as a psychiatric diagnosis.

As in any historical research on drinking and mental health, methodological problems restrict what can be gleaned from the available primary sources about people's perceptions in contrast to their behaviours; about doctors' theories versus their medical practices; and in regard to theories about alcohol consumption and its effects in contrast to what was actually happening and experienced at the time. Furthermore, pre-twentieth-century statistics are not always reliable, the reported incidence of drink-related mental health concerns does not equate with the actual frequency of these events, and the effects of moonshining and home brews in contrast to adverse health impacts resulting from 'officially' produced alcohols are difficult to ascertain. While these issues have been raised in some of the chapters in this book, certain topics have been omitted because of the ambition to focus on as yet under-researched fields, like, for example, drinking in colonial and Eastern European countries, rather than deal with hitherto well-covered themes, such as the impact of the world wars and the roles of the intemperance movement, prohibition and conceptions of alcohol as a public health issue in the wake of WHO interventions during the period after World War II.[43]

Alcohol consumption, psychiatry and society historicised

The chapters in this book are arranged chronologically to facilitate the temporal mapping of shifting medical and psychiatric trends in the interpretation and treatment of alcohol-related issues at different localities. They focus on medical, political and socio-cultural debates, conflicts and processes of negotiation about drunkenness and alcohol abuse in a variety of geographical and temporal spaces, ranging from the anglophone world of the early modern era to colonial Africa, East Asia and the Pacific to the post-communist states of Eastern Europe towards the end of the twentieth century. Individual authors assess a variety of historical sources, including official, semi-official and secret service publications; medical textbooks, journal articles, dissertations and institutional records; newspaper reports, journal articles and religious texts; and the websites and documents of self-help organisations. Methodologically they are united by the ambition to firmly locate medical ideas and practices regarding alcohol consumption within their specific social, cultural and political historical contexts as well as identify the global scientific developments and flows of knowledge that had a bearing on them.

The authors discuss the relationship between alcohol, psychiatry and society and identify how cultural, political and social factors underpinned both medical and public attitudes towards alcohol, and how these attitudes changed over time. Some chapters focus on the characteristics of debates and discourses within the framework of specific nation states. They examine aspects such as the popular resonance of mythological imagery about alcohol within a specific cultural setting (Greece) and the varied impact of missionary endeavours and colonial politics on alcohol policies, medical perspectives and different colonial populations' perceptions of drunkenness (Algeria, Nigeria, Fiji Islands) as well as the resulting social and political conflicts (Algeria). In other chapters, the employment of a comparative approach allows the identification of similarities and differences in the global transfer and local diversification of European-bred ideas on the causes, effects and treatments of alcohol-related conditions in relation to neighbouring countries (Chile and Brazil), whilst the contrasting strategies pursued by medical actors within particular countries that have commonly been considered totalitarian (such as Czechoslovakia and Yugoslavia) accentuate the limits of political streamlining and Orwellian doublethink. Overall, questions concerning the causation of alcohol-related conditions have been answered in astoundingly diverse ways for the different geo-cultural and historical contexts.

David Korostyshevsky's chapter on early modern perceptions of drunkenness and alcohol-related diseases (Chapter 1) shows that a new medical paradigm emerged in England and the British Atlantic world from the eighteenth century onwards, rather than, as has commonly been assumed, during the nineteenth century. An iatromechanical focus in learned medicine integrated the traditional concepts of constitutional health, resulting in a medical paradigm that was based on a material vision of the body as a mechanical, hydraulic machine. Within this new framework, distilled spirits became substances that were assumed to mechanically alter healthy 'fibrous tension', exerting a deleterious effect on body and mind. As a consequence, learned doctors began to focus on the intrinsic qualities of different alcohol substances.

In chronological terms, Korostyshevsky sets the stage for the subsequent chapters in this book but also challenges medical historiography. Medical historians have hitherto mainly concentrated on alcohol, drinking and temperance during the modern period, to the detriment of investigations into pre-modern medical understandings. Historiography, Korostyshevsky argues, has been dominated by a quest to locate the historical origins of modern concepts such as 'alcoholism' and 'addiction', and has been overly focused on the perceived shift from religio-moral constructions of drunkenness as sin to science-based categories of disease. Conceiving of the early modern period merely as a part of the prehistory of 'alcoholism' fails to fully contextualise and historicise the role of medical ideas in the conceptualisation of alcohol and drunkenness of this particular period.

Taking early modern concepts on their own, context-specific terms, rather than as forerunners of, or as inferior to, later ideas, Korostyshevsky engages with the mechanical explanations of drunkenness promoted by natural philosophers, popular health writers and clergymen, showing how distilled spirits were pathologised as poisonous substances. Their physical effects were seen to translate into cognitive changes, altered behaviour, loss of control and, ultimately, 'vice' and disease. On account of the blurred boundaries between the physical, psychological and moral, the distinction between the effects of alcoholic substances and the individual's responsibility for the correct way of living became complicated.

Ricardo Campos (Chapter 2) locates the Spanish discourse of the last quarter of the nineteenth century on alcohol and drinking at the juncture where 'vice' and disease met. He examines the related medical and psychiatric discourses between 1870 and 1920, with an emphasis on the characteristics of the latter. During the earlier period, Spanish psychiatrists did not engage with alcohol-related problems and degeneration theory in the same way their colleagues did, for example in France, Germany and Britain. Nor were they at the forefront in the fight against alcoholism alongside their fellow Spanish hygienists and social medicine practitioners. This is surprising, because French psychiatric traditions and degeneration theories were well received in other European countries (such as Greece) and even in the former Spanish colony of Brazil. Until the mid-1890s 'alcoholism' and 'alcohol insanity' were consequently rarely diagnosed in Spain. Campos suggests that this indifference towards and even rejection of degeneration theory in relation to alcohol was partly due to the fact that private institutions, designed for paying clientele, dominated the field of psychiatry at the time, making doctors hesitant to avail themselves of explanatory paradigms that employed negative rationales in regard to the causation and prognosis of their clients' conditions.

The negative signposting inherent to degenerationism was used by Spanish psychiatrists primarily in courts of justice. Only from around 1895 onwards did Spanish psychiatrists begin to subscribe to the tenets of degeneration theory and to engage with alcohol as a medical problem along the lines established by French psychiatry. According to Campos, the interpretation of degenerationism in Spanish psychiatry never assumed the socially discriminative and racially discrediting tone evident in other national contexts. Psychiatrists in Spain focused on the effects of alcohol misuse on individuals and their families.

Mauricio Becerra Rebolledo (Chapter 3) assesses medical developments in the former Spanish and Portuguese colonies of Chile and Brazil during the nineteenth century. His focus is on the flow of ideas to South America from Europe, in particular from France and Germany. Employing a comparative approach, Rebolledo maps the similarities in the adoption of specific European nosologies, diagnostics and therapies, as well as differences in the ways particular European-bred ideas were modified and adapted to very different local conditions in the two South American countries. The cases of Chile and Brazil show that there was no one single 'South American blueprint' in regard to the flow of psychiatrists' ideas about alcohol consumption and their approaches to alcohol misuse. Neither was it necessarily the case that the psychiatric ideas prevalent or developed in the former colonisers' countries would become the standard models for independent nations: doctors in Chile and Brazil looked to France and Germany rather than Spain and Portugal for medical inspiration, education and training. What is more, consumer preferences for, and marketing of, particular alcoholic beverages were closely related to the specifics of agricultural production in these countries, such as grapes in Chile, for wine, and sugar cane in Brazil, for rum.

By the end of the nineteenth century, the use of alcoholic beverages was likened to a social disease that affected the working classes and hence the progress and modernisation of industrialising societies, with the medical establishment assuming a predominant role in the limitation of the affliction and the design of public control policies. The diagnostic category that emerged in medical discourses was 'alcoholism', framed as a mental illness via the notions of 'alcoholic psychosis' and *delirium tremens*, which operated as an articulating nexus in the relationship between excessive drinking and madness. In both countries the framing of alcoholism as a diagnostic category contributed to the pathologisation of alcohol consumption and the institutionalisation of psychiatry as a medical science and field of diagnostic competence and therapeutic intervention. At the end of the nineteenth century, and in sharp contrast to Spain, 'alcoholism' was the most prevalent diagnostic category in psychiatric institutions in Chile and Brazil, subsequently underpinning intense campaigns of social hygiene.

Jacqueline Leckie, Simon Heap and Nina S. Studer show for colonial Fiji, Nigeria and Algeria respectively that drinking and legal access to alcohol were seen as entitlements of 'race', while drunkenness was at the same time considered as a negative attribute of the 'white man's civilisation' and indicative of moral failing. Within colonial contexts, 'race' was intertwined with the consumption of alcohol in varied and complex ways. Leckie (Chapter 4) explores the entanglement of the local and the global regarding ideas and policies concerning alcohol and its misuse. She identifies also the related discourses that were imbued with ideas of race, and reflected assumptions about degeneracy, entitlement and civilisation among Fiji's plural indigenous and immigrant communities of indigenous Fijians, Indo-Fijians, other Pacific Islanders and Europeans. Conceptions of alcoholic insanity and 'race' were transferred to Fiji from Britain, other colonies and the USA. Mental hospital records revealed that before World War II, 'alcoholic insanity' was overwhelmingly considered to be the burden of the white man.

This gendered and ethnic attribution changed after the war, when increasing numbers of Indo-Fijians but fewer Fijians than Europeans were diagnosed with alcohol-related mental disorders. The global forces of war had brought change – all lubricated by drink. Leckie shows that the global flow of alcohol across cultures was deeply embedded in assumptions of race and that power dynamics, especially those between coloniser and colonised, are central to an understanding of past patterns of alcohol consumption.

Heap (Chapter 5) contrasts the meanings of alcohol consumption and misuse among Nigerian communities with those of European expatriate communities. He highlights the detrimental impact of European alcohol imports on Nigerian communities, in particular in the southern regions of the country, focusing on colonial and missionary debates on the merits of the wider availability of strong alcohol and its differential impact on Africans and Europeans. The case of colonial Nigeria reveals that commercial and political factors were greatly implicated in the reported increase of alcohol consumption and alcohol abuse. The Atlantic slave trade encouraged consumption of imported distilled spirits, as slaves were exchanged for rum and whisky. Strong liquor became a socially prestigious commodity, a transitional currency and a powerful catalyst for trade. The liquor trade continued even after the end of the slave trade, reaching large volumes in the second half of the nineteenth century in the wake of the expansion of British control. While the newly created British colony of Northern Nigeria became a prohibition zone for imported alcohol in 1900, liquor constituted the most significant import in terms of volume and value in the provinces of Southern Nigeria.

Debates over the physical and psychological problems caused by the consumption of spirits became a key battleground in the late nineteenth and early twentieth centuries. Liquor trade critics argued that as brewed forms of alcohol had been available in precolonial times, the much more potent imported spirits would cause widespread drunkenness, alcoholism and death. Others pointed to racial differences in the psychological and physiological effects of alcohol, suggesting that Nigerians were physically stronger than Europeans and hence were able to drink more alcohol without ill effects. Europeans, on the other hand, were seen to suffer from the debilitating local climate and frequent bouts of ill-health, which made their lives particularly trying and made them prone to consuming too much alcohol on a regular basis.

Jasmin Brötz (Chapter 6) explores why the debate on alcohol misuse resurfaced in Germany around 1900, long after having been a controversial issue in the early nineteenth century. After the earlier campaigns against hard liquor, a call not just for temperance but for complete abstinence emerged around 1880. Even moderate drinking was frowned upon by medical experts and the general public, as this was believed to be the route to excessive drinking. Brötz focuses on newly emerging science-based concepts of alcohol misuse, such as those promulgated by the well-known psychiatrists Auguste Forel, of Switzerland, and the prominent German psychiatrist Emil Kraepelin. Both protagonists provided expert knowledge and saw 'alcoholism' as inheritable and also as a mental illness. Brötz argues that increased interest in alcoholism was based on the idea of rationalisation as a process that changed society. The anticipated realisation of reason was regarded both as an unavoidable, almost natural process and as a potential for human action.

Alongside eugenicist ideals of 'forming the nation' by means of birth control and of raising the efficiency of economic production through rationally planned and regulated working processes, the interest in 'healing the nation' from alcoholism fitted in squarely with the self-perception of Germany as a modern, progressive and rationalised society. As in many other countries, in this discourse, inheritable degeneration through alcoholism was feared, economic losses due to alcoholism were accurately calculated, and, especially before World War I, alcohol was considered to be a factor that had the potential to compromise Germany's competitiveness among the nations. The healing of the individual was expected to lead to the healing of the collective (later on referred to as the *Volkskörper*). Brötz also highlights early twentieth-century concerns about the detrimental effects of modernity on individuals, which were regarded as a cause of the preponderance of alcoholism in society.

Alcohol was so culturally embedded in certain societies that its use within mental hospitals was widespread among both staff and patients. In mid-nineteenth-century Germany, for example, patients engaged in work were sometimes offered alcohol as an add-on to payment.[44] As Konstantinos Gkotsinas shows in Chapter 7, in twentieth-century Greek institutions, too, patients' total abstinence from alcohol was not always prescribed by psychiatrists. In Greece, physicians turned their attention to the problem of alcohol-induced diseases at the turn of the twentieth century, despite the economic benefits of alcohol to Greek society in terms of trade and tax revenue and its social and cultural practices. Gkotsinas maps the competing discourses surrounding alcoholism in a 'wet culture'. During the 1903 Pan-Hellenic Medical Conference held in Athens, most speakers emphasised that alcohol causes health damage. Only a few delegates claimed that alcohol could not be considered a poison but should in fact be seen as nutrition. In the following years, Greek psychiatrists were divided between proponents of total abstinence and advocates of moderate use, who also made a distinction between fermented and distilled beverages. Eventually, Greek psychiatrists came to perceive 'immoderate' alcohol consumption as a pathology. Gkotsinas highlights the importance of transnational networks to treatment at the Athens lunatic asylum, which was mainly influenced by French and German approaches.

Nina S. Studer focuses on psychiatric theories in colonial Algeria during the three decades preceding its independence from France in 1962 (Chapter 8). During this period proponents of the influential psychiatric school of thought known as the *École d'Alger* (1925–62) were engrossed in debates about Algerians' allegedly inherent 'primitivism', Muslims' reported propensity to become violently insane and suppositions that the North African brain could not develop to the French level of civilisation and, hence, that their assimilation was bound to fail. As Algeria became increasingly earmarked for European settlement, assimilation constituted a potent issue with regard to colonial interests. Yet, at the same time, colonial governance was based on the precepts of the French *mission civilisatrice* and its allegedly positive effects, one of which was considered to be the refinement of North Africans' taste and the development of a cultured palate for the consumption of French wine, the quintessence of civilised, cosmopolitan drinking.

As alcohol consumption increased among the colonised, so did reports of drunkenness and alcohol misuse among formerly – allegedly – abstaining Algerian Muslims. This put the spotlight on two major problems in relation to alcohol within a colonial context. First, French civilisation and its culturally desirable habits seemed to contribute to, if not cause, undesirable alcohol-related problems that had severe health and social control implications, in the shape of a reported rise in alcoholism and drink-related violence. Second, because an Orientalist conception of Muslims as teetotallers, by force of their religious creed, was common among both French colonial psychiatrists and a wider European public, the allegedly observed loss of inhibition to drinking alcohol was construed as a 'new' phenomenon, for which the French as well as Muslims' lack of moderation were to blame. Although French settlers in Algeria were often portrayed as lacking moderation in their alcohol consumption and criticised for this by the metropolitan French, against the background of racial prejudice and colonial power interests, it was drunkenness among the colonised that was seen to be particularly dangerous, as alcohol was thought to lead to social upheaval.

Akira Hashimoto (Chapter 9) focuses on a non-colonial context. He examines the development of medical and social approaches to alcohol misuse in post-World War II Japan. During this period, the country's consumption of alcohol escalated considerably, as a result of economic growth, increase in national income and Westernisation of lifestyle. Alcohol consumption peaked in the mid-1990s, but has declined since then. Until the second half of the twentieth century, alcohol abuse did not elicit much government and medical attention in Japan, with only a small number of alcoholic patients being reported in the official records before World War II.

Hashimoto examines Japanese notions of alcohol misuse and how doctors drew on Western theories and treatments, while developing their own culturally congruent brands of therapeutic intervention. He discusses both hospital-centred medical approaches and patients' and their families' initiatives in dealing with alcohol-related problems, such as Alcoholics Anonymous (AA), Danshukai and Naikan. These approaches were influenced by Western psychotherapeutic practices to varying extents. For example, Danshukai, the most popular network of self-help groups in Japan, was originally inspired by Alcoholics Anonymous and North American concepts of group therapy. In Danshukai, family participation and support were considered to be of immeasurable value in establishing and maintaining abstinence. Naikan, an individual psychotherapy approach inspired by Buddhist values, was from the 1970s employed in the treatment of alcohol-related conditions. It became integrated into Japanese psychiatry and soon was found also in other Asian countries, Europe and the USA.

The role of self-help and group therapy approaches in the treatment of alcohol misuse is also at the centre of analysis in two of the three chapters on former communist Eastern European nations, by Mat Savelli and Adéla Gjuričová. Savelli (Chapter 10) explores the origins of the 'Hudolin Club' phenomenon. Unlike its more famous cousin, Alcoholics Anonymous, Hudolin Clubs or 'Clubs of Treated Alcoholics' combined the rehabilitation of former alcoholic patients in patient- and doctor-led therapeutic groups with public education about alcoholism. The initiative was based on the efforts of a group of physicians connected to Vladimir Hudolin and his Zagreb clinic, who sought out a new form of treatment to handle the burgeoning alcohol problem in Communist Yugoslavia. Savelli shows that health experts identified both popular attitudes about drinking and the consequences of industrialisation and modernisation as causes for the alarming increase in alcohol-related illnesses during the 1950s and 1960s. Although the Yugoslav health system substantially increased its treatment capacity between the 1960s and 1980s, alcoholism remained the seventh most commonly treated medical problem.

Despite the political and ideological restrictions characteristic of communist states, the Hudolin movement succeeded in providing self-directed treatment options for alcoholic patients and in establishing strong ties with Western colleagues, such as Maxwell Jones and Joshua Bierer, who developed the concepts of 'therapeutic communities' and 'social psychiatry' in Britain. Hudolin also managed to integrate the work of competing Western psychotherapeutic schools of thought into his practice, establishing professional links with prominent protagonists of the psychoanalytic movement, namely the London-based psychoanalysts Wilfred Bion and S.H. Foulkes, a German émigré. The clubs also helped shape the efforts of the social psychiatry movement in Yugoslavia. The political developments from 1991 onwards and the dissolution of the Yugoslav Federation, as well as the death of Hudolin in 1996, proved disruptive to the clubs' innovative initiatives within the various regions of the former Yugoslavia. However, Hudolin's legacy endured, and by the twenty-first century thousands of Hudolin Clubs existed in over thirty countries across four continents.

Like Savelli's chapter, Adéla Gjuričová's chapter on Communist Czechoslovakia (Chapter 11) focuses on the period after World War II, when alternatives to the traditional treatment of alcoholism were sought after by health professionals. Despite the limitations suffered by socially and psychologically oriented therapeutic approaches on account of their perceived challenge to Communist political principles and established party hierarchies, the treatment of alcohol addiction enjoyed a dynamic development from the late 1940s onwards. Gjuričová examines the generally conservative and repressive context of psychiatric care in the country within which the psychiatrist Jaroslav Skála and his colleagues succeeded in developing an alternative, non-Pavlovian and non-biological method of doctor-led group therapy that included alcoholics and their families. In contrast to earlier academic work that tended to focus on abuses of psychiatric patients within communist-ruled states, Gjuričová argues that, in regard to the treatment of alcoholism, individual doctors managed to maximise their professional opportunities despite central state-imposed political limitations, succeeding, like Hudolin in Yugoslavia, in establishing a level of professional exchange between domestic debates on alcohol and Western ideas and practices. Nonetheless, a certain distance from Western templates such as the anti-psychiatry movement was retained as Skála developed a therapeutic model in its own right. Skála and his colleagues made use of detoxification units or 'drunk tanks' for patients suffering from alcoholism and established a semi-official system of psychotherapy training. Between the 1950s and the 1970s a network of about 200 specialised counselling and advice centres was established.

In contrast to the apparent permeability of central state-enforced limitations on psychiatric theories and practices in Czechoslovakia and Yugoslavia, Christian Werkmeister's chapter (Chapter 12) highlights the punitive and segregationist measures enforced on alcoholics in Soviet Russia. Werkmeister focuses on the two decades preceding Gorbachëv's policy of *glasnost* or openness in the Soviet

Union. While there was a spike in international interest in the fate of political prisoners confined in Soviet psychiatric institutions during the 1970s, still little is known about the medical treatment of alcoholics behind the Iron Curtain.

Heavy drinking has been widely considered to be characteristic of Russian culture. However, it was not until the establishment of the Soviet Union that the state condemned the 'drinker's disease' of the Tsarist era as a crime, considering it backward, anti-Soviet and alien to an enlightened and liberated society. Yet, like the criminalisation of drinkers, the establishment of a biologically focused clinical psychiatry under the Soviet regime had grave consequences for people diagnosed as alcoholics. People were often institutionalised at the first sign of drunkenness, which often followed a tip-off by neighbours or by line managers at work, or criminalised on the exhibition of alcohol-related disorderly behaviour, and forced to undergo treatment. Alcoholics were sent for harsh treatment to various types of institutions, such as psychiatric hospitals, prisons and work colonies. They were deprived of their citizens' rights, were forced to perform compulsory labour and – even after their release – remained subject to surveillance and further episodes of forced hospitalisation and involuntary treatment. Werkmeister's chapter shows the interrelationship between the Soviet project of ideologically streamlining the population and the role of science and medicine in forcefully readjusting those who were perceived to deviate from the politically prescribed social and behavioural norms.

As the chapters in this volume show, the quests for a definitive nosology of alcohol-related diseases, and for therapeutic strategies and public health measures that enable national governments to effectively deal with drunkenness and alcohol misuse, were characterised by heated debate and locality-specific decision-making. There is no one single story of the 'birth of alcoholism as a disease', nor one single history of how alcohol was represented as a medical, moral and political problem.

Despite similarities around the globe, alcohol consumption in its varied guises and the medical responses to it are profoundly context-sensitive and need to be closely historicised. Whether one believes the American statesman Thomas Jefferson (1743–1826), who is reported to have claimed that 'Beer, if drank with moderation, softens the temper, cheers the spirit, and promotes health', or the English clergyman Robert South (1634–1716), for whom 'Abstinence is the great strengthener and clearer of reason', there appeared to be a consensus that excessive drinking was – and is – a scourge of society and a cause of ill-health, even if such a consensus was not reached simultaneously across the globe and different or even diverging reasons were applied in different localities.[45]

Notes

1 Eubulus described the effects of the successive consumption of between one and ten kraters of diluted wine when Dionysus presides as symposiarch: 'I mix three kraters only for those who are wise. / One is for good health, which they drink first. / The second is for love and pleasure. / The third is for sleep, and when they have drunk it those who are wise wander homewards. / The fourth is no longer ours, but belongs to arrogance. / The fifth leads to shouting. / The sixth to a drunken revel. / The seventh to black eyes. / The eighth to a summons. / The ninth to bile. / The tenth to madness, in that it makes people throw things.' R.L. Hunter (ed.), *Eubulus: The Fragments* (Cambridge: Cambridge University Press, 1983), 186. See also Christopher C.H. Cook and Helen Tarbet, 'Classically intoxicated: correlations between quantity of alcohol consumed and alcohol related problems in a classical Greek text', *British Medical Journal*, 335, no. 7633 (2007), 1302–4. In the Greco-Roman medical corpus, black bile was thought to lead to introspection, sentimentality and lethargic melancholy; yellow bile to aggressivity, irascibility and choleric melancholia or mania.

2 James McHugh, 'Alcohol in pre-modern South Asia', in H. Fischer-Tiné and J. Tschurenev (eds), *A History of Alcohol and Drugs in Modern South Asia: Intoxicating Affairs* (London: Routledge, 2014), 29–44.

3 William F. Bynum, 'Cronic alcoholism in the first half of the 19th century', *Bulletin on the History of Medicine*, 17, no. 2 (1968), 160–85.

4 Ibid., 160; Roy Porter, 'The drinking man's disease: the "pre-history" of alcoholism in Georgian Britain', *British Journal of Addiction*, 80 (1985), 385–96; Jonathan Reinarz and Rebecca Wynter, 'The spirit of medicine: the use of alcohol in nineteenth-century medical practice', in S. Schmid and B. Schmidt-Haberkamp (eds), *Drink in the*

Eighteenth and Nineteenth Centuries (London: Pickering and Chatto, 2014), 121–41; S.E. Williams, 'The use of beverage alcohol as medicine, 1790–1860', *Journal of Studies on Alcohol*, 41, no. 5 (1980), 543–66. J. Nicholls, *The Politics of Alcohol: A History of the Drink Question in England* (Manchester, Manchester University Press, 2009); V. Berridge, *Demons: Our Changing Attitudes to Alcohol, Tobacco, and Drugs* (Oxford: University Press, 2013); Alice Mauger, 'Alcoholism, medicine and psychiatry in Ireland, c. 1890–1921', in Steven J. Taylor and Alice Brumby (eds), *Healthy Minds in the Twentieth Century* (Basingstoke: Palgrave Macmillan, 2019), 17–52; Peter MacCandless, 'Curses of civilisation: insanity and drunkenness in Victorian Britain', *British Journal of Addiction*, 80 (1985), 385–96; Patricia E. Prestwich, 'Drinkers, drunkards and degenerates: the alcoholic population of a Parisian asylum, 1867–1914', *Social History*, 27, no. 54 (1994), 321–35.

5 In Britain, the Scottish physician Thomas Trotter (1760–1832) developed similar ideas around the same time. Griffith Edwards, 'Thomas Trotter's "Essay on Drunkenness" appraised', *Addiction*, 107, no. 9 (2012), 1562–79.

6 Quoted in H.G. Levine, 'The discovery of addiction: changing conceptions of habitual drunkenness in America', *Journal of Studies on Alcohol*, 39, no. 1 (1978), 143–74, at p. 168.

7 Roy Porter, *Health for Sale: Quackery in England, 1660–1850* (Manchester: Manchester University Press, 1989): Amelia Bonea, Melissa Dickson, Sally Shuttleworth and Jennifer Wallis, Anxious *Times: Medicine and Modernity in Nineteenth-Century Britain* (Pittsburgh: University of Pittsburgh Press, 2019).

8 In contrast, amrita or sudha, the mythical nectar of Gods (the Greeks' Ambrosia), bestowed higher levels of knowledge and power and was the imaginary drink of choice reserved exclusively for the elite; only ordinary castes were not allowed to imbibe a wide range of man-made drinks. McHugh, 'Alcohol in pre-modern South Asia'; James McHugh, Sidhu: the sugar cane 'wine' of ancient and early medieval India', *History of Science in South Asia*, 8 (2020), 36–56; James McHugh, 'Varieties of drunk experience in early medieval South Asia', *Journal of South Asian Studies*, 43, no. 2 (2020), 345–53; Arkotong Longkumer, 'Rice-beer, purification and debates over religion and culture in north-east India', *South Asia: Journal of South Asian Studies*, 39, no. 2 (2016), 444–61.

9 Michael Dietler, 'Alcohol: anthropological/archaeological perspectives', Annual Review of Anthropology, 35 (2006), 229–49, at 232. See also M. Dietler, 'Theorizing the feast: rituals of consumption,

commensal politics and power in African contexts', in M. Dietler and B. Hayden (eds), *Feasts: Archeological and Ethnographic Perspectives on Food, Politics and Power* (Washington DC and London: Smithsonian Institution Press, 2001), 65–114.

10 M. Dietler, 'Feasting and fasting', in Timothy Insoll (ed.), *Oxford Handbook of the Archaeology of Ritual and Religion* (Oxford: Oxford University Press, 2012), 179–94; Polly Wiessner and Wulf Shieffenhovel (eds), *Food and the Status Quest: Interdisciplinary Perspectives* (Oxford and New York: Berghahn, 1996).

11 For further reflections on historiography and methodology, see A. Digby, W. Ernst and P.B. Mukharji (eds), *Crossing Colonial Historiographies: Histories of Colonial and Indigenous Medicines in Transnational Perspective* (Cambridge: Cambridge Scholars, 2010).

12 Elvin Morton Jellinek, *The Disease Concept of Alcoholism* (New Haven, CT: Hillhouse Press, 1960); Peter Conrad, 'Medicalization and social control', *Annual Review of Sociology*, 18 (1992), 209–32; Johan Edman, 'Alcohol consumption as a public health problem 1885–1992', in Johannes Kananen, Sophy Bergenheim and Merle Wessel (eds), *Conceptualising Public Health: Historical and Contemporary Struggles over Key Concepts* (London: Routledge, 2018), 135–55; Johan Edman, 'A medical challenge: the alcohol disease in Sweden 1946–1955', *Social History of Medicine*, 33, no. 1 (2020), 224–46; Carl May, 'Habitual drunkards and the invention of alcoholism: susceptibility and culpability in nineteenth century medicine', *Addiction Research*, 5 (1997), 169–87; William L. White, 'The rebirth of the disease concept of alcoholism in the 20th century', *Counselor*, 1 (2000), 62–6.

13 See, for example, Dietler, 'Alcohol: anthropological/archaeological perspectives'.

14 Waltraud Ernst (ed.), *Alcohol Flows across Cultures: Drinking Cultures in Transnational and Comparative Perspective* (London: Routledge, 2020).

15 L.A. Schmidt and R. Room, 'Alcohol and inequity in the process of development: contributions from ethnographic research', *International Journal of Alcohol and Drug Research, 1*, no. 1 (2012), 41–55; Nance Wilson et al., 'Adolescent alcohol, tobacco, and marijuana use: the influence of neighborhood disorder and hope', *American Journal of Health Promotion*, 20, no. 1 (2005), 11–19; Dietler, 'Alcohol: anthropological/archaeological perspectives'; Patricia E. Prestwich, 'Female alcoholism in Paris, 1870–1920: the response of psychiatrists and of families', *History of Psychiatry*, 14, no. 3 (2003), 321–36.

16 Mary Douglas, *Constructive Drinking: Perspectives on Drink from Anthropology* (Cambridge: Cambridge University Press, 1987).
17 See for example, R. Gordon, D. Heim and S. MacAskill, 'Rethinking drinking cultures: a review of drinking cultures and a reconstructed dimensional approach', *Public Health*, 126, no. 1 (2011), 3–11; Michael Savic et al., 'Defining "drinking culture"', *Drugs: Education, Prevention and Policy*, 23, no. 4 (2016), 270–82; P. d'Abbs, 'Reform and resistance: exploring the interplay of alcohol policies with drinking cultures and drinking practices', *Contemporary Drug Problems*, 42, no. 2 (2015), 118–29; R. Room and K. Mäkelä, 'Typologies of the cultural position of drinking', *Journal of Studies on Alcohol*, 61, no. 3 (2000), 475–83; H. Keane, 'Intoxication, harm and pleasure: an analysis of the Australian National Alcohol Strategy', *Critical Public Health*, 19, no. 2 (2009), 135–42.
18 Gordon, Heim and MacAskill, 'Rethinking drinking cultures'; Rahul Rao, 'Alcohol misuse and ethnicity: hidden populations need specific services – and more research', *British Medical Journal*, 332, no. 7543 (2006), 682.
19 A. Ritter, 'Where is the pleasure?' *Addiction*, 109 (2014), 1587–8.
20 Institute of Alcohol Studies, *The Cost of Alcohol to Society*, October 2020, p. 2, www.ias.org.uk/wp-content/uploads/2020/12/The-costs-of-alcohol-to-society.pdf (accessed 15 May 2021). For England and Wales, the most widely cited figure dates from 2003, when the Cabinet Office estimated the costs of drinking to have been £21 billion, excluding any personal impact. Ibid., 11. In 2018 the World Health Organization suggested that worldwide, three million deaths every year resulted from harmful use of alcohol, representing 5.3 per cent of all deaths. World Health Organization, Alcohol', factsheet, https://www.who.int/news-room/fact-sheets/detail/alcohol (accessed 15 May 2021).
21 Gretchen Pierce and Áurea Toxqui (eds), *Alcohol in Latin America: A Social and Cultural History* (Tucson: University of Arizona Press, 2014); Deborah Toner, *Alcohol and Nationhood in Nineteenth-Century Mexico* (Lincoln: University of Nebraska Press, 2016); Erica Wald, 'Governing the bottle: alcohol, race and class in nineteenth century India', *Journal of Imperial and Commonwealth History*, 46, no. 3 (2018), 397–417; H. Fischer-Tiné and J. Tschurenev (eds), *A History of Alcohol and Drugs in Modern South Asia: Intoxicating Affairs* (London: Routledge, 2014), 29–44; Harald Fischer-Tiné, '"The drinking habits of our countrymen": European alcohol consumption and colonial power in British India', *Journal of Imperial and*

Commonwealth History, 40, no. 3 (2012), 383–408; Eric Engstrom and Ivan Crozier, 'Race, alcohol and general paralysis: Emil Kraepelin's comparative psychiatry and his trips to Java (1904) and North America (1925)', *History of Psychiatry*, 29, no. 4 (2018), 263–81; Gerard Sasges, *Imperial Intoxication: Alcohol and the Making of Colonial Indochina* (Honolulu: University of Hawaii Press, 2017); Nandini Bhattacharya, 'The problem of alcohol in colonial India (c. 1907–1942)', *Studies in History*, 33, no. 2 (2017), 187–212.

22 Enrico Petrilli and Franka Beccaria, 'The Italian "alcohol question" from 1860 to 1930: two opposing scientific interpretations', *International Journal of Alcohol and Drug Research*, 4, no. 1 (2015), 37–43.

23 P.C. Mancall, *Deadly Medicine: Indians and Alcohol in Early America* (Ithaca: Cornell University Press, 1997); V.B. Stolberg, 'A review of perspectives on alcohol and alcoholism in the history of American health and medicine', *Journal of Ethnicity in Substance Abuse*, 5, no. 4 (2006), 39–106; M.J. Sargent, 'Heavy drinking and its relation to alcoholism – with special reference to Australia', *Australian and New Zealand Journal of Sociology*, 4 (1968), 146–57; Victorian Government, *Victoria's Alcohol Action Plan 2008–2013: Restoring the Balance* (Melbourne: Victorian Government, 2008); Maggie Brady, *Teaching 'Proper' Drinking? Clubs and Pubs in Indigenous Australia* (Canberra: ANU Press, 2017); P.C. Mancall, Paul Robertson and Terry Huriwai, 'Maori and alcohol: a reconsidered history', *Australian and New Zealand Journal of Psychiatry*, 34, no. 1 (2000), 129–34; T. Huriwai, 'Re-enculturation: culturally congruent interventions for Maori with alcohol-and drug-use-associated problems in New Zealand', *Substance Use and Misuse*, 37 (2002), 1259–68; J. Partanen, *Sociability and Intoxication: Alcohol and Drinking in Kenya, Africa, and the Modern World* (Helsinki: Finnish Foundation for Alcohol Studies, 1991); David Kalema et al., 'Alcohol misuse, policy and treatment responses in Sub-Saharan Africa: the case of Uganda', *Drugs: Education, Prevention and Policy*, 22, no. 6 (2015), 476–82.

24 W. Ernst, *Mad Tales from the Raj* (London: Routledge, 1991); J. Sadowsky, *Imperial Bedlam: Institutions of Madness in Colonial Southwest Nigeria* (Berkeley and Los Angeles: University of California, 1999).

25 Royal Commission on the Sanitary State of the Army in India, report (London: Eyre and Spottiswoode for HMSO, 1863), p. lix. For 2017 in the UK see https://alcoholchange.org.uk/alcohol-facts/fact-sheets/

drinking-trends-in-the-uk (accessed 4 February 2022). See also Hannah Ritchie and Max Roser (2018) – 'Alcohol consumption' (2018), *OurWorldInData.org*, https://ourworldindata.org/alcohol-consumption' (accessed 16 May 2021).

26 Royal Commission, report, xvii.

27 On case studies involving alcohol and mental illness, see W. Ernst, 'On being insane in alien places: case histories from British India, *c.* 1800–1930', in Marjory Harper (ed.), *Migration and Mental Health* (London: Palgrave Macmillan, 2016), 61–84. See also Wald, 'Governing the bottle'.

28 On transnational flows of ideas and practices in psychiatry, see W. Ernst and T. Müller (eds), *Transnational Psychiatries: Social and Cultural Histories of Psychiatry in Comparative Perspective, c. 1800–2000* (Cambridge: Cambridge Scholars, 2010; 2015 2nd ed.).

29 J.E. Dhunjibhoy, 'A brief resume of the types of insanity commonly met with in India, with a full description of "Indian hemp insanity" peculiar to the country', *Journal of Mental Science*, 76 (1930), 254–64, at 256.

30 Alexander William Overbeck-Wright, *Lunacy in India* (London: Bailliere, Tindall and Cox, 1921), 131.

31 Dhunjibhoy, 'Indian hemp insanity', 256.

32 Overbeck-Wright, *Lunacy in India*, 131.

33 Cecil A. Moore, *Backgrounds of English Literature, 1700–1760* (Minneapolis: University of Minnesota Press, 1953), 176. On the English Malady, see V. Skultans, *English Madness: Ideas on Insanity, 1580–1890* (London: Routledge and Kegan Paul, 1979).

34 George Luis Le Sage, quoted in Moore, *Backgrounds of English Literature*, 183.

35 George Cheyne, *An Essay of Health and Long Life* (London: Strahan & Leake, 1724).

36 For a publication by a physician around this time, see Benjamin Ward Richardson, *Diseases of Modern Life* (1882). See also Amelia Bonea, Melissa Dickson, Sally Shuttleworth and Jennifer Wallis, *Anxious Times: Medicine and Modernity in Nineteenth-Century Britain* (Pittsburgh: University of Pittsburgh Press, 2019).

37 John O'Brien, *States of Intoxication: The Place of Alcohol in Civilisation* (London: Routledge, 2018).

38 Sebastian Conrad, 'Enlightenment in global history: a historiographical critique', *American Historical Review*, 117, no. 4 (2012), 999–1027; Lukas Rieppell, Eugenia Leann and William Deringer (eds), 'Science and capitalism: entangled histories', *Osiris*, 33 (2018) [whole issue].

39 W. Ernst and B.J. Harris (eds), *Race, Science and Medicine, 1700–1960* (London: Routledge, 1999); Rohan Deb Roy, 'Science, medicine and new imperial histories', *British Journal for the History of Science*, 45, no. 3 (2012), 443–50; Paul A. Gilbert and Sarah E. Zemore, 'Discrimination and drinking: a systematic review of the evidence', *Social Science and Medicine*, 161 (2016), 178–94.

40 The impact of these theories on tropes about alcohol insanity and alcoholism will be discussed in relation to Germany, Fiji, Spain, Chile, Brazil and Algeria in this book. See also Stephen Jay Gould, *The Mismeasure of Man*, rev. and expanded edn, with a new introduction (New York: W.W. Norton, 2018); Mary Gibson, 'Forensic psychiatry and the birth of the criminal insane asylum in modern Italy', *International Journal of Law and Psychiatry*, 37, no. 1 (2014), 117–26; Ian Dowbiggin, 'Degeneration and hereditarianism in French mental medicine 1840–1890: psychiatric theory as ideological adaptation', in William F. Bynum, Roy Porter and Michael Shepherd (eds), *The Anatomy of Madness*, vol. 1: *People and Ideas* (London and New York: Tavistock Publications, 1985), 188–232; Ian R. Dowbiggin, *Keeping America Sane: Psychiatry and Eugenics in the United States and Canada, 1880–1940* (Ithaca: Cornell University Press, 1997); Paul Hoff, 'Kraepelin and degeneration theory', *European Archives of Psychiatry and Clinical Neuroscience*, 258, no. 2 (2008), 12–17.

41 Pam Lock, 'The habitual drunkard in Victorian fiction and culture' (PhD dissertation, University of Bristol, 2019); An Vleugels, *Narratives of Drunkenness: Belgium, 1830–1914* (London: Pickering and Chatto, 2013).

42 For gender-based drinking patterns, see: S. Eriksen, 'Alcohol as a gender symbol', *Scandinavian Journal of History*, 24, no. 1 (2010), 45–73. See also Bonea et al., *Anxious Times*, ch. 4, 'The woman secret drinker in the late nineteenth-century press', 119–48.

43 On prohibition, see Mark L. Schrad, *Smashing the Liquor Machine: A Global History of Prohibition* (Oxford: Oxford University Press, 2020).

44 As part of work therapy, patients sometimes even worked in breweries' beer gardens. See Thomas Müller, 'Between therapeutic instrument and exploitation of labour force: patient work in rural asylums in Württemberg, c. 1810–1945', in W. Ernst (ed.), *Work, Therapy, Psychiatry and Society, c. 1750–2010* (Manchester: Manchester University Press, 2016), 220–37, at 224; Around 1840, patients of Zwiefalten asylum who supervised other patients were also offered

beer. See Rudolf Camerer and Emil Krimmel, *Geschichte der Königl. Württembergischen Heilanstalt Zwiefalten 1812–1912* (Stuttgart: Greiner and Pfeiffer, 1912), 25–6.

45 Thanks to Jane Freebody for alerting us to these evocative quotes, which, alas, appear to be spurious, with sources unidentified.

1

Corrupting the body and mind: distilled spirits, drunkenness and disease in early modern England and the British Atlantic world

David Korostyshevsky

In 1545 the anonymous author of *An Inuectiue ageinst Glotony and Dronkennes* lamented that drinking 'empoysoned the bodie', wounding 'mortally both the Body and Soule'.[1] Supported by the title's concern with excessive eating and drinking, this statement situated drunkenness within long-standing beliefs linking intoxication with the loss of appetite control and poor health. Early modern English vernacular health guides, which recapitulated learned medical theories about health and disease for popular audiences, applied the Galenic concept of non-naturals to constitute drunkenness as the result of excessive consumption, an aberration of natural behaviours such as eating and drinking, that destroyed the constitution and brought about chronic diseases.[2]

During the eighteenth century, a new medical paradigm emerged, a material vision of the fibre body as a mechanical, hydraulic machine. This theory provided a conceptual framework that medical writers used to materialise distilled spirits as poisonous substances that exerted a deleterious agency upon the body and mind by mechanically altering healthy fibrous tension. Where sixteenth- and seventeenth-century authors focused on the ill effects of excessive drinking, eighteenth-century medical materialists focused a new attention on the effects of the liquors themselves. Circulating in the English Atlantic world, these new medical understandings of intoxication pathologised drunkenness and distilled spirits and, by the early nineteenth century, alcohol. Although the drunkard remained a loathsome and pitiful character, he was no longer solely to blame for his diseases. Distilled spirits, taken initially by choice, eventually degraded the drinker's physical ability to resist.

The historiography of alcoholism is characterised by a quest to locate the historical origins of modern addiction concepts, the formation of which represents a medicalisation of drunkenness from sin to disease.[3] Medicalisation, as defined by the sociologist Peter Conrad, is 'a process by which nonmedical problems become defined and treated as medical problems'.[4] Led by Harry Levine, many scholars initially credited Benjamin Rush (1746–1813), an early American physician, with discovering addiction.[5] Reacting against this American exceptionalist interpretation, the British and Canadian historians Roy Porter, Jessica Warner and, more recently, James Nicholls argued that the concept of addiction has an early modern, European genesis.[6] Although the 'medical writers of Georgian England' understood 'that heavy alcohol consumption was often responsible for ill-health and disease, and ... was one of the triggers of madness', Porter wondered, 'was habitual drunkenness itself seen as a disease?'[7] Whether they located its origins in the early modern period or at the turn of the nineteenth century, these scholars did not question the existence of addiction as an ontological, medically definable pathology.

Since 2000, cultural and linguistic studies have demonstrated that 'alcoholism' and 'addiction' are modern concepts that did not enter common usage until the turn of the twentieth century, both in the UK and in the USA.[8] Consequently, early modernists like Phil Withington and a constellation of scholars including David Clemis are leaving behind rhetorically burdened concepts like drugs and addiction to focus instead on 'intoxication', a concept that 'invites consideration of all consumptive experiences and practices involving intoxicants'.[9] The realisation that alcoholism is a modern socio-medical construction, not an ontological entity waiting to be discovered, has inspired some renewed interest in the language of addiction and its medical framings in the early modern period.[10] However, research focused on early modern medical understandings of intoxication remains sparse in comparison to the attention devoted to drinking, temperance and prohibition in the nineteenth and twentieth centuries.[11]

Moreover, the medicalisation of compulsive drinking from sin to disease remains centre stage. Clemis, for example, works to locate the formation of distinctly 'medical expertise with respect to chronic drinking', which he argues did 'indeed [emerge] later in the eighteenth century' only after new developments in 'neurological theory ... encouraged chronic drinking to be approached without reference to moral agency and the language of sin and vice'.[12] But Clemis also points out 'that the moral and the medical were not' easily 'distinguished' during the seventeenth and eighteenth centuries, an outcome of 'wider ideas' developed by theologians, clergymen and other intellectuals who 'did not readily disentangle the body, mind and soul'.[13] In a period in which modern professional boundaries between physicians, clergymen and other popular health writers were not yet drawn, physicians often acted as moralists while clergymen practised or wrote about medicine. I argue that the ways in which early modern writers understood the effects of the drink itself challenges Clemis's conclusion 'that discussion of purely medical aspects of drunkenness and habitual drinking could never be seen as determining the moral agency of the drunkard'.[14]

I work to close the enduring gap between the medical and the moral in early modern addiction studies by anchoring this analysis within another vein of recent intoxication scholarship that situates drinking as a component of sociability within an emerging eighteenth-century public sphere.[15] Just as the consumption of intoxicants was a public activity, so too was the circulation of ideas, including medical ones, about the dangers of drinking. Therefore, in this chapter, I study popular health guides aimed at the reading public as well as medical treatises, which were produced by physicians for physicians. Read together, these sources reveal that compulsive drinking had acquired a distinctly medical dimension before the turn of the nineteenth century even if it was also regarded as a moral failure. And during the second half of the eighteenth century, medical understandings of distilled spirits circulated in the British Atlantic world, where they would inspire early American temperance reformers in the early nineteenth century.

I also examine changing medical characterisations of the intoxicant as well as the intoxication it produces. Until the last decades of the eighteenth century, Clemis writes, 'the problem of why alcohol produced certain behaviour' or 'how drinking became habitual' was dealt with by 'moralists, clergy, and occasionally, jurists, but seldom physicians', who had failed to 'provide a compelling explanation of why people became chronic drinkers'.[16] However, popular health guides produced between the sixteenth and eighteenth centuries tell a different story. Written by physicians, clergymen and learned non-specialists, these health guides reveal an early interest in the effects of the drink itself, which was explained in terms of prevailing medical theory. Before mechanical medicine, the effects of drinks like wine, including its capacity to rob men of their reason and agency, were described in terms of humoral medicine. As distilled liquors became commonly used commodities, their destructive effects were explained in iatromechanical terms that dominated eighteenth-century medical theory.

Moving beyond the quest to locate an early modern medicalisation of alcohol addiction, I argue that an intersection of medical, religious and popular writers pathologised drunkenness by focusing on the injurious physical effects of the drink. The pathologisation of distilled spirits and, later, all forms of alcohol as physical poisons underpinned the configuration of compulsive drinking as an aberration of health even if it was not fully recognised or treated as a disease and laid the conceptual foundations for modern medical understandings of alcoholism.

Intoxication and popular medical knowledge, *c.* 1500–1700

In the early modern period, medical explanations of drunkenness and its negative physical consequences appeared most often in vernacular health guides, a genre of popular medical literature that exploded in England during the sixteenth and seventeenth centuries. Elizabeth Lane Furdell explains that 'Printers, publishers, and booksellers' became specialists 'in medical works', joining learned and irregular practitioners alike in England's diverse, and often fractious, medical marketplace and transforming 'health care literature into a genre unto itself'.[17] The production of health guides generated further 'public demand for ever more information, discussion, and advice about sickness and well-being'.[18] More importantly, this growing genre was printed in vernacular English, which made it accessible by any literate person who could get a copy of the book. The number of medical texts available to the lay public dramatically expanded from the sixteenth century onwards. According to Andrew Wear, such health guides transmitted long-standing learned concepts of preventative medicine to 'readers who were then expected to apply it themselves'.[19]

Vernacular health guides and learned medical texts alike emphasised Galenic understandings of the body, which had changed little since late Antiquity.[20] Wear writes that early modern medical literature organised 'most aspects of life' according to the concept of 'the six non-naturals', which had become 'canonical categories around which advice on the preservation of health was based'.[21] First described by the second-century Greco-Roman physician Galen in *Ars medicina*, the six non-naturals included '(1) air, (2) food and drink, (3) sleep and waking, (4) movement and rest, (5) retention and evacuation including sexual activity, and (6) the passions of the soul or the emotions'.[22] In early modern health guides, the first two non-naturals became the most important determinants of health, with special emphasis on diet.[23] It was in this category that drinking and drunkenness fell. Because non-naturals like eating and drinking were factors over which an individual ostensibly had control, early modern English preventative medicine continued to assign moral meaning to health. Abuse of the non-naturals was a sin against the natural laws of life, made manifest by the chronic diseases that resulted. Linking the state of the body to whether a person engaged in right living associated disease with sin, while health represented a person's goodness. As a result, the medical descriptions of intoxication acquired a distinctly moral tone, blurring the boundary between sin and disease and complicating historiographical narratives about the medicalisation of excessive drinking into addiction.[24]

Before the emergence of psychiatry as a medical speciality during the nineteenth century, the popular health guides genre developed at a time when English society paid increased attention to the maladies of the mind and their bodily causes. Even though asylums such as Bethlem Hospital date back to the fifteenth century, according to historians like Roy Porter, psychiatry did not come 'of professional age' until the mid-nineteenth century, 'when medical superintendents ("alienists") banded together to form specialized organizations'.[25] Nevertheless, mental afflictions, which had traditionally been associated with spiritual deviance or disturbance, were increasingly viewed within the context of health and medicine, a trend exemplified by Robert Burton's immensely popular *Anatomy of Melancholy* (1621). For Burton (1577–1640), mental afflictions like folly, madness and melancholy were conditions of the body as well as of the mind, rooted in the prevailing Galenic physiology.[26] A little over a century later, the elite physician and popular health writer George Cheyne (1671–1743) continued this tradition with the popular *The English Malady* (1733), in which he argued that mental affliction was a problem to which English people were especially prone.[27]

For most of the sixteenth and seventeenth centuries, before the democratisation of distillation and the commodification of its products, only fermented beverages like wine, beer, ale and cider (in all their varieties) appeared as subjects of discussion in health guides. While most health writers agreed that clean water was the most healthful thirst quencher, fermented beverages such as wine, beer and ale were regarded as both nutritive and medicinal. What drew health writers' ire was that these drinks had become the subject of popular consumption, a context that invited overuse. It was excessive drinking, intemperance in its classical definition, anything immoderate that imbalanced the humours, that they believed was harmful to the body. Acknowledging its health benefits when used moderately and under medical direction, the physician William Bullein (1515–1576) wrote that when 'dronken with excesse', wine 'is a poyson mooste venemous'.[28] Another health writer, Henry Wingfield, a Puritan minister, explained that 'wyne drunke superfluouse doth hurte the liuer, the brayne, and the senewes', causing 'crampes, palseies, apaplexies, & oftentimes … sodayne death'. Moreover, the bodily harm caused by too much wine also debilitated the drinker's mind. 'Drunkennes' induced 'a grosse and thycke fume' that, ascending to the 'brayne', debilitated mental function by covering 'the places where reason and memorie lyeth'.[29] These forms of early modern medical knowledge about drunkenness were often reproduced in a growing literature of sixteenth- and seventeenth-century treatises dedicated solely to drunkenness.[30]

The connection between drunkenness, degraded constitutions and chronic disease was even more clearly articulated by the end of the seventeenth century. The influential physician Thomas Sydenham (1624–1689) described how improper habits of life affected the body. Although he broke from the medical establishment of his day, Sydenham's explanation of the link between drunkenness and chronic disease nevertheless reflected enduring Galenic understandings of the body. Chronic diseases like gout were caused by poorly digested morbific matter that accumulated, slowly poisoning the body. '[C]ontinual Errors in the ... Non-naturals, especially in Meat and Drink' caused 'indigestion of the Humours', leading to a host of 'Chronical Diseases' such as gout, dropsy and rheumatism. Moreover, 'Surfeiting and Drunkenness', along with a sedentary mode of life, wore the body out, 'subvert[ing]' and 'destroy[ing]' its constitution, which began as a 'pristine and natural Oeconomy of the Body'.[31] Unlike the health guides of the preceding centuries, Sydenham's detailed discussion about how lifestyle could induce debilitating chronic diseases would shape growing social concerns about drinking in England.

While Sydenham's understanding of drunkenness was buried in his broader discussion of chronic diseases like gout, one of his contemporaries, Everard Maynwaringe (1629–1713), applied this medical knowledge directly to the medical problems of drunkenness.[32] Demonstrating their growing status as objects of commercial consumption, Maynwaringe now included distilled products like brandy, whisky and aquavit alongside traditional beverages like wine. Warning that distilled drinks were rapidly becoming 'in fashion', Maynwaringe warned his readers that they were 'pernicious Drinks to use commonly', destructive to 'Health, and opposite to long Life'.[33] Reflecting on the medical consequences of drunkenness regardless of the beverage that induced it, Maynwaringe acknowledged that while getting drunk was not fatal, it was the establishment of a habit or lifestyle of drinking that slowly harmed and killed the drinker. Outside medicinal use prescribed by a physician, 'Drink exceeding its measure to excess; is no longer a refreshment', but a 'degenerate condition ... of *body* and *mind*' – so much so, Maynwaringe argued, that no 'difference' could be found between '*sickness* and *drunkenness*', for 'Drunkenness' had 'all the requisites to constitute a Disease'. The inability of the 'faculties' of the body and mind to perform their 'free and regular functions' after drinking constituted the '*symptoms* and *diagnostick signs*, of an acute Disease'.[34] While drunkenness was frequently compared to disease in a metaphorical sense in sixteenth- and seventeenth-century sermons and pamphlets, Maynwaringe's statement is one of the earliest articulations of the idea that drinking too much could be a disease.

Like Sydenham, Maynwaringe understood that the 'degenerate Chyle' created by drinking too much 'do accumulate', laying 'the foundation of many *chronick diseases*' that 'subvert the aeconomy and government of humane Nature' and 'ruine the Fabrick of mans body'. Maynwaring divided the 'ill effects' of drunkenness into three categories. First, the excessive use of intoxicating beverages disordered the '*natural tone of the stomach*', which in turn deranged its ability to digest food properly. Second, Maynwaring argued that, if this was repeated for long enough, digestive ability could be permanently destroyed. Too much 'degenerate Chyle ... produced' by improper digestion conferred upon the body an '*unwholesome corpulency*' and '*catchectick plenititude*'.[35] Finally, 'intemperate drinking' draws the 'whole body' into a '*degenerate* state', characterised finally by an '*imbecility of the Nerves*'.[36]

By describing drunkenness as a disease in the literal sense, Maynwaringe presaged the growing focus on the substance causing intoxication, the intoxicant, that would come to define medical discourses about drunkenness during the eighteenth century. 'Drunkenness being a Raging Distemper' was 'denominated and distinguished from other sicknesses' because it had an obvious material cause, '*Drink*'.[37] Maynwaringe's statements demonstrate that by the end of the seventeenth century, English physicians had developed distinctly medical explanations of drunkenness as a function of the negative effects of the drink itself on the body and mind. These effects were explained in terms of the dominant Galenic humoral understanding of the body. The commercialisation of distilled spirits, the development of medical frameworks to understand drunkenness and the growing emphasis on the material causes of drunkenness would become mainstream medical thought during the medical Enlightenment in the century that followed.

Mechanical medicine and the Gin Craze, *c.* 1700–1760

During the first half of the eighteenth century, the rising consumption of distilled spirits, particularly in London, England's urban centre and one of Europe's largest cities, inspired social, medical and political anxiety that historians have dubbed the Gin Craze. The democratisation of distillation through the publication of vernacular manuals, royal encouragement of a domestic distilling industry and the growth of an impoverished urban underclass resulted in dramatic increases in the common consumption of distilled spirits that had previously been the rare medicinal product of alchemical laboratories.[38] During this period, the interest of physicians, natural philosophers and clergymen in the medical consequences of drunkenness on individuals as well as the body politic increased. The physical destruction wreaked by drinking on individual bodies, they worried, would lead to an irreversible physical and moral degradation of the labouring classes and elites alike, weakening the nation. Their configuration of drinking as an economic, social and political threat drew heavily upon medical explanations of the effects of drunkenness on the body and mind.

The Gin Craze coincided with a period of significant changes in medical theories about the body and its functions. By the early 1700s, learned medical men believed that the physical body was composed of a series of interwoven fibres. While this idea had also been a part of Western medical thought at least since Galen, the idea that these fibres interacted with each other in a mechanical way was new. The advent of microscopy in the mid-seventeenth century enabled the observation of tissues at a level of magnification that made it appear that the whole body was made of fibres, not just muscles. Envisioning a 'fibre body', these early Enlightenment physicians believed that interwoven fibres formed the fundamental building blocks of the corporeal human form.[39] The emergent view that the body was physically composed of a multitude of fibres was further materialised by the application of Newtonian natural philosophy, which applied mechanical explanations of motion to medicine – an Enlightenment project known by historians as medical materialism or iatromechanism.[40]

The mechanical fibre body paradigm was operationalised for the medical profession by Herman Boerhaave (1668–1738), an influential Dutch medical teacher in Leiden, at the turn of the eighteenth century.[41] Boerhaave 'proposed that physical systems throughout the body comprised an integrated, balanced whole in which pressures and liquid flows were equalised and everything found its own level'.[42] These fluid flows were regulated by the tension in the solid fibres containing them. Boerhaave wrote that the 'Body consists of two parts, *Solids* and *Fluids*' and '*Health* consists *in an equal motion of the Fluids, and an equal resistance of the Solids in every part*'. If this tension was imbalanced in either direction, disease resulted. By extension, food and drugs, many of which had entered common use through the influence of chemical medicine on popular practices, 'are ... *mechanical* instruments ... by means of which' the physician could manipulate the body's fibrous tension. 'Every Medicine produces its effects *mechanically*' by 'changing ... the figure, motion and bulk of' the matter composing the body.[43] He classed intoxicating drinks among those substances that acted directly on the body's fibres by virtue of their acridity, a physical property denoting that the particles possessed sharp or pointed edges that poked or lacerated the fibres.[44]

Iatromechanical visions of the fibre body, however, did not displace older medical theory. Instead, as Porter points out, the 'old humoral emphasis on balance' was 'preserved but translated into mechanical and hydrostatic terms'.[45] Likewise, the emphasis on the individual's responsibility for maintaining preventative health based on the non-naturals – especially eating and drinking – never changed. Channelling Sydenham, whom he regarded as equal only to Hippocrates, Boerhaave believed that corrupted, chronic disease-causing matter could be 'bred in the Body' via 'Air, Meat, Drink, Sauces, medicines, or Poisons'.[46] Similarly, one of his most influential students, the Edinburgh physician and instructor William Cullen (1710–1790), who transmitted Boerhaave's views into the English-speaking medical world via the medical school in Edinburgh, wrote in his discussion of dyspepsia that 'sedative or narcotic substances', including tea, coffee, tobacco, ardent spirits and opium, all possessed the ability to disorder the fibrous tension. An 'indolent and sedentary life', especially if accompanied by excessive 'venery' and '[f]requent intoxication', Cullen wrote, disordered alimentary and nervous function, eventually debilitating the body's constitution.[47]

As in the preceding centuries, new medical knowledge generated by men like Boerhaave and Cullen circulated freely in health guides, which remained as popular as ever. Mechanical explanations of the body and its interaction with food, drink and medicines was quickly adopted by popular medical writers. For example, the physician Thomas Short (1690–1772) wrote several guides specifically focusing on food and drink that explained the effects of distilled spirits within an iatromechanical framework. 'All Spirits cause Drunkenness', Short wrote, by causing an 'Overfusion of the Fluids, and the Distention of their containing Vessels'. The spirituous '*Spicula*' worked by 'darting into and pricking the relaxed Vessels ... till the Person becomes paralytic, lethargic, apoplectic, convulsed, stupid, &c.'[48] He further supported his assessments by citing medical materialists.[49] Within the context of Gin Craze anxieties, medical writers mobilised the fibre body paradigm to explain drunkenness. Mechanical explanations of how intoxication harmed the fibre body materialised the intoxicant, in this case, distilled spirit, as a discrete substance to which physicians and clergymen attached notions of physical and mental harm.

One of the most prolific of these writers was George Cheyne. Born in Scotland, Cheyne went to the medical school in Edinburgh, where he studied with Archibald Pitcairn (1652–1713), a dedicated early medical Newtonian. Like his mentor, Cheyne may have also spent some time in Leiden. In 1701 Cheyne began his career in London, joining the Royal Society the following year, and became acquainted with Newton himself. However, enjoying a lifestyle of urban luxury customary in the metropolis left him severely overweight and prone to illness. These circumstances prompted him to move his practice to Bath, a town associated with healing, in 1718. Treating the various afflictions of the English social elite who congregated there, Cheyne advocated a lifestyle of moderation and a vegetarian diet, which he regarded as having restored his own ill health. It was during his career in Bath that he wrote his most popular works on the preservation of health, *An Essay on Health and Long Life* (1724) and *An Essay on Regimen* (1740). Both became some of the period's best sellers, were reprinted in multiple editions and were often cited by English-speaking physicians well into the nineteenth century.[50] It was in these health guides that Cheyne adopted the mechanical fibre body paradigm to discuss the effects of drunkenness. He concluded that, because they hardened, constricted and solidified the body's fibres, '*Spirituous* Liquors, are really *Poison* to' the 'Constitution', which, once destroyed, took on a now familiar slew of chronic diseases, including gout, rheumatism, apoplexy and various nervous maladies.[51]

While Cheyne did not devote an entire treatise to drunkenness specifically, his contemporary Stephen Hales (1677–1761), a clergyman and natural philosopher, did just that. A studious Cambridge man, Hales became a member of the Royal Society in 1717 and the perpetual curate (a kind of parish priest in the Church of England) of Teddington. In this bucolic town located a day's carriage ride west of London, Hales became a polymathic researcher, with interests ranging from astronomy and botany to the distillation of seawater and ventilation of air to improve conditions aboard ships in the Royal Navy. Hales also became interested in what he called statics, measuring the pressure of fluids within plants and animals, a project that was informed by his interest in medical materialism and the social context of the Gin Craze.[52] These investigations included testing the effects of distilled spirits on the body's tissues.

In 'Experiment XV', Hales described his efforts to determine the effect of various fluids, specifically brandy and water, on bodily tissues. Taking 'a young spaniel dog' that 'had bled to death by having his jugular veins cut', Hales opened its body cavity and applied various fluids to the digestive organs, determining their effect on the tissue by measuring the displacement of their volume in a marked glass tube that he had inserted into the aorta.[53] On the basis of such studies, Hales concluded that 'brandy contracts the fine capillary arteries of the guts', but 'that water soon relaxes them again', a finding that confirmed that distilled spirits harmed the body, while water was healthy.[54] Moreover, he sought to educate the public about the results of the 'Experiments' he had 'purposely made, with Brandy, on … Animals' by publishing *A*

Friendly Admonition to the Drinkers of Gin, Brandy, and Other Distilled Spirituous Liquors in 1733, the height of the Gin Craze.[55] The pamphlet would be reprinted in multiple editions in the decades that followed, often at times of peak concern about drinking.

While many Gin Craze writers continued to lament that drunkenness destroyed an individual's morality and, thereby, society more generally, Hales made, according to Patrick Dillon, one of the first 'detailed medical case[s] against the abuse of spirits'[56] by marshalling the explanatory power of the popular fibre body paradigm. By 'frequently contracting and shrivelling, and then soon after relaxing' the fibres of the body, Hales wrote, distilled liquors 'weaken and wear out the Substance and Coats of the Stomach, on which they … immediately prey, every time they are drank'. Liquor destroyed the 'habituate[d]' drinker's 'Appetite and Digestion', 'dr[ied] up, and spoil[ed] the Nerves', making them 'insensible', and hurt 'the very fine Blood-Vessels, especially where their Fibres are most tender, as in the Brain; whereby they spoil the Memory and intellectual Faculties'. Together, these effects destroyed 'the natural Temper', the constitution, of the body.[57]

Using the terminology of Boerhaave's medical materialism, Hales explained in later editions of the *Friendly Admonition* that distilled liquors had these unhealthy effects because of their physical properties, their 'harsh, fiery and acrimonious Nature'.[58] These deleterious physical and mechanical properties convinced Hales that 'these *spirituous Liquors* … are … direct *Poison to human Bodies*', an argument that would became a defining feature of nineteenth-century toxicology manuals and temperance discourses.[59] By focusing on the physical properties of distilled spirit, Hales helped cement the notion that drunkenness and its chronic consequences were the distinctly physical result of spirit ingested into the body, rendering a substance that had hitherto been considered *aqua vitae*, the water of life, as a poison. And further demonstrating the interplay between elite medical theories and popular health discourses, Hales cited widely read physicians like Thomas Short and George Cheyne frequently in his discussion of intoxication.

Hale's ideas were readily adopted by some of his fellow clergymen, most notably Thomas Wilson (1703–1784). Wilson became a friend of Hales through the Society for the Promotion of Christian

Knowledge, a moral reform organisation in which both men participated. The son of the elder Thomas Wilson (1663–1755), who had served as the well-respected Bishop of Sodor and Man, Wilson moved to London to launch his clerical career in the 1730s, the height of the Gin Craze. Searching for worthy causes to adopt, he was inspired by Hales and his work on drunkenness. In 1736 he published his own book, *Distilled Spirituous Liquors the Bane of the Nation*, which drew heavily upon Hales's arguments. His analysis of the physical effects of liquor was 'grounded upon the Experiments of a very Curious Gentleman', most probably Hales, 'to whom the learned World, and especially the Physicians have been indebted'. If that was not convincing enough to the reader, Wilson also 'had the Opinion of two or three eminent Physicians in Town' and cited the work of other medical men, especially George Cheyne.[60]

Literal medical explanations of drunkenness were often applied to society, which was envisioned as a metaphorical body. Comparing the spread of drunkenness to contagion and plague, Wilson called it a spreading 'INFECTION', a 'Great Injury' that 'accrues to the Publick, by making and vending such Quantities of Distilled Spirituous Liquors'.[61] Drunkenness laid 'the Foundation of Distempers, which will be handed down to their posterity; so that in a Generation or two We shall not have People able to do the Servile Offices, or to cultivate our Lands'.[62] The success of English society depended on the health of the '*Bodies* of Men', which 'are without doubt the most valuable *Treasure* of a Country'. Drunkenness among 'the *ordinary People*' caused particular concern because they 'are as serviceable to the Commonwealth as the *Rich*'. For 'if they are *able* to work, or are *employed* in honest Labour and useful Arts; and such being more in Number', they 'do more contribute to the Nation's *Wealth* than those of *higher Rank*'.[63] By afflicting all classes, the physical and social disease of drunkenness threatened the national body politic.

By the end of the eighteenth century, the link between poison, distilled spirits and chronic disease – understood within the frame of the fibre body – had become unassailable medical knowledge for a small but growing cohort of Edinburgh-trained physicians. Men like Anthony Fothergill (1732–1813), John Coakley Lettsom

(1744–1815) and Thomas Trotter (1760–1832) agreed that the longer and more frequently they were ingested, distilled spirits degraded the body's natural health, debilitating the drinker's physical, mental and moral capacities.[64] The most influential of these, Thomas Trotter, who became an esteemed naval physician, recognised that 'independent of its intoxicating quality', distilled spirits possessed 'a chemical operation in the human body' that acts deleteriously 'upon the fibers'.[65] That 'our intellectual part' could 'be disturbed, and so completely deranged' by the physical consequences of drunkenness Trotter declared to be 'a fact sufficiently established to be universally admitted'.[66]

Transatlantic circulations, *c.* 1750–1820

An awareness of distilled spirits and drunkenness expressed in terms of medical materialism was not confined to Britain. Ideas expressed by writers like Cheyne and Hales crossed the Atlantic via growing networks within which letters, books and other printed materials circulated between learned men. Through his work with the Society for the Promotion of Christian Knowledge, Hales became closely associated with efforts to establish the penal colony of Georgia. On 30 May 1733, he bequeathed to the trustees of the colony a donation of religious texts, including 200 copies of his newly printed *Friendly Admonition to Drinkers of Brandy* for shipment across the Atlantic.[67] Several decades later, in 1758, Hales wrote a letter to 'several Governors in America' that summarised his arguments about distilled spirits, which was published, along with extracts from his writings on distilled liquors, in the *New American Magazine*. It made an impression, for a 1759 pamphlet, condensed as 'The pernicious practice of dram-drinking', began with the remark that 'it hath been thought expedient to cause a Number of' additional copies 'to be reprinted, and dispersed gratis amongst the Inhabitants ... of New-Jersey'.[68]

These initial circulations of Stephen Hales's research into New Jersey and Georgia found a fertile home in Philadelphia during the second half of the eighteenth century. In this period, Philadelphia became one of North America's most prosperous cities, a port that received goods, ideas and knowledge from across Britain's growing empire. The city's elites, including a growing number of learned physicians, saw themselves as members of a Republic of Letters, a network of personal relationships and epistolary correspondence that transmitted medical, scientific and philosophical knowledge in both directions across the Atlantic.[69] The integration of Philadelphia into transatlantic commercial and intellectual networks made it particularly receptive to English medical ideas, theories and practices. If North America became, in the words of Helen Brock, a 'Western outpost of European medicine', Philadelphia became its leading *entrepôt* of medical knowledge.[70]

It was within this context that Anthony Benezet (1713–1784), a French Huguenot-turned-Quaker, became interested in the social, medical and moral problems of drunkenness. Born into a Protestant family in Catholic France, Benezet emigrated and became a Quaker before finally settling in Philadelphia in 1731. He is primarily remembered as an educator and abolitionist.[71] Interested in solving what he considered the most pressing problems of his time, Benezet was also inspired by Hales's work on drunkenness. Worried about 'the dreadful havock made by the excessive use of distilled spirituous liquors in' the English colonies, he was moved to 'insert in one of the almanacks an extract of what had been written on that subject by Dr. Hales'.[72] In 1774 he published his own essay on the matter. Although Benezet was not a physician, his essay relied almost exclusively on early eighteenth century British and European medical sources. Much of the essay consisted of large direct quotes reproduced from learned medical authorities like Stephen Hales as well as writers from the ever-popular health guide genre such as Thomas Short and George Cheyne. Like his Gin Craze contemporaries, Benezet focused primarily on the problems that intoxication posed to bodies and minds and on how, in turn, their consequences threatened society more generally.

Benezet's influence would inspire another Philadelphian, Benjamin Rush (1746–1813), a signatory of the Declaration of Independence, a physician and social reformer and the first American citizen to write about the medical consequences of drunkenness. Rush's *Inquiry into the Effects of Ardent Spirits upon the Body and Mind*, first published in 1784, recapitulated several centuries of early modern English medical knowledge about drunkenness.[73] Rush's book was reprinted in multiple editions during the nineteenth century (see Figure 0.1), and his interest in the medical aspects of drunkenness and his reform impulse would inspire several generations of American and British temperance activists of all stripes.[74]

The growing concern about distilled spirit during the eighteenth century, not just the state of drunkenness and the drunkard as an individual, redefined 'alcohol' as a term which gradually came to signify the discrete chemical substance within fermented and distilled beverages directly responsible for the physical and mental effects of drunkenness and its chronic consequences. Traditionally, 'alcohol' derived from an Arabic alchemical term that signified any subtle material and, later, any distillate more generally.[75] Thus during the Gin Craze, distilled spirits would have been understood as a type of alcohol. And while wine, beer, ale, cider and other fermented beverages were understood to possess the ability to bring about drunkenness, distilled spirits were understood as a separate substance, changed from its original form by the process of distillation itself. Writers like Hales and Wilson expressed this understanding when they described the effects of drinking distilled spirits because of them having been 'inflamed by repeated Distillations'.[76] Hales later wrote that distilled spirits contained 'pernicious, burning, caustick salts' that had been produced 'by the action of fire on them in distillation'.[77]

However, the growing association of distillation with drinking and new chemical understandings of fermentation meant that the term 'alcohol' increasingly indicated a discrete chemical substance, a product of sugar fermentation, within all intoxicating drinks.[78] Physicians gradually adopted this view. For example, Thomas Trotter wrote that the 'inebriating quality of all liquors ... depends upon the alkohol which they contain', a 'word ... of Arabic origins' meaning 'the *pure spirit* separated by repeated distillations from all grosser matter'.[79] Similarly, the physician and natural philosopher Erasmus Darwin considered a whole range of fermented and distilled drinks, including 'rum, brandy, gin, whisky, usquebaugh, wine, cyder, beer, and porter' to be forms of 'alcohol'.[80] Although the Swiss naturalist and chemist Nicolas-Théodore de Saussure (1767–1845) determined the exact chemical composition of alcohol in 1804, the differences between fermented and distilled beverages remained unsettled until the work of the English chemist William Thomas Brande (1788–1866) during the early nineteenth century.[81]

Born into a family of apothecaries in London, Brande trained as a physician and initially intended to practise medicine. After meeting Humphry Davy (1778–1829) and attending his lectures, Brande became interested in chemistry. He began his career with a study that established once and for all that alcohol was a discrete chemical substance in all intoxicating drinks, and for which he was awarded the Royal Society's highest honour, the Copley Medal.[82] Publishing his findings in the *Philosophical Transactions of the Royal Society of London* in 1811, Brande criticised the 'commonly received opinion, that the alcohol obtained by the distillation of wine, does not exist ready formed in the liquor' but is formed by the 'operation' of distillation.[83] Conducting a series of experiments in which he altered various distillation parameters, Brande concluded that alcohol was present in the whole range of fermented and distilled beverages; distillation simply concentrated the spirit that fermentation had formed. He closed the article with a table listing the popular drinks at the time, including the percentage of alcohol each contained.[84] Cutting through debates about what exactly alcohol was, Brande's findings resonated with temperance reformers, many of whom were physicians. By the 1830s, fermented drinks like beer, wine and cider were soon thought to be as harmful as distilled spirits. Popularised by the Englishman Joseph Livesey, teetotalism – the total abstinence from all intoxicating drinks – would become temperance orthodoxy on both sides of the Atlantic Ocean.[85]

Conclusion

The pathologisation of distilled spirits, which emphasised their deleterious agency on the physical body, also fostered new attention on the loss of control that so often seemed to accompany heavy drinking. As Jessica Warner discovered, seventeenth-century writers frequently recognised that drunkenness was a difficult sin to quit and used the language of disease to describe it.[86] In a 1609 sermon, the preacher John Downame (1571–1652) employed the metaphors of slavery and feudal allegiance to describe the loss of control to which drinkers often succumbed. The 'drunkard by his much tipling maketh himselfe a slaue to his vice', Downame wrote, 'and by long custome bringeth superfluitie into vrgent necessitie', which reigned over the body as a lord over his vassals. Drunkenness was first 'committed, then practised, and often practise bringeth custome, and custome becommeth a second nature, and hath in it the force of a law which must be obeyed, not in courtesie, but vpon necessitie' until drinkers 'bring themselues to such an vnsatiable thirst, that they cannot sit without the cup at their elbow'.[87]

During the eighteenth century, writers still denounced the inability to control one's consumption of intoxicating drinks as a personal failure of self-control and willpower, but they increasingly recognised that once the drinking commenced, distilled spirits gradually degraded the body's physical health – which was required for mental function, morality and willpower – using a mixture of religious concepts, medical knowledge and the metaphor of slavery to describe the process of habituation. The 'bewitching Naughtiness in these Fiery Liquors', wrote Stephen Hales, caused 'a Man's Will and Affections' to become so 'depraved' that he becomes 'delighted with this worst of Slavery', a condition analogous to that of a 'Madman'.[88] Similarly, George Cheyne wrote, 'Drops beget Drams, and Drams beget more Drams, 'till they come to be without Weight and without Measure'.[89] This understanding informed the work of physicians in the second half of the eighteenth century like John Coakley Lettsom. '[W]hen the indulgence in spirituous liquors is rendered habitual', Lettsom wrote, 'it is extremely difficult to overcome'. The 'debility and tremors of the body' and the 'horrid ... despondency of the mind after the exhilarating effects of these liquors have subsided' made it very difficult to 'vanquish this habit' of taking the 'delusive poison'.[90] In North America, Benjamin Rush wrote that drunkenness and its consequences represented 'a disease induced by an act of vice'.[91] In his final work, *Medical Inquiries and Observations, upon the Diseases of the Mind* (1812), Rush explained, 'The use of strong drink is at first the effect of free agency', but once a 'habit' formed, continual drinking became 'necessity'.[92]

But does the continuity between such statements really represent an early modern concept of alcoholism and addiction, as Roy Porter and Jessica Warner posited? Even though the modern recognition of alcoholism as a form of addiction did not really take hold until the second half of the nineteenth century, the development of the understanding that distilled spirits degraded the power of will reveals that the pathologisation of intoxication was part of a broader medicalisation of right living in the early modern period that preceded the development of modern addiction concepts. As Andrew Wear writes, the 'sense of moral imperative' associated with health advice lends support to the argument that the very specific and detailed advice given on diet and on healthy places in which to live was a form of medicalisation, 'a process in which 'physicians were trying to bring ways of living, and indeed, the whole world, under medical scrutiny and control'.[93] Although 'this process had limited success', a 'medical view of the environment and of diet was shared across literate culture, even if the knowledge was not always acted upon'.[94] Thus in the early modern period, drunkenness was pathologised as a cause of grievous diseases. Gradually, distilled spirits and, later, the alcohol within them, and their ability to cause drunkenness were pathologised as substances poisonous to the body and mind.

The increased attention to the physical properties of distilled spirits during the eighteenth century and the emergence of the modern definition of alcohol in 1811 ascribed a new degree of agency to the intoxicating beverages themselves. While these discourses remained very much concerned with the drunkard's individual responsibility for his condition, the new focus on distilled spirits and alcohol pathologised drinking in ways that became useful to emerging temperance movements and the budding nineteenth-century psychiatric profession alike. By the 1820s to 1830s, the idea that alcohol was a discrete chemical substance in all intoxicating drinks was expressed by temperance writers on both sides of the Atlantic, who routinely included Brande's chart in their publications and transformed the traditional meaning of temperance as moderation to total abstinence, eventually calling for the complete prohibition of all alcoholic drinks.[95] Just as Thomas Wilson had called distilled liquors the bane of the nation, so too in the nineteenth century, temperance reformers united against King Alcohol and Demon Rum, personifications of the intoxicating substance itself. Intemperance had become all but synonymous with excessive alcohol use during the first decades of the nineteenth century. In 1849 the Swedish physician Magnus Huss coined the term 'alcoholism', a lexical construction in which the medical condition described was now named directly after the substance causing it.[96] Even though the term was slow to catch on, not entering more common usage until the turn of the twentieth century, its emergence demonstrates the degree to which alcohol had become materialised and pathologised by the mid-nineteenth century.

Early modern medical writing about intoxication, therefore, demonstrates that drunkenness had acquired distinctly medical characteristics before the emergence of psychiatry during the nineteenth century. Translating traditional Galenic and humoral medicine into Enlightenment terms, medical materialism provided a new framework for explaining how breaking the rules of right living brought about debility and disease by emphasising physical causes, specifically the effects of distilled spirits on the body and mind. The mechanical explanations of drunkenness promoted by natural philosophers like Stephen Hales, popular health writers like George Cheyne and clergymen like Thomas Wilson pathologised distilled spirits as poisonous substances whose physical effects translated into mental changes, altered behaviour and, ultimately, a loss of control that resembled sin and disease simultaneously. Moreover, medical explanations were adopted by clergymen, who used them both literally and metaphorically. Neither disease nor addiction in the modern sense, the effect of distilled spirits and intoxication was nevertheless explained within medical frameworks that supported traditional denunciations of drunkenness as a vice or sin. A growing sense that distilled spirits possessed physical properties that caused a loss of control over appetite blurred the boundary between disease and sin, complicating the distinction between the physical effects of distilled spirit and an individual's responsibility for right living once craving rendered drinking a necessity.

Notes

1 *An Inuectiue ageinst Glotony and Dronkennes* (London: Printed by Richard Lant and Richard Bankes, 1545), 7r.

2 Historians conventionally call the period from *c.* 1500 to 1800 the early modern period. Andrew Wear, *Knowledge and Practice in English Medicine, 1550–1680* (Cambridge: Cambridge University Press, 2000); Elizabeth Lane Furdell, *Publishing and Medicine in Early Modern England* (Rochester: University of Rochester Press, 2002).

3 Within a vast historical literature on alcoholism, see especially Jean-Charles Sournia, *A History of Alcoholism*, trans. Nick Hindley and Gareth Stanton (Cambridge: Basil Blackwell, 1990); Mariana Valverde, *Diseases of the Will: Alcohol and the Dilemmas of Freedom* (Cambridge: Cambridge University Press, 1998); Peter Ferentzy, 'From sin to disease: differences and similarities between past and current conceptions of chronic drunkenness', *Contemporary Drug Problems*, 28, no. 3 (1 September 2001), 363–90; Sarah W. Tracy, *Alcoholism in America: From Reconstruction to Prohibition* (Baltimore: Johns Hopkins University Press, 2005); Matthew Warner Osborn, *Rum Maniacs: Alcoholic Insanity in the Early American Republic* (Chicago: University of Chicago Press, 2014).

4 Peter Conrad, *The Medicalization of Society: On the Transformation of Human Conditions into Treatable Disorders* (Baltimore: Johns Hopkins University Press, 2007), 4.

5 An influential early essay supporting this view is Harry G. Levine, 'The discovery of addiction: changing conceptions of habitual drunkenness in America', *Journal of Studies on Alcohol*, 39, no. 1 (1978), 143–74.

6 Roy Porter, 'The drinking man's disease: the "pre-history" of alcoholism in Georgian Britain', *British Journal of Addiction*, 80, no. 4 (December 1985), 385–96; Jessica Warner, '"Resolv'd to drink no more": addiction as a preindustrial construct', *Journal of Studies on Alcohol*, 55, no. 6 (1994), 685–91; James Nicholls, 'Vinum Britannicum: the "drink question" in Early Modern England', *Social History of Alcohol and Drugs*, 22, no. 2 (2008), 190–208.

7 Porter, 'The drinking man's disease', 385.

8 Virginia Berridge, Jennifer Walke and Alex Mold, 'From inebriety to addiction: terminology and concepts in the UK, 1860–1930', *Social History of Alcohol and Drugs*, 28, no. 1 (2014), 88–106; William L. White, 'The lessons of language: historical perspectives on the rhetoric

of addiction', in Sarah W. Tracy and Caroline Jean Acker (eds), *Altering American Consciousness: The History of Alcohol and Drug Use in the United States, 1800–2000* (Amherst: University of Massachusetts Press, 2004), 33–60.

9 Phil Withington, 'Introduction: cultures of intoxiation', *Past & Present*, 222, supplement 9 (1 January 2014), 14. See also Jonathan Herring et al. (eds), *Intoxication and Society: Problematic Pleasures of Drugs and Alcohol* (Macmillan International Higher Education, 2012).

10 On the language of addiction in the early modern period, see especially Jose Murgatroyd Cree, 'Protestant Evangelicals and addiction in Early Modern English', *Renaissance Studies*, 32, no. 3 (2018), 446–62. A landmark study about the contributions of medical professionals to temperance reform, albeit in nineteenth-century America, is Osborn, *Rum Maniacs*. The role of physicians in early modern English discourses about compulsive drinking is also a key feature of James Nicholls, *The Politics of Alcohol: A History of the Drink Question in England* (Manchester: Manchester University Press, 2011), 59–72.

11 See especially David Clemis, 'medical expertise and the understandings of intoxication in Britain, 1660–1830', in Jonathan Herring et al. (eds), *Intoxication and Society: Problematic Pleasures of Drugs and Alcohol* (New York: Palgrave Macmillan, 2013), 33–51.

12 Clemis, 'Medical expertise', 34.

13 Clemis, 'Medical expertise', 35.

14 Clemis, 'Medical expertise', 35.

15 See especially Susanne Schmid and Barbara Schmidt-Haberkamp (eds), *Drink in the Eighteenth and Nineteenth Centuries* (Abingdon: Routledge, 2014).

16 Clemis, 'Medical expertise', 35–36.

17 Furdell, *Publishing and Medicine in Early Modern England*, 28.

18 Furdell, *Publishing and Medicine in Early Modern England*, 28.

19 Wear, *Knowledge and Practice in English Medicine*, 154; Furdell, *Publishing and Medicine in Early Modern England*, 3.

20 Clemis, 'Medical expertise', 34–6; Wear, *Knowledge and Practice in English Medicine*; Furdell, *Publishing and Medicine in Early Modern England*, 3–4.

21 Wear, *Knowledge and Practice in English Medicine*, 156.

22 Wear, *Knowledge and Practice in English Medicine*, 156.

23 Wear, *Knowledge and Practice in English Medicine*, 154–6; Furdell, *Publishing and Medicine*, 3.

24 Clemis, 'Medical expertise', 34–6; Wear, *Knowledge and Practice in English Medicine*, 155, 178–84. See also Rosenberg (ed.), *Right Living*.

25 Roy Porter, *Madness: A Brief History* (Oxford: Oxford University Press, 2003), 153.
26 Robert Burton, *The Anatomy of Melancholy* (Oxford: Printed by John Lichfield and James Short, for Henry Cripps, 1621); D.C.T. Cox-Maksimov, 'Burton's *Anatomy of Melancholy: Philosophically, Medically and Historically*: part 1', *History of Psychiatry* 7, no. 26 (1 June 1996), 203; D.C.T. Cox-Maksimov, 'Burton's *Anatomy of Melancholy: Philosophically, Medically and Historically*: part 2', *History of Psychiatry*, 7, no. 27 (1 September 1996), 349.
27 George Cheyne, *The English Malady: Or, A Treatise of Nervous Diseases of All Kinds* (London: Printed for G. Strahan in Cornhill, and J. Leake at Bath, 1734).
28 William Bullein, *A Newe Booke Entituled the Gouernement of Healthe* (London: Printed by Ione Day, 1558), p. cx.
29 Henry Wingfield, *A Compendious or Short Treatise, Gathered out of the Chyefe and Principall Authors of Phisycke Conteynyuge Certeyne Preceptes Necessary to the Preseruacion of Healthe, and Longe Continuaunce of the Same* (London: Printed by Robert Stoughten, 1551), ch. 6. For a similar description, see Andrew Boorde, *Compendyous Regyment or a Dyetary of Helth* (London, 1547), chs IX–X.
30 For example, see George Gascoigne, *A Delicate Diet, for Daintiemouthde Droonkardes Wherein the Fowle Abuse of Common Carowsing, and Quaffing with Hartie Draughtes, Is Honestlie Admonished* (London: Printed by John Charlewood for Richard Ihones, 1576), 12v; John Downame, *Foure Treatises Tending to Disswade All Christians from ... Swearing, Drunkennesse, Whoredome, and Briberie* (London: Imprinted by Felix Kyngston, for William Welby, 1609), 94–8, 109, 125–6; Richard Rawlidge, *A Monster Late Found Out and Discovered: Or, The Scourging of Tiplers, the Ruine of Bacchus, and the Bane of Tapsters* (Amsterdam, 1628), 1; Thomas Heywood, *Philocothonista, or, The Drunkard, Opened, Dissected, and Anatomized* (London: Printed by Robert Raworth; and are to be sold at his house neere the White-Hart Taverne in Smithfield, 1635), 84; Richard Younge, *The Drunkard's Character, or, A True Drunkard with Such Sinnes as Raigne in Him* (London: Printed by R. Badger, for George Latham, 1638), 27, 40.
31 Thomas Sydenham, *The Whole Works of That Excellent Practical Physician, Dr. Thomas Sydenham, the Third Edition, Corrected from the Original Latin, by John Pechey of the College of Physicians in London* (London: Printed for R. Wellington, at the Dolphin and Crown, at the West-End of St. Pauls Church-Yard, 1701), 362, 364.

32 On Maynwaringe and his career, see Jonathan Barry, 'The "compleat physician" and experimentation in medicines: Everard Maynwaring (c. 1629–1713) and the Restoration debate on medical practice in London', *Medical History*, 62, no. 2 (April 2018), 155–76.
33 Everard Maynwaringe, *The Method and Means of Enjoying Health, Vigour, and Long LIfe* (London: Printed by J.M. for Dorman Newman, at the Kings-Arms in the Poultrey, 1683), 120–1.
34 Maynwaringe, *The Method and Means*, 124–5.
35 Maynwaringe, *The Method and Means*, 130. Italics in original text.
36 Maynwaringe, *The Method and Means*, 134. Italics in original text.
37 Maynwaringe, *The Method and Means*, 125. Italics in original text.
38 On the Gin Craze, see Patrick Dillon, *Gin: The Much Lamented Death of Madam Geneva* (Boston: Justin, Charles & Co., 2004); Jessica Warner, *Craze: Gin and Debauchery in an Age of Reason* (New York: Four Walls Eight Windows, 2002). On the commercialisation of distillation, see also Tillmann Taape, 'Distilling reliable remedies: Hieronymus Brunschwig's *Liber de arte distillandi* (1500) between alchemical learning and craft practice', *Ambix*, 61, no. 3 (1 August 2014), 236–56.
39 Hisao Ishizuka, '"Fibre body": the concept of fibre in eighteenth-century medicine, c. 1700–40', *Medical History*, 56, no. 4 (2012), 562–84; Hisao Ishizuka, 'Visualizing the fibre-woven body: Nehemiah Grew's plant anatomy and the emergence of the fibre body', in Matthew Landers and Brian Muñoz (eds), *Anatomy and the Organization of Knowledge, 1500–1850* (London: Pickering & Chatto, 2012), 113–28; Guenter B. Risse, 'Medicine in the Age of Enlightenment', in Andrew Wear (ed.), *Medicine in Society: Historical Essays* (Cambridge: Cambridge University Press, 1992), 149–95.
40 In a vast literature on medicine during the Enlightenment, see especially Robert E. Schofield, *Mechanism and Materialism: British Natural Philosophy in an Age of Reason* (Princeton: Princeton University Press, 2015); Andrew Cunningham and Roger K. French (eds), *The Medical Enlightenment of the Eighteenth Century* (Cambridge: Cambridge University Press, 1990); Harold John Cook, *Matters of Exchange: Commerce, Medicine, and Science in the Dutch Golden Age* (New Haven, CT: Yale University Press, 2007), 226–66, 378–409.
41 G.A. Lindeboom, *Herman Boerhaave: The Man and His Work* (London: Methuen & Co. Ltd, 1968); Andrew Cunningham, 'Medicine to calm the mind: Boerhaave's medical system, and why it was adopted in Edinburgh', in Andrew Cunningham and Roger K. French (eds), *The Medical Enlightenment of the Eighteenth Century* (Cambridge:

Cambridge University Press, 1990), 40–66; Rina Knoeff, *Herman Boerhaave (1668–1738): Calvinist Chemist and Physician* (Amsterdam: Koninklijke Nederlandse Akademie van Wetenschappen, 2002); Allen G. Debus, *The Chemical Promise: Experiment and Mysticism in the Chemical Philosophy, 1550–1800 – Selected Essays of Allen G. Debus* (Sagamore Beach, MA: Science History Publications, 2006), 487–96; John C. Powers, *Inventing Chemistry: Herman Boerhaave and the Reform of the Medical Arts* (Chicago: University of Chicago Press, 2012).

42 Roy Porter, 'Medical science', in Roy Porter (ed.), *The Cambridge History of Medicine* (Cambridge: Cambridge University Press, 2006 [2001]), 143.

43 Herman Boerhaave, *A Treatise on the Power of Medicines*, trans. John Martyn (London: Printed by C. Jephson for John Wilcox, and James Hodges, 1740), 11–13. Italics in original text.

44 Boerhaave, *A Treatise on the Power of Medicines*, 45, 50, 96–7.

45 Porter, 'Medical science', 143.

46 Herman Boerhaave, *Boerhaave's Aphorisms: Concerning the Knowledge and Cure of Diseases* (London: Printed for B. Cowse, and W. Innys, in St. Paul's Church-Yard, 1715), 278.

47 William Cullen, *First Lines of the Practice of Physic*, 4th edn, corrected and enlarged, vol. 3 (Edinburgh: Printed for C. Elliot, 1784), 224–6.

48 Thomas Short, *Discourses on Tea, Sugar, Milk, Made-Wines, Spirits, Punch, Tobacco, &c.: With Plain and Useful Rules for Gouty People* (London: Printed for T. Longman, in Pater-noster-row; and A. Millar, in the Strand, 1750), 172.

49 Short, *Discourses on Tea*, 185–7.

50 Anita Guerrini, *Obesity and Depression in the Enlightenment: The Life and Times of George Cheyne* (Norman: University of Oklahoma Press, 2000).

51 George Cheyne, *An Essay on Regimen* (London: Printed for C. Rivington, in St. Paul's Church-yard; and J. Leake, Bookseller in Bath, 1753), 67–8.

52 A.E. Clark-Kennedy, *Stephen Hales*, reprint (Cambridge: Cambridge University Press, 2015 [1929]); 'The life of Dr. Stephen Hales', in *British Biography: Or, an Accurate and Impartial Account of the Lives and Writings of Eminent Persons in Great Britain and Ireland*, vol. 9 (London: R. Goadby, 1778), 214–25; Anita Guerrini, *Experimenting with Humans and Animals: From Galen to Animal Rights* (Baltimore: Johns Hopkins University Press, 2003), 57–60.

53 Stephen Hales, *Statical Essays: Containing Hæmastatics; or, An Account of Some Hydraulic and Hydrostatical Experiments Made on the Blood and Blood-Vessels of Animals*, 3rd edn, vol. 2 (London, 1769), 123–4.
54 Hales, *Statical Essays*, vol. 2, 124.
55 Stephen Hales, *A Friendly Admonition to the Drinkers of Brandy, and Other Distilled Spirituous Liquors* (London: Printed for Joseph Downing, 1733), 4.
56 Dillon, *Gin*, 100.
57 Hales, *Friendly Admonition*, 4.
58 Stephen Hales, *A Friendly Admonition to the Drinkers of Gin, Brandy, and Other Distilled Spirituous Liquors*, 5th edn (London: Printed for B. Dodd, Bookseller to The Society for promoting Christian Knowledge, at the Bible and Ket in Ave-Mary Lane, near Stationers Hall, 1754), 10.
59 Hales, *Friendly Admonition* (1733), 14.
60 Thomas Wilson, *Distilled Spirituous Liquors the Bane of the Nation* (London: Printed for J. Roberts in Warwick Lane, 1736), 28.
61 Wilson, *Distilled Spirituous Liquors*, i–ii.
62 Wilson, *Distilled Spirituous Liquors*, ii.
63 Wilson, *Distilled Spirituous Liquors*, 42. Italics in original text.
64 Clemis, 'Medical Expertise', 44–7; Griffith Edwards, 'Thomas Trotter's "Essay on Drunkenness" appraised', *Addiction*, 107, no. 9 (September 2012), 1562–79; Anthony Fothergill, *An Essay on the Abuse of Spirituous Liquors* (Bath: Printed by R. Cruttwell, 1796); John Coakley Lettsom, *History of Some of the Effects of Hard Drinking*, 6th edn (London: Printed by W. Darton and Co., 1791); Thomas Trotter, *An Essay, Medical, Philosophical, and Chemical, on Drunkenness, and Its Effects on the Human Body*, 4th edn (London: Longman, Hurst, Rees, and Orme, 1810).
65 Trotter, *An Essay*, 68.
66 Trotter, *An Essay*, 53.
67 Stephen Hales, *A Sermon Preached before the Trustees for Establishing the Colony of Georgia in America* (London: Printed for T. Woodward, 1734), 61.
68 Stephen Hales, *The Pernicious Practice of Dram-Drinking* (Woodbridge, NJ: Printed by James Parker, 1759), 1.
69 Gilman Marston Ostrander, *Republic of Letters: The American Intellectual Community, 1776–1865* (Madison: Madison House, 1999), ch. 3; Gary B. Nash, *First City: Philadelphia and the Forging of Historical Memory* (Philadelphia: University of Pennsylvania Press, 2006); Trevor Burnard, 'The British Atlantic', in Jack P. Greene and

Philip D. Morgan (eds), *Atlantic History: A Critical Appraisal* (Oxford: Oxford University Press, 2008), 111–36; Mark A. Peterson, 'Theopolis Americana: The city-state of Boston, the Republic of Letters, and the Protestant International, 1689–1739', in Bernard Bailyn and Patricia L. Denault (eds), *Soundings in Atlantic History: Latent Structures and Intellectual Currents, 1500–1830* (Cambridge, MA: Harvard University Press, 2009), 329–70.

70 Helen Brock, 'North America, a western outpost of European medicine', in Andrew Cunningham and Roger K. French (eds), *The Medical Enlightenment of the Eighteenth Century* (Cambridge: Cambridge University Press, 1990), 194–216. See also Lisa Rosner, 'Thistle on the Delaware: Edinburgh medical education and Philadelphia practice, 1800–1825', *Social History of Medicine*, 5, no. 1 (1 April 1992), 19–42.

71 Maurice Jackson, *Let This Voice Be Heard: Anthony Benezet, Father of Atlantic Abolitionism* (Philadelphia: University of Pennsylvania Press, 2009).

72 Anthony Benezet, *The Potent Enemies of America Laid Open: Being Some Account of the Baneful Effects Attending the Use of Distilled Spirituous Liquors, and the Slavery of the Negroes* (Philadelphia: Printed by Joseph Crukshank, 1774), 3.

73 See especially the fourth edition, Benjamin Rush, *An Inquiry into the Effects of Ardent Spirits upon the Human Body and Mind*, 4th edn (Philadelphia: Printed for Thomas Dobson, 1808); Nicholls, 'Vinum Britannicum'; Nicholls, *The Politics of Alcohol*, 64–5; Osborn, *Rum Maniacs*, 13–44.

74 For interpretations of Rush's central role in inspiring temperance reformers, see especially Brian Harrison, *Drink and the Victorians: The Temperance Question in England, 1815–1872* (Pittsburgh: University of Pittsburgh Press, 1971); Norman H. Clark, *Deliver Us from Evil: An Interpretation of American Prohibition* (New York: W.W. Norton & Company, 1976); William J. Rorabaugh, *The Alcoholic Republic: An American Tradition* (New York: Oxford University Press, 1981); Ian R. Tyrrell, *Sobering Up: From Temperance to Prohibition in Antebellum America, 1800–1860* (Westport: Greenwood Press, 1979); Jack S. Blocker, *American Temperance Movements: Cycles of Reform* (Boston: Twayne Publishers, 1989); Thomas R. Pegram, *Battling Demon Rum: The Struggle for a Dry America, 1800–1933* (Chicago: Ivan R. Dee, 1998).

75 Seth C. Rasmussen, *The Quest for Aqua Vitae: The History and Chemistry of Alcohol from Antiquity to the Middle Ages* (Cambridge:

Springer, 2014), 2–7; Robert J. Forbes, *Short History of the Art of Distillation: From the Beginning to the Death of Cellier Blumenthal* (Leiden: E.J. Brill, 1948), 47.

76 Both authors used the same phrase. Hales, *Friendly Admonition* (1733), 14; Wilson, *Distilled Spirituous Liquors the Bane of the Nation*, 37.

77 Hales, *The Pernicious Practice of Dram-Drinking*, 5.

78 See especially the work of the French chemist Antoine Laurent Lavoisier, *Elements of Chemistry*, trans. Robert Kerr (Edinburgh: W. Creech, 1790), 130–1; Aaron J. Ihde, *The Development of Modern Chemistry*, rev. edn (New York: Dover Publications, 2012), 79–80.

79 Trotter, *An Essay*, 42–3. Italics in original.

80 Erasmus Darwin, *Zoonomia; Or, The Laws of Organic Life*, vol. 1 (Dublin: Printed for P. Byrne, and W. Jones, 1794), 353.

81 Ihde, *The Development of Modern Chemistry*, 177. Clemis, 'Medical expertise', 44.

82 Elizabeth Haigh, 'William Thomas Brande and the chemical education of medical students', in Roger French and Andrew Cunningham (eds), *British Medicine in an Age of Reform* (New York: Routledge, 2005 [1991]), 185–6.

83 William Thomas Brande, 'Experiments to ascertain the state in which spirit exists in fermented liquors: with a table exhibiting the relative proportion of pure alcohol contained in several kinds of wine and some other liquors', *Philosophical Transactions of the Royal Society of London*, 101 (1811), 337.

84 Brande, 'Experiments to ascertain', 345–6.

85 Annemarie McAllister, 'The alternative world of the proud non-drinker: nineteenth-century public displays of temperance', *Social History of Alcohol and Drugs*, 28, no. 2 (Summer 2014), 161–79; Harrison, *Drink and the Victorians*, 103–20; Blocker, *American Temperance Movements*, 21–5.

86 Warner, 'Resolv'd to drink no more'.

87 Downame, *Foure Treatises*, 93–94; see also 111–12.

88 Hales, *Friendly Admonition* (1754), 11–12. Italics in original text.

89 George Cheyne, *An Essay of Health and Long Life* (London: Printed for George Strahan, at the Golden Ball over-against the Royal Exchange in Cornhill; and J. Leake, Bookseller at Bath, 1724), 52.

90 Lettsom, *History of Some of the Effects of Hard Drinking*, 11–12.

91 Benjamin Rush, *An Inquiry Into the Effects of Ardent Spirits upon the Human Body and Mind* (Boston: James Loring, 1823), 29.

92 Benjamin Rush, *Medical Inquiries and Observations, upon the Diseases of the Mind* (Philadelphia: Grigg & Elliot, 1835), 264.

93 Wear, *Knowledge and Practice in English Medicine*, 155.
94 Wear, *Knowledge and Practice in English Medicine*, 155.
95 On Brande's influence in the USA, see Rorabaugh, *The Alcoholic Republic*, 101–02; Blocker, *American Temperance Movements*, 23.
96 Tracy, *Alcoholism in America*, 41.

2

Alcoholism, degeneration, madness and psychiatry in Spain, 1870–1920

Ricardo Campos

Between 1870 and 1920 Spanish doctors' perspectives on alcoholism were directly influenced by French and to a lesser extent British, German and Italian scientific research.[1] In general, Spanish medical studies dedicated to alcoholism did not demonstrate doctrinal originality, nor did they have an original empirical basis, as evidenced in the use and systematic analysis of statistics from other countries to support their claims. This doctrinal dependence on foreign research affected the nature of the work focusing on alcoholism, which consequently had an evident propagandistic and informative tone, making it difficult to distinguish from the writings and lectures of non-medical, anti-alcohol propagandists.[2]

In general, medical studies focused on warning the population of the dangers of excessive consumption of alcohol regarding health, morals, social order and race. This created a dual perspective of alcoholism within the medical-social field: as a vice and a disease.[3] Alcoholism was associated with a lack of morality, deviant behaviour – such as crime, sexual promiscuity, prostitution and vagrancy – and misery. Since alcoholism was also seen to be a social plague, a connection began to be established between alcohol and other diseases such as syphilis, tuberculosis and madness.

In this regard, studies on alcoholism and anti-alcohol attitudes differed little from the international publications of the time, and the appearance of alcoholism in degeneration theory strengthened the view of drunkenness and alcoholism as vice and disease. This trend began to crystallise in Spain in the 1890s, coinciding with a period of significant social and economic change and the loss of its last colonies in 1898, and after a brief war with the USA plunged the country into a crisis that was interpreted by elites as a symptom of deep decline.[4] The biological determinism of degenerationism – the idea that it was based on heredity – had a substantial influence on anti-alcohol discourse in such a context, reinforcing the association of alcohol with vice and disease: alcoholism appeared to be the cause and product of degeneration. Additionally, the importance given to the idea that alcoholism was hereditary created a nihilistic attitude towards the issue, which in turn led the anti-alcohol struggle to propose the implementation of preventive measures, essentially suggesting that treating hereditary alcoholism would be unsuccessful. Nevertheless, Spanish psychiatrists played a secondary role in the development of this anti-alcohol corpus, which was led by doctors and hygienists with no psychiatric training. This fact is striking, and the possible causes of their reticence should be analysed.

The purpose of this chapter is to analyse psychiatrists' positions on alcoholism at this time and explain why they did not play a leading role in the fight against alcoholism together with hygienists and social doctors. An explanation given by some authors is that alcoholism is a difficult disease to catalogue and cure, a fact which may have led many psychiatrists to pay little attention to it.[5] However, from the many sources that I have studied I have inferred that there are deeper issues relating to the clinical approach to alcoholism and psychiatrists' professional priorities, ingrained in the social weakness of the discipline of psychiatry at that time.[6] I will work from the hypothesis that psychiatry during this period was still constructing itself as a profession and was focusing on other priorities that would legitimise it publicly as a field in itself, such as psychiatric expertise in major criminal cases. Psychiatrists' interest in alcoholism was reduced to psychiatric clinical symptoms, in that alcoholism was considered a cause of 'alcohol madness': alcoholism was not, at this point, considered from a social perspective by psychiatrists.

On this basis, this chapter analyses alcoholism in psychiatric publications and the clinical perspective of the disease, within the context of hereditary alcoholism advocated by degenerationism, as well as changes that occurred after 1900. The period of analysis of this work begins in 1870, when the term 'alcoholism' was used for the first time in Spanish medical literature. It concludes in 1920, when the journal *Archivos de Neurobiología* (Archives of Neurobiology) was founded and the movement of mental hygiene began. In the new context of mental hygiene that developed during the 1920s and 1930s, psychiatric discourses and practices began to focus on the prevention of mental illness.

Medicine and alcoholism: the discreet role of psychiatrists

From the mid-nineteenth century, Spanish medicine described immoderate consumption of alcohol as a social and health problem associated with profound changes emerging from industrialisation. The first hygienist doctors noted the significant consequences that these transformations had on the life of the popular classes, and especially among the emerging working class. In this new context, traditional patterns of consumption and production of alcoholic beverages changed, and alcohol began to be perceived not only as a vice and a danger to the social order, but also as a social disease closely linked to the working class and their miserable living and working conditions. In the mid-nineteenth century, Spanish doctors believed that alcoholism was mainly sociological and moral and could thus not be treated clinically. An important addition to Spanish scientific data was the late and incomplete incorporation of *Alcoholismus chronicus* by Magnus Huss (1807–1890), published in Swedish in 1849 and translated into German in 1852.[7]

In this sense, the delay in the use of the term 'alcoholism' in Spanish studies is striking.[8] Coined by the Swedish doctor to define a new disease, used by French alienism since the 1850s,[9] and incorporated and reinterpreted by Benedict Augustin Morel (1809–1873) in his formulation of degeneration theory in 1857,[10] the term was not used in Spain until the 1870s. One of the first authors to do so was Pedro Felipe Monlau (1808–1871) in the third edition of his work *Elementos de higiene pública* (Elements of Public Hygiene), published in 1871. Unlike the two previous editions of that book (1847 and 1862), the third edition included the terms 'alcoholism' and 'alcoholic' to refer to both the excessive consumption of alcohol and its effects on health and the intoxicated subject.[11] Despite the modern terminology, medicine continued to incorporate social prejudices towards drinkers, which in turn influenced new scientific parameters, meaning that an alcoholic came to be defined as a medicalised drunk, and alcoholism as a vice and social plague rather than as a disease. In this sense, the substitution was never complete, and the old and new terminologies were interchangeable for decades, as is evidenced by the 1914 publication of a book entitled *Borrachos* (Drunkards) that attempted to clarify and define the use of those terms.[12]

The late use of the term 'alcoholism' points to Spanish doctors' unawareness – until the last quarter of the nineteenth century – of the innovative work on alcoholism being published abroad. It also shows that until then there was no clear appreciation that the consumption of alcoholic beverages could be a disease in itself. A greater understanding and knowledge of alcoholism from works published abroad, especially in France, and a reception of degenerationism contributed to the terminological change and, to a lesser extent, a conceptual change; despite the biological determinism that permeated degeneration theory, the nature of alcoholism as a social plague began to be emphasised, paradoxically, as it was now believed to be hereditary.

Degenerationism was very well received by social doctors and hygienists as a medical-sociological theory to explain the collective evils of society.[13] Their support for an interventionist approach to the population's physical and moral environment, especially in the case of the working class, fitted well with the ideas of degenerationism and the interpretation of alcoholism based on that theory. Familiar with social problems and committed to their solution, doctors and social hygienists interpreted degeneration and alcoholism as a collective issue, and the clinical and individual aspects of degeneration were quietly ignored. They gave vital importance to the consequences of alcoholism for the human species and the necessity of imposing a moral intervention on the population.

In this context, psychiatrists' minimal role in the anti-alcohol struggle is striking. Despite their familiarity with alcohol-dependent patients admitted to psychiatric institutions, their writings on the subject were scarce and focused on the clinical symptoms related to the mental health of the alcohol-dependent patient, avoiding social-medical discourse that emphasised the nature of alcoholism as a social plague. In their publications, psychiatrists of the time tried to define alcoholism, as well as its clinical evolution and its different phases, using both the literature and theories of the time and their daily practice in asylums. The resulting scientific production, however, was unoriginal, borrowing heavily from foreign literature, especially French publications.

There was, in my view, a contradiction between theory and conceptualisation on the one hand and practical application on the other. The former was characterised by unoriginality (although psychiatric theories did raise some interesting points such as rejecting – or questioning the importance of – degeneration theory and the role of hereditary alcoholism). In regard to the latter, cases of alcoholism were presented in medical journals to illustrate and construct a scientific discourse based on clinical observation. But beyond these published case studies, research into clinical cases from asylum settings showed a fissure between theoretical and practical facets, as is evidenced by the low percentage of admissions due to alcoholism in psychiatric institutions and the absence of therapy reflected in the medical records.[14]

For example, between 1857 and 1928, from 2,314 medical records, the Santa Isabel National Asylum diagnosed a total of seventy-eight cases of alcoholism, thirty-three of them as first diagnoses, forty-three as second and two as third.[15] Between 1900 and 1931, there were thirty-four cases of alcoholism, ten as second diagnoses: 3.2 per cent of the total number of patients.[16] In the case of the Sant Boi de Llobregat Asylum (Barcelona), the figures were higher, reaching 6.7 per cent of the patients admitted between 1885 and 1939.[17] In 1917 Salvador Vives, director of the Salt Asylum (Girona), said that of the 525 patients admitted, twenty were alcoholics (3.8 per cent), excluding those who consumed excessive amounts of alcohol because of the mental illness they suffered.[18]

Why did psychiatrists remain in the shadows? What motivated their seeming disinterest in the theory of degeneration, despite it being well received by their medical colleagues? If doctors and hygienists openly interpreted alcoholism as a collective issue associated with degeneration, why did psychiatrists focus on the clinical aspects of alcoholism and prioritise them over an approach that focused on population issues?

Some authors have suggested that the disinterest of psychiatry towards alcoholism was rooted in the resistance of the disease to therapeutic advances.[19] The moral considerations involved – namely that alcohol consumption was considered a vice – may have been responsible for psychiatrists' lack of attention to alcoholism, and the prioritisation of less socially pejorative pathologies.[20] Although this idea is partially true, both psychiatrists' relative disinterest towards alcoholism and the contradictions noted above directly relate not only to clinical factors, but also to the institutionalisation of psychiatry as a medical speciality – a slow and hesitant movement in Spain during the nineteenth century. As will be shown below, Spanish psychiatrists were not interested in the theory of degeneration until the 1890s. Therefore, up to that point, their interpretation of alcoholism was not degenerationist and was limited to a clinical and individual focus. From the 1890s, and especially after the trauma of the 1898 war against the USA, they began to pay more attention to degenerationism and included it in their explanations of alcoholism.

Psychiatry and degeneration: an ambiguous relationship

In 1876 Juan Giné y Partagás (1836–1903), director of the Nueva Belén Asylum (Barcelona), published his *Tratado teórico-práctico de freno-patología o Estudio de las enfermedades mentales* (Theoretical-Practical Treatise on Phreno-Pathology or The Study of Mental Illnesses),[21] which is considered the first Spanish book on the subject of psychiatry. It recognised the role of biological heredity as an individual predisposing cause to mental illness, including alcoholism. Closely following the ideas of Auguste Voisin (1829–1898), Giné noted that 'the alcoholic habits of parents' produced a predisposition to mental disorders in their children, especially if those parents 'were under the influence of alcohol at the time of intercourse'.[22] However, despite declaring himself a somaticist and positivist, Giné was reluctant to recognise the influence of heredity within the framework of degeneration theory as formulated by Morel in 1857, as he considered it to be 'inapplicable as a diagnostic guide'.[23] He distanced himself from degenerationism because of clinical reasons, but also because of the theoretical influence of Joseph Guislain (1792–1860) and others related to the hesitant development of psychiatry as an institution in Spain.[24]

Giné was not the only psychiatrist who distanced himself from degeneration theory. His disciple Arturo Galcerán y Granés (1850–1919) paid scant attention to it until the twentieth century. Neither Galcerán's articles in the *Revista Frenopática Barcelonesa* (Barcelona Phrenopathy Journal) published during the 1880s, nor his book *Neuropatología y psiquiatría generales* (General Neuropathology and Psychiatry) published in 1895, addressed the issue.[25] This omission is most surprising in the case of the latter: the theory of degenerationism had been updated by Valentin Magnan (1835–1916) and Paul Maurice Legrain (1860–1939) in the years preceding the publication of Galcerán's book, and that same year Magnan's *Les degenerés* was published.[26] Further to this, José María Esquerdo (1842–1912), director and owner of the Carabanchel Asylum (Madrid) and promoter of a large group of psychiatrists in Madrid, did not use degenerationism in his clinical practice either.

Despite this, these authors and their disciples openly supported degenerationism when they intervened as experts in the courts of justice. Their expert psychiatric reports on criminals on trial meticulously described family trees showing the apparent importance of biological heredity in the spread of madness and of 'degenerative' symptoms throughout the family.[27] They also meticulously referred to the physical and mental symptoms of the accused in order to show that their criminal act was determined by the mental illness they suffered and provoked by being born into a 'degenerate' family. Why were psychiatrists so inconsistent in their use of degenerationism? Why was it left out in clinical practice but used in psychiatric expertise? Included among the clinical reasons that psychiatrists themselves gave, flexibility towards degenerationism served a political and social strategy to support the legitimisation of psychiatry.

During the first half of the nineteenthth century, healthcare in Spain was marked by the attempt to replace the private charity system of the Ancien Régime with one in line with liberalism that recognised charity as an obligation of the state. The process was complicated on account of the political instability of the country (French invasion, independence of the American colonies, civil war between absolutists and liberals) and the economic bankruptcy of the state. From 1843 onwards, a period of political stability began that allowed the liberal reforms and the debate on the care of the mentally ill to be tackled. In order to solve the economic crisis of the charitable institutions, organise healthcare and solve the problem of begging, the Law of Beneficence was passed in 1849. For the care of the insane, the creation of a network of six model asylums was envisaged, although economic difficulties did not allow it to be developed, and it was limited to the creation of the National Asylum of Santa Isabel in Leganés. Although the state assumed its obligations with regard to care, the law enshrined the principle of the subsidiary nature of public care, assuming a mixed management formula that allowed the development of a private network of lunatic asylums.

The 1849 Law of Beneficence consecrated a double welfare model of madness. On the one hand, it created a public healthcare model that was more social than medical, and did not receive sufficient funding for the number of people in need of help. On the other, it also set up a private healthcare network, located mainly in Catalonia and Madrid, which played a fundamental role in the development of psychiatry as a scientific discipline.[28]

The purpose of private centres was to attract clients with solid purchasing power. Thus medical directors' discourse, regardless of their beliefs on mental illness, emphasised the scientific nature of psychiatry, the curability of mental illness, the therapeutic virtues of their establishments and these establishments' high success rates.[29] Although they defended the somatic origins of mental illness and the importance of biological heredity in its genesis, an acceptance of degenerationism – associated with incurability – in the clinical setting would conflict with the economic and scientific interests of private institutions. However, the objectives of psychiatrists in a legal context differed. The necessity for their expert opinions had opened an important opportunity for the public and official legitimisation of their profession: they were the only experts able to define whether defendants were truly 'mad' or not.

In judicial courts, psychiatrists were not asked to ascertain whether madness was curable or not, but to defend and consolidate the figure of the alienist as an ally of public order.

Therefore the rejection of or indifference to degenerationism as an explanatory model of mental illness and in turn alcoholism had, in those years, a combination of clinical and socio-professional motivations. However, from the 1890s Spanish psychiatry did eventually begin to assimilate degenerationism, albeit with certain peculiarities, which affected the interpretation of alcoholism as a fundamentally clinical and individual phenomenon.

The psychiatric clinic and hereditary alcoholism

In his 1876 treatise, Giné addressed alcoholism from a triple perspective: as a cause of madness, as a madness and as a vice. A concern that the effects of alcoholism could be confused with symptoms of other mental pathologies was central to his work. He thus wrote that the injuries typical of 'confirmed alcoholism' included alcohol insanity, alcoholic epilepsy and chronic alcoholism. The latter included general paralysis, dementia and alcoholic pseudo-pellagra. He went on to describe the symptoms that accompanied each of the injuries, comparing them with other mental pathologies in an attempt to clarify differences and establish a correct diagnosis. Giné was also very aware of the existence of drinkers who had previously suffered from mental illness – as a consequence of either biological heredity or what seemed to be an alcohol-related monomania or dipsomania[30] – who should not be confused with those inclined, voluntarily or by habit, to drink.

Despite these detailed descriptions of clinical symptoms and comparisons with other pathologies, moral and social considerations were also present in his arguments. Consequently, he thus associated drunkenness with a licentious life and considered it a degrading vice that caused disorder, abandonment of obligations and laziness,[31] which especially affected the working classes, 'who could not resist' the influence of alcohol 'as a restorative diet'.[32]

Despite this, alcoholism was not one of psychiatry's central concerns during the next two decades. José María Esquerdo's most well-known work concerned certain psychiatric reports and documents related to crime. Alcoholism had a notable presence only in psychiatric reports on the defendants' family backgrounds and in work on criminality. In this context, it was always presented as the cause of hereditary madness and degeneration. The 1881 psychiatric report that Esquerdo wrote on José Garayo, known as 'El Sacamantecas', accused the latter of murdering, raping and disembowelling several women, and diagnosed him as an imbecile and as suffering from moral insanity.[33] A reconstruction of Garayo's family tree was used as evidence to suggest that alcoholism was predominant in the family as a cause of madness and degeneration: Garayo was the son of an alcoholic, the brother of two alcoholic women and the father of an alcoholic child. Moreover, in 1894 Giné published a report, endorsed by fourteen other doctors, stating that alcoholism was prevalent in the genealogical background of Samuel Willie, an English businessman based in Barcelona who murdered his associates and was diagnosed as a degenerate by heredity. Willie's maternal grandfather had habitually abused alcohol, it was suggested, because he suffered from some kind of madness that impelled him to drink.[34]

In 1888 Victoriano Garrido, a disciple of Esquerdo, published his book *La cárcel o el manicomio* (Prison or Asylum), in which he used openly degenerationist and Lombrosoesque positions in order to defend the idea that insanity and crime were linked.[35] He included alcoholism in his chapter on impulsive madness, warning of the devastating effects the hereditary degenerateness of alcoholics could have on the human race: 'From drunken parents come epileptic children, neuropaths, unstable beings, of little moral sense, with early tendencies for vice and crime'; he added that alcoholics were 'monstrous excrescences of a sick society, disgusting dross born in the rot of vice'.[36] Following Morel, Garrido further argued that 'deviation from the normal type of the human species' is born 'from causes that threaten the natural growth of organisms, and in particular the intemperance or abuse of beverages'.[37] Nonetheless, Garrido's perspective was exceptional, and his frightening messages about the effects of alcoholism on the human race did not correspond to the rather moderate and distant tone of most psychiatrists.

In 1893 Vicente Ots (1863?–1906) strongly criticised Spanish psychiatry's lack of knowledge regarding alcoholism. He noted that, unlike those in other countries, Spanish asylums almost never diagnosed alcohol insanity even though 'many of the mentally ill' had symptoms that suggested they were suffering from it. According to Ots, this was because of the 'scarce classification of diseases' available for diagnosis, limited to the paralytic, epileptic, hysterical madness and imbecility, such that many mental dispositions were left out, among them alcohol insanity. To address this, Ots suggested studying the types of alcohol insanity more closely, which, in his opinion, had increased exorbitantly as a consequence 'of dominant mercantilism'.[38]

Ots also noted that alcoholism was difficult to diagnose because it shared symptoms with other forms of mental illness. In his opinion, 'degenerative syndromes and stigmas of alcoholism as defined by Magnan' were difficult to distinguish from each other and tended to be 'be identified as the same kind of illness', and that it would require detailed observational clinical study to tell them apart.[39] Ots's article presented several clinical cases with different varieties of alcohol insanity: dipsomania, alcoholic maniacal excitement, alcoholic mania, alcoholic epileptic madness, alcoholic pseudo-paralysis and a final form that, according to Ots, produced symptoms that could be related 'to both alcoholism and degeneration' and which presented in difficult-to-diagnose degenerated individuals. Ots noted that if the individual was observed during periods of calm, their 'somatic and psychological analysis' was used to deduce that they were degenerates. However, the diagnosis could change if they were examined in a state of alcoholic intoxication. Here, they would be likely to be diagnosed with toxic insanity[40]

Ots had absolute belief in degenerationism and thus analysed alcoholism through that perspective. Within this standpoint, however, he was limited to the individual and a clinical setting and so was unable to associate alcoholism with the degeneration of the human race as a whole, as the social-medical field had done. This perspective was evident in other works by Ots, such as his book *Neurosis y degeneración* (Neurosis and Degeneration, 1897), where he advocated a clinical approach to the issue in order to create

> solid and lasting consensus to finally settle the hypotheses, theories and doctrines – that incessantly encroach on our scientific domain – by attempting to explain and reveal the most ignored phenomena occurring in the organisation of the human organism.[41]

Speculation on the social aspects of degeneration fell outside his interpretations and would form part of what he called 'legal degeneration that included 'criminals, vagabonds and prostitutes'.[42] The moderation in the language used here contrasted with the tone used in a conference on alcoholism he gave to socialist workers, where he used all the clichés associated with degenerationism: 'Children conceived during the drunkenness of either a man or a woman are born idiots, imbeciles, deaf-dumb, crazy, stunted, sickly, epileptic or unable to live properly.'[43]

In general, psychiatrists were very cautious with therapy because, despite using certain treatments to facilitate patients' abstinence, they used to rely exclusively on patients' complete isolation. But there were also psychiatrists, such as Timoteo Sanz, who were optimistic about the possibility of treating alcoholics,[44] and in Sanz's case this was despite being a supporter of the theories of heredity and degeneration. Sanz thought that the negative regression of the human race was not unavoidable, as was argued by Morel and other psychiatrists, because there were *regenerative* elements present in the environment that cushioned and corrected the 'pathological energies' contracted through heredity.[45] Thus he distanced himself from the nihilistic idea that the implacable laws of heredity would lead to the total degradation of the human species. This therapeutic optimism was reflected in the articles he published in 1895, where the cases of alcoholism he presented, including those with a hereditary background of the disease, were cured.[46]

In the social-medical field, theoretical links between alcoholism and degeneration grew rapidly during the second half of the 1890s. In addition to scientific justifications for degenerationism, the political and cultural climate of the country was characterised by what was perceived as a generalised decadence – the consequence of a significant political crisis, a military defeat against the USA in 1898 and the subsequent loss of Cuba, Puerto Rico and the Philippines – which was fundamental to the growth in popularity of degeneration theory. From this crisis emerged a 'Regenerationist' movement which penetrated the entire ideological spectrum.[47] The presuppositions of degeneration theory, in both its scientific and its cultural interpretations, offered a social-biological explanation for the ills that the country was suffering, and warned of national decadence. In such a context, at the end of the century, anti-alcohol medical discourse became radicalised and unashamedly adopted degenerationism and the idea that alcoholism was hereditary. Warnings about the dangers that alcoholism entailed for 'the race' multiplied and were central to medical-social discourse and to anti-alcohol, non-medical propaganda.[48]

Psychiatrists also began to show greater interest in degeneration and the effects of alcoholism on the population, although in a more careful manner. José María Escuder (1852–1923) stated in 1895 that 'a town full of drunks paves the way for a generation of imbeciles, fools or evildoers'.[49] In his text, alcoholism was not exclusively an individual problem but took on a social dimension that affected society as a whole and the future of the race. Shortly afterwards, Mateo Bonafonte (1862–1940), a psychiatrist at the Zaragoza asylum, defended the link between 'the development of alcoholism and mental derangement', pointing to the increase of 'degenerative insanity', to the detriment of 'pure' psychoses, and as a result of 'habits and customs inherent to modern civilisation and widely developed vices and diseases'.[50] For Bonafonte, alcoholism was a symptom of degeneration that had a strong hereditary nature.

To illustrate this point, Bonafonte used the case study of Ada Jurke, an alcoholic vagabond whose offspring over time had produced 106 illegitimate children, 142 beggars, 64 vagrants living in homeless shelters, 81 prostitutes and 76 convicted criminals, all of them, according to Bonafonte, degenerate.[51] He also used Legrain's research, especially *Dégénérescence sociale et alcoolisme* (Social Degenerationism and Alcoholism) to demonstrate the devastating effect that alcoholism had had on hereditary alcoholics. Bonafonte's conclusion from analysing this data was that alcohol was a toxin, producing 'degenerative states' that were transmitted by heredity.[52] The social dimension of the problem was thus outlined by Bonafonte, who proposed preventative action with regard to the popular classes, who he considered to be ravaged by hereditary alcoholism and degeneration, and educating them. In his work, he attributed the triumph of Germany over France in 1870 and of the USA over Spain in 1898 to racial and cultural superiority. However, that same year another psychiatrist, Joaquín Martínez Valverde (1862–1902), addressed alcoholism in strictly clinical terms, describing its phases and insisting on the difficulties of differential diagnosis, without referring to hereditary alcoholism or degenerationism.[53] The tension between the two approaches was thus still in existence at the beginning of the twentieth century.

Nonetheless, the importance given to hereditary factors in an explanatory model of alcoholism was similar in extent to the acceptance of degenerationism by Spanish psychiatry. In 1905 Luis Martín Isturiz (1863–1944), director of the asylums in Palencia, published his doctoral thesis, in which, from a strictly clinical perspective, he analysed the causes and forms of nervous and mental illnesses produced by alcohol intoxication. In this thesis he also argued that alcoholism was the main cause of degeneration, weakening the human body and 'transmitting morphological anomalies to the embryo that are then translated into offspring in neurotic or degenerative manifestations'.[54] Although his work focused on clinical aspects, he also showed a concern about the effects of alcoholism on the population by indicating its influence on the degeneration of the race. In this sense, the *Revista Frenopática Española* (Spanish Phrenopathy Journal) published articles that were in line with degenerationism and went beyond the clinical framework.

Thus Francisco Ferrer wrote in the journal in 1908 that alcoholism was 'an important factor in the individual decline of the race and one of the immediate causes of crime',[55] Ramón Álvarez Gómez (1870–?), studied a case of a dipsomaniac who had 'symptoms of physical and psychological degeneration',[56] and A. F. Victorio attributed a fundamental role to hereditary alcoholism in the aetiology of 'many nervous and mental conditions'.[57] Other articles were published, usually by foreign publicists, which had a similar tone and a view of alcoholism that was similar to that of a social plague.[58]

The journal also published psychiatric and expert reports on individuals who were considered degenerate and whose family history contained alcoholics.[59] There was the case of a patient accused of terrorist attacks who was diagnosed as degenerate, whose father was a drinker and whose grandfather was known as the Rey del alcohol' (King of Alcohol).[60] The link between revolution, terrorism, degeneration and alcoholism had been popular in the degenerationist and anti-alcohol literature since the Paris Commune in 1871.[61] In his 1920 book *Los degenerados en sociedad* (The Degenerates in Society), the director of the Santa Isabel National Asylum, José Salas y Vaca (1877–1933), argued that in the most advanced political organisations 'there are always fools' who are clearly degenerate, and alcoholics who lead the masses to commit seditious and criminal acts.[62]

However, in 1919 the director of the asylum in Salt (Girona), Salvador Vives (1886–1965), questioned the commonly accepted knowledge of hereditary alcoholism. From the responses of fifty-nine doctors to a survey sent to the 247 doctors practising in the province of Girona, the purpose of which was to gather data to investigate whether there was a direct relationship between alcoholism and defective procreation, Vives concluded that it was not

> possible to form a definite answer – be it either negative or positive – on the role that alcoholism plays as a hereditary factor in psychopathies and, therefore, on the influence of hereditary alcoholism on our mentally ill population.[63]

Vives was therefore of the opinion that the effects of alcoholism on offspring were far from known and required more in-depth studies, and he accused anti-alcohol publicists of simplifying the question:

> It is probable that the problem of inherited alcoholism is not as simple as the anti-alcohol reformers pretend it to be, not as clear as it seems, and much less resolved than it appears to be in most treatises on psychiatry and abnormal childhood.[64]

The use of the concepts of degenerationism and hereditary alcoholism is very evident among psychiatrists from 1898 onwards, when the explanation of the loss of the last colonies in the wake of the Spanish defeat during the war against the USA in terms of biological and cultural decadence favoured the spread of degenerationism. However, the clear link between alcoholism, degeneration and racial decadence was established by hygienists, who were more accustomed than psychiatrists to thinking in terms of 'collective health'. Psychiatrists were more cautious and focused on the clinical aspects of hereditary alcoholism and degeneration. From 1910 onwards, however, there was greater interest in the social dimension of alcoholism. In 1911 Arturo Galcerán y Granés gave a speech in which he stressed the importance of psychiatry in the fight against social diseases and vices.[65] Salas y Vaca was also concerned about the social consequences of racial degeneration and decadence, proposing educational and social measures to help prevent it. From the 1920s onwards, within the framework of the mental hygiene movement and with a new generation of psychiatrists as protagonists, concern for the consequences of mental illness on the population as a whole became part of their priorities. In this new context, which is beyond the scope of my analysis, the discourse about the prevention of mental illness and eugenic reflections became central.

Alcoholism, a voluntary disease

When the psychiatric texts on alcoholism being published during this period are analysed, an important tension regarding its aetiology emerges. The individual is essential in this categorisation, because alcoholism was declared to be either a disease or a vice depending on the individual's involuntary or voluntary intentions. Despite both origins coexisting in permanent dialogue in the psychiatric discourse of the time, the involuntary type seems to have been given more weight. The two main forms of involuntary alcoholism described by psychiatrists were dipsomania and heredity alcoholism, which were both part of general alcohol insanity.

Dipsomania was a recurring theme. Classified among mental dispositions, it was said to be characterised by fits of insanity that pushed the individual to consume uncontrollable amounts of alcohol.[66] It was thought at that time that its main difference from alcoholism, understood to be a vice, was that the dipsomaniac patient lacked will while the alcoholic, unless having acquired the disease hereditarily, drank for pleasure and vice. Giné included dipsomania alongside impulsive monomanias, in the same list as homicidal and incendiary monomanias and kleptomania. For him, dipsomania was characterised by 'a morbid impulse that creates an irresistible urge to abuse alcohol', not to be confused 'with a fondness for drinking that is frequently seen at the beginning of mania and general paralysis: in the former, fondness for alcohol is a mere symptom, whereas in the latter, it constitutes the whole disease.'[67] He warned that neither should it be confused with alcohol insanity, which was 'a mental disorder symptomatic of alcoholism'.[68] Dipsomania was also distinguished from drunkenness in that the latter was 'a degrading vice' and the former 'a true mental affliction'.[69]

The idea that dipsomania marked the limits between illness and vice was maintained during the period. Ots commented that the 'dipsomaniac patient differs completely from the depraved drinker' because, according to him, the former only got drunk when 'compelled by obsessive urges', while the drunk imbibed alcohol 'at any opportunity'.[70] Thus, noted another author, the dipsomaniac patient is 'a madman who drinks because he is mentally ill, while the alcoholic is a degraded being who is responsible for his own madness'.[71] Another characteristic attributed to the dipsomaniac patient by such authors was that after consuming alcohol they felt shame and remorse for their behaviour.

But this apparent consensus on dipsomania was not in fact a consensus at all. Although most authors noted that alcoholism was a mental affliction, in cases where there was a hereditary background to the disease, there were nuances in the arguments put forward. In 1920 José Salas y Vaca considered that dipsomania was a closed circle, because the 'alcoholic ended up being dipsomaniac' and 'dipsomania leads to intoxication'.[72] From this reasoning, this author differentiated between the patient who was dipsomaniac by habit and the patient who was constitutionally so. The first was a 'normal individual' who became a dipsomaniac 'because they began being an alcoholic', while the latter was a degenerate and felt irresistible impulses towards drinking.[73] For Vaca, the latter had no possible cure while the former was 'susceptible to returning to reason' if they were isolated and abstained from drinking.[74]

The underlying issue was whether alcoholism was a disease of will or one of intoxication. According to Abdón Sanchez-Herrero

(1875–1934), the differences between the alcoholic and the dipsomaniac patient were negligible because 'the will of both is weak, their capacity to resist evil, minimal'.[75] Gimeno Riera (1877–1945), director of the Zaragoza asylum, linked dipsomania 'to neuropathic heredity' that weakened the will and led the subject to commit immoral acts, such as the 'immoderate and constant use' of alcohol.[76]

Along with the idea that alcoholism and dipsomania were the result of previous, usually inherited, mental illness, psychiatrists also focused on acquired or voluntary alcoholism. They concurred in defining alcoholism as a process of voluntary intoxication caused by the habitual consumption of alcohol. This perception opened the door to the consideration of alcoholism, especially in its acute phase, as a degrading vice. In this interpretation, acute alcoholism was not strictly thought of as a disease but as a fleeting alcoholic intoxication, the effects of which disappeared with the elimination of alcohol from the body, just like some temporary mental illnesses might. Chronic alcoholism, on the other hand, was defined as permanent intoxication arising from habit and 'an acquired need', and as sharing symptoms with other mental illnesses.[77]

Another aspect of the relationship between mental illness and alcoholism that concerned doctors was moral insanity. Defined by J.C. Prichard, moral insanity was characterised by the loss of moral feelings without the faculties of intelligence being affected.[78] Alarm over the high number of crimes committed under the influence of drunkenness was widespread among psychiatrists and many diverse anti-alcohol propagandists. Moral insanity was seen as an important link between alcoholism, mental illness and criminality. Martínez Valverde considered that it was transmissible by heredity and typical of degenerates.[79] At the end of the 1880s, Victoriano Garrido warned that alcoholism 'disturbs and disorders' the moral element of humankind, and gives rise to offspring 'of little moral sense, with early tendencies to vice and crime'.[80]

In addition, one of the characteristics of chronic alcoholism was said to be 'general mental weakness involving stultification and anaesthesia of the moral sense, and racing thoughts, with rapid enactment of these thoughts in action, which often makes the patients frightening'.[81] This moral anaesthesia was also described from a perspective that was not necessarily degenerationist, an example of which is the work published by Prosper Despine (1812–1892) in 1871.[82] From the field of criminal anthropology, Rafael Salillas (1854–1923) addressed the issue in a session of the Criminology Laboratory group; he carried out an in-depth analysis of a case of alcoholism and moral insanity exposed by Morel in his *Traité des dégénérescences* (Treatise of Degeneration).[83]

Conclusions

As noted at the beginning of this chapter, the purpose of this study was to analyse Spanish psychiatry's position towards alcoholism. Unlike psychiatry in other countries, psychiatry in Spain did not seem to be particularly interested in alcoholism during the last quarter of the nineteenth century, which seems paradoxical given the enormous influence that degeneration theory was having on the construction of anti-alcohol discourse. Clinical and theoretical reasons formed the basis of the rejection or indifference towards degenerationism, as the psychiatrists themselves acknowledged. But there were also professional reasons for this which were related to the development of psychiatric care. The existence of private institutions had a significant influence on the hesitant use of degeneration theory: in establishments designed for a paying clientele, it was deemed important that clients heard only optimistic messages regarding the successful treatment of mental illness. In the courts of justice, however, the discourse was different, and degenerationism was readily used in psychiatric expert reports. This dual approach was in response to different strategies of professionalising the psychiatric field, and psychiatrists did not hesitate to adapt their discourse to different contexts as needed.

In contrast to the way that other medical sectors interacted with the anti-alcohol struggle, the field of psychiatry did not fully exploit degenerationism in the study of alcoholism. It was only from the 1890s, in the context of political and social crisis enveloping Spain – interpreted by many in the country as a crisis caused by utter decadence – that psychiatrists began to accept degeneration theory to a greater extent and to implement it in their clinical practice regarding alcoholism. But their interpretation of degenerationism never had the social and racial tone used by their medical colleagues. Far from the apocalyptic hysteria that biological heredity determinism evoked, with the associated dangers that alcoholism and degeneration brought to the country as a whole, psychiatrists focused on the individual and family consequences of hereditary alcoholism, causing more flexible positions to be adopted. Interestingly, psychiatrists addressed alcoholism as both the cause and the consequence of madness. Reflections on dipsomania, alcohol insanity and moral insanity emphasised the different clinical symptoms of each, but above all they testify to the dual conceptual categorisation of alcoholism as both vice and disease.

This chapter has provided a chronological account that ends shortly before the emergence of the mental hygiene movement that reached its highest peak in the 1920s and 1930s. The impact this movement had on the development of psychiatry in that particular social context was extensive, to the point that reforms in psychiatric care undertaken during the Second Republic (1931–39) were conducted by practising psychiatrists themselves, who became part of the apparatus of the state. Principles advocating prevention and prophylaxis of mental illness were fundamental to the thinking behind these reforms. This new context had direct consequences with regard to psychiatric perspectives on alcoholism, a topic I hope to investigate in a future study.

Notes

Acknowledgements: This work has been done in the framework of the research projects HAR2015–66374-r (MINECO-FEDER) and RTI2018–098006-B-I00 (Ministerio de Ciencia, Innovación y Universidades de España- FEDER).

1 R. Campos Marín, *Alcoholismo, medicina y sociedad en España (1876–1923)* (Madrid: Consejo Superior de Investigaciones Científicas, 1997).

2 An example, among many others, is A. Muñoz Ruiz de Pasanis, *Alcoholismo: su influencia en la degeneración de la raza latina* (Madrid: Giné Carrión, 1906).

3 H. Bernard, 'Alcoolisme et antialcoolisme en France au XIXe siècle (autour de Magnus Huss)', *Histoire, économie et société*, 1984, no. 4, 622–3.

4 S. Balfour, *The End of the Spanish Empire 1898–1923* (Oxford: Clarendon Press, 1997); J. Álvarez Junco, 'La nación en duda', in J. Pan-Montojo (ed.), *Más se perdió en Cuba. España, 1898 y la crisis de fin de siglo* (Madrid: Alianza Editorial, 1998), 405–75.

5 L. Bach and F. Freixa, 'Problema del tratamiento psicosocial del enfermo alcohólico', in M.A. Gassull (ed.), *La enfermedad alcohólica* (Barcelona: Químicos Unidos, 1978), 269; P. Fouquet and M. Borde, *Le roman de l'alcool* (París: Seghers, 1986), 158–9; A. Rey González, *Estudios médico-sociales sobre marginados en la España del siglo XIX* (Madrid: Ministerio de Sanidad y Consumo, 1990), 24–5.

6 R. Huertas, *Organizar y persuadir. estrategias profesionales y retóricas de legitimación de la medicina mental española (1875–1936)* (Madrid: Frenia, 1997), 131–44.

7 For the first medical elaborations of alcoholism as a disease, see W.F. Bynum 'Chronic alcoholism in the first half of the 19th century?', *Bulletin of the History of Medicine* 42, no. 2 (1968), 160–85. Regarding the impact of Huss's work had on French psychiatry, see Bernard, 'Alcoolisme et antialcoholisme en France'; C. Quétel and J-Y. Simon, 'L'aliénation alcoolique en France (XIXe siècle et 1ère moitié du XXe siècle)', *Histoire, économie et société*, 1988, no. 4, 507–33.

8 While the impact of French alienists on Spanish psychiatry in general was considerable, the term 'alcoholism' was not adopted by Spanish psychiatrists in relation to degenerationism until the end of the nineteenth century. This is in stark contrast to the relatively early integration of both the French term and concept into psychiatric discourse in Brazil and Chile, as shown by Mauricio Becerra Rebolledo in his chapter in this volume (see Chapter 3).

9 Bernard, 'Alcoolisme et antialcoholisme en France.

10 R. Huertas, 'Madness and degeneration, II: alcoholism and degeneration', *History of Psychiatry*, 4, no. 13 (1993), 1–21.

11 P.F. Monlau, *Elementos de higiene pública o, Arte de conservar la salud de los pueblos, completamente nueva por la refundición total de su plan y texto* (Madrid: Moya y Plaza, 1871), 322–7.

12 P. Artés, *Borrachos. Etiología, síntomas, diagnóstico, pronóstico y tratamiento* (Alicante: Papelería, Librería y Tipografía San José, 1914).

13 On this subject see D. Pick, *Faces of Degeneration: A European Disorder, c. 1848–c. 1918* (Cambridge: Cambridge University Press, 1989).

14 It is difficult to refer to compare admission statistics to those from other countries. Didier Nourrisson points out for the French case that in 1877, according to Louis Lunier, 10 per cent of admissions to asylums were due to alcoholism. He also points to statistics provided by Senator Claude des Vosgues which indicated that between 1861 and 1865, admissions due to alcoholism were 9.79 per cent, and between 1881 and 1885 they reached 14.42 per cent. However, these rates are difficult to compare with the Spanish ones as they refer to the country as a whole, whereas in the Spanish case I have used those of two institutions.

15 E. Mollejo Aparicio, 'Evolución de los criterios diagnósticos y terapéuticos en el Hospital Psiquiátrico de Leganés (1852–1936)' (PhD dissertation, Universidad de Salamanca, 2001), 519.

16 R. Candela Ramírez, 'El Manicomio Nacional de Leganés en el primer tercio del siglo XX (1900–1931): organización asistencial, aspectos demográficos, clínicos y terapéuticos de la población internada' (PhD dissertation. Universidad Complutense de Madrid, 2017), 405.

17 P. Antón Fructuoso, *Almacén de razones perdidas. Historia del Manicomio de Sant Boi* (Barcelona: Editorial Científico-Médica, 1982), 196–216.

18 S. Vives, 'Psicopaties i alcoholisme a les comarques gironines', in *Tercer congres de metges de llengua catalana*, vol. 2 (Barcelona: Imprenta Badía, 1919), 261–2.

19 Fouquet and Borde, *Le roman de l'alcool,* 158–9.

20 Bach and Freixa, 'Problema del tratamiento psicosocial', 269.

21 J. Giné y Partagás, *Tratado teórico-práctico de freno-patología o Estudio de las enfermedades mentales fundado en la clínica y la fisiología de los centros nerviosos* (Madrid: Moya y Plaza, 1876).

22 Giné, *Tratado teórico-práctico*, 222: 'los hábitos alcohólicos de los padres … se hallaban bajo la acción del alcohol en el momento de la cópula fecundante'. All translations are by the author. See A.F. Voisin, *L'alcoolisme et la séquestration des aliénés* (Paris: Impr. de E. Donnaud, 1872).

23 Giné, *Tratado teórico-practico*, 240: 'inaplicable como guía de diagnóstico'.

24 The work of Joseph Guislain had an important influence on Giné and other psychiatrists such as José María Esquerdo; the latter sponsored in 1881 the translation into Spanish of his *Leçons orales sur les phrénopathies, ou Traité théorique et pratique des maladies mentales: cours*

donné à la clinique des établissements d'aliénés à Gand (Paris: J.B. Baillière, 1852). Regarding the work published by Giné see A. Dieguez, 'El problema de la nosografía en la obra psiquiátrica de J. Giné y Partagás', *Asclepio*, 50, no. 1 (1998), 199–221.

25 A. Galcerán y Granés, *Neuropatología y psiquiatría generales* (Barcelona: Imp. C.P. Caridad, 1895).

26 R. Huertas, 'Madness and degeneration, I: from "fallen angel" to mentally ill', *History of Psychiatry*, 3, no. 12 (1992), 403–11; R. Campos Marín, J. Martínez-Pérez and R. Huertas, *Los ilegales de la naturaleza. Medicina y degeneracionismo en la España de la Restauración (1876–1923)* (Madrid: CSIC, 2000).

27 J. Varela and F. Álvarez-Uría (eds), *El cura Galeote, asesino del Obispo de Madrid-Alcalá. Proceso médico-legal, reconstruido y presentado por Julia Varela y Fernando Álvarez-Uría* (Madrid: La Piqueta, 1979); R. Campos Marín, 'Criminalidad y locura en la Restauración. El proceso del cura Galeote (1886–1888)', *Frenia*, 3, no. 2 (2003), 111–45.

28 J.M. Comelles, *La razón y la sinrazón. Asistencia psiquiátrica y desarrollo del Estado en la España contemporánea* (Barcelona: Promociones y Publicaciones Universitarias, 1988), 42–100; Huertas, *Organizar y persuadir*, 169–80.

29 O. Villasante and R. Huertas, 'El manicomio del Dr. Esquerdo: entre la promoción empresarial y la legitimación científica', *Siso/saúde*, 32 (1999), 27–34.

30 Giné, *Tratado teórico-práctico*, 456.

31 Giné, *Tratado teórico-práctico*, 236.

32 Giné, *Tratado teórico-práctico*, 463: 'que no pueden oponer ... una alimentación restauradora'.

33 J.M. Esquerdo, 'Locos que no lo parecen. Garayo El Saca-mantecas', *Revista de medicina y cirugía prácticas*, 5, no. 112 (1881), 154–9.

34 J. Giné y Partagás, *Dictamen médico-legal que en el proceso Samuel Willie unánimemente han emitido los peritos nombrados por el Ministerio Fiscal, la acusación privada y la defensa* (Barcelona: Imprenta de la Casa Provincial de la Caridad, 1894), 18.

35 V. Garrido, *La cárcel o el manicomio. Estudio médico legal sobre la locura* (Madrid: Administración Casa Editorial de don José María Faquineto, 1888), 19.

36 Garrido, *La cárcel o el manicomio*, 203, 204:'De padres borrachos, hijos epilépticos, neurópatas, seres inestables, de poco sentido moral, con tendencias precoces para el vicio y el crimen'; 'excrecencias monstruosas de una organización enferma, escorias repugnantes nacidas en el pudridero del vicio'.

37 Garrido, *La cárcel o el manicomio*, 204: 'la desviación del tipo normal de la especie humana ... de causas que atentan contra el crecimiento natural de los organismos, y en particular de la intemperancia o el abuso de bebidas'.
38 V. Ots y Esquerdo, 'Locura alcohólica', *El Siglo Médico*, 40, no. 2065 (1893), 470–2: 'a la pobreza de la clasificación de enfermedades ... del mercantilismo dominante'.
39 Ots y Esquerdo, 'Locura alcohólica', 471:'síndromes degenerativos de Magnan y las manifestaciones alcohólicas ... filiarlos únicamente a una sola clase de enajenación'.
40 V. Ots y Esquerdo, 'Locura alcohólica', *El Siglo Médico*, 40, no. 2066 (1893), 487.
41 V. Ots y Esquerdo, *Neurosis y degeneración* (Madrid: Administración de la Revista de Medicina y Cirugía Prácticas, 1897), 5: 'única base sólida y duradera, sobre la cual pueden asentarse a perpetuidad las hipótesis, teorías o doctrinas, que incesantemente invaden los dominios de nuestra ciencia, tratando de explicar o demostrar los más ignorados fenómenos que en la organización humana puedan ocurrir'.
42 Ots y Esquerdo, *Neurosis y degeneración*, 5: 'criminales, vagamundos y prostitutas'.
43 V. Ots y Esquerdo, 'Factor social del alcoholismo. Conferencia dada en el Centro de Sociedades Obreras de Bilbao el 5 de diciembre de 1901 por Vicente Ots y Esquerdo', *La lucha de clases*, 17 May 1902. 'En el alcoholismo sucede todo lo contrario. Cuantos hijos se engendran durante las embriaguez, sea del hombre o de la mujer, nacen idiotas, imbéciles, sordo-mudos, locos, raquíticos, enfermizos, epilepticos o incapacitados para poder vivir.'
44 T. Sanz y Gómez, 'Clínica de psiquiatría. Locura alcohólica. Curación', *El Siglo Médico*, 42, no. 2142 (1895), 25–6; no. 2143 (1895), 42–4.
45 T. Sanz y Gómez, ' Problemas médico-sociales. Regenerados y degenerados', *El Siglo Médico*, 38, no. 2016 (1892), 519: 'energías patológicas'. When Sanz refers to the term 'regenerative' he is optimistic about the possibilities of healing. He looks on the possibility that environmental factors act over the biological and hereditary factors, allowing the regeneration of the alcoholic patient.
46 Sanz y Gómez, 'Clínica de psiquiatría', 25–6 and 42–4.
47 Regenerationism (*Regeneracionismo*) was an intellectual, social and political movement in late nineteenth-century and early twentieth-century Spain. It sought to create an objective and scientific study of the causes of Spain's decline as a nation and to suggest remedies. Regenerationism penetrated across the entire political spectrum of the

country, from the socialist left to the extreme right. For further information see S. Balfour, 'Riot, regeneration and reaction: Spain in the aftermath of the 1898 disaster', *Historical Journal*, 38, no. 2 (1995), 405–23; J. Varela Ortega, 'Aftermath of splendid disaster: Spanish politics before and after the Spanish American War of 1898', *Journal of Contemporary History*, 15, no. 2 (1980), 317–44.

48 Campos, Martínez and Huertas, *Los ilegales de la naturaleza*.

49 J.M. Escuder, *Locos y anómalos* (Madrid: Establecimiento Tip. Sucesores de Rivadeneyra, 1895), 215: 'un pueblo de borrachos prepara una generación de imbéciles, de insensatos o malvados'.

50 M. Bonafonte Nogués, *Degeneración y locura* (Zaragoza: Tipografía de Manuel Ventura 1900), 74, 75: 'el desarrollo del alcoholismo y la alienación mental'; 'locuras degenerativas'; 'hábitos y costumbres inherentes a la moderna civilización y de vicios y enfermedades desarrolladas en alto grado'.

51 Bonafonte, *Degeneración y locura*, 73. This data was taken from the work of the German psychiatrist Carl Wilhem Pelman, although he is not mentioned. The same case would be reviewed in a brief note in a well-known psychiatric journal: 'Dinastía alcohólica', *Revista Frenopática Española*, 19 (1904), 205.

52 Bonafonte, *Degeneración y locura*, 75: 'estados degenerativos'.

53 J. Martínez Valverde, *Guía del diagnóstico de las enfermedades mentales con nociones sobre la terapéutica, deontología y medicina legal frenopáticas* (Barcelona: José Espasa Editor, 1900), 245–8.

54 L. Martín Istúriz, *Memoria sobre la influencia etiológica del alcohol en la génesis de los procesos mentales* (Palencia: Abundio Z. Meléndez, 1905): 'transmitirse al embrión las anomalías morfológicas que después se traducen en la descendencia por estigmas neurósicos o degenerativos'.

55 J.F. Ferrer, 'Profilaxis social contra el alcoholismo', *Revista frenopática española*, 71 (1908), 327: 'un factor importante de la decadencia individual de la raza y una de las causas inmediatas de la criminalidad'.

56 R. Álvarez Gómez Salazar, 'Las dipsofugas de los degenerados', *Revista frenopática española*, 64 (1908), 109–15: 'síntomas de degeneración física y psíquica'.

57 A.F. Victorio, 'Notas de psiquiatría clínica. Las psicosis alcohólicas', *Revista frenopática española*, 44 (1906), 231–2: 'muchas afecciones nerviosas y mentale'.

58 For example: J. Ingenieros, 'La alienación mental y el delito. La condena de enfermos irresponsables', *Revista frenopática española*, 58 (1907), 305–10; A. Ley, 'Alcoholismo y criminalidad', *Revista Frenopática*

Española, 94 (1910), 314–17; V. Delfino, 'Alcohol y trabajo', *Revista frenopática española*, 116 (1912), 238–42.

59 D. Ruiz, 'El crimen de un Werther de aldea', *Revista Frenopática Española*, 110 (1912), 48.

60 Dr. Bravo Moreno and Dr. Roig y Boet, 'Dictamen acerca el Estado de las facultades mentales de J.A., procesado por los atentados terroristas', *Revista Frenopática Española*, 68 (1908), 230.

61 F. Dumolin, 'Le débat sur l'alcoolisme après la Commune (1871–1887)' (PhD dissertation, Université de Paris X. Nanterre, 1979); D. Nourrisson, *Le buveur du XIXème siècle* (Paris: Albin Michel, 1990), 210–15. For the Spanish case see Campos, Martínez and Huertas, *Los ilegales de la naturaleza*.

62 J. Salas y Vaca, *Los degenerados en sociedad* (Madrid: Imprenta y Librería de Nicolás Moya, 1920), 36–7: 'figuran siempre sujetos tarados'.

63 'posible formar un concepto preciso, ni en un sentido afirmativo ni en un sentido negativo, sobre el papel que corresponde al alcoholismo como factor hereditario en las psicopatías y, por lo tanto, sobre la influencia de la herencia alcohólica en nuestra proporción de alienados': S. Vives, *El alcoholismo en la provincia de Gerona. (Resultados de una encuesta)* (Gerona: Viuda e hijo de Franquet y Serra, 1919), 8.

64 Vives, *El alcoholismo en la provincia de Gerona*, 5–8: 'Es infinitamente probable que el problema de la herencia alcohólica no es tan simple como lo pretenden la mayoría de los reformadores antialcohólicos, ni tan claro y mucho menos resuelto como aparece en la mayoría de los tratados de psiquiatría y de infancia anormal.'

65 A. Galcerán y Granés, 'Sociedad de Psiquiatría y Neurología de Barcelona. Discurso inaugural', *Revista Frenopática Española*, 99 (1911), 85–94.

66 A. Sánchez Hernández, 'Un dipsomaniaco', *El Siglo Médico*, 52, no. 2715 (1905), 833.

67 Giné, *Tratado teórico-práctico*, 456: 'la impulsión morbosa que crea inclinación irresistible a abusar de las bebidas alcohólicas … con la afición a la bebida que frecuentemente se observa al principio de la manía y de la parálisis general: en estas, la afición alcohólica es un mero síntoma; en aquella, constituye toda la enfermedad'.

68 Giné, *Tratado teórico-práctico*, 456: 'el trastorno mental sintomático del alcoholismo'.

69 Giné, *Tratado teórico-práctico*, 456: 'un vicio degradante … una verdadera alienación mental'.

70 Ots y Esquerdo, 'Locura alcohólica', 471: 'dipsómano difiere completamente del vicioso bebedor ... que les invade un acceso ...cuantas veces encuentran ocasión de beber'.
71 Sánchez Hernández, 'Un dipsomaniaco', 833.: 'un loco que bebe porque está enajenado, mientras que el alcohólico es un ser degradado que se enajena'.
72 Salas y Vaca, *Los degenerados en sociedad*, 30: 'alcohólico termina en dipsomaniac patient ... dipsomanía conduce a la intoxicación'.
73 Salas y Vaca, *Los degenerados en sociedad*, 30: 'individuo normal ... porque empezó siendo alcohólico'.
74 Salas y Vaca, *Los degenerados en sociedad*, 30: 'susceptible de volver a su razón'.
75 A. Sánchez-Herrero, ' Los alcoholizados', *El Siglo Médico*, 61, no. 3175 (1914), 659: 'ambos tienen la voluntad decaída, una capacidad de resistencia a su mal minima'.
76 J. Gimeno Riera, 'Un caso de dipsomanía', *Revista Frenopática Española*, 96 (1910), 360: 'a la herencia neuropática ... uso inmoderado y constante'.
77 Muñoz Ruiz de Pasanis, *Alcoholismo*, 62: 'una necesidad adquirida'.
78 J.C. Prichard, *A Treatise on Insanity and Other Disorders Affecting the Mind* (London: Sherwood, Gilbert and Piper, 1835), 6; J.C. Prichard, *On the Different Forms of Insanity, in Relation to Jurisprudence* (London: Hippolyte Bailière Publisher, 1842), 33.
79 J. Martinez Valverde, *Guía del diagnóstico de las enfermedades mentales con nociones sobre la terapéutica, deontología y medicina legal frenopáticas* (Barcelona: José Espasa Editor, 1900), 325.
80 Garrido y Escuin, *La cárcel o el manicomio*, 203: 'perturba y desordena ... de poco sentido moral, con tendencias precoces al vicio y el crimen'.
81 Martinez Valverde, *Guía del diagnostico*, 247: 'la debilidad psíquica general con embrutecimiento y anestesia del sentido moral, y movilidad de ideas con paso rápido de éstas a la acción, lo que les hace temibles siempre a éstos enfermos'.
82 P. Despine, *Le démon alcool, ses effets désastreux sur la moral sur l'intelligence et sur la phisique. Moyens d'y porter remède* (Paris: F. Savy, 1871), 45.
83 R. Salillas, 'Laboratorio de Criminología. Alcoholismo y locura moral. (Nota del Sr Salillas)', *Revista General de Legislación y Jurisprudencia*, 96 (1900), 449–55.

3

From nutrition to powerful agent of degeneration: alcohol in nineteenth-century Chile and Brazil

Mauricio Becerra Rebolledo

This chapter focuses on the ways in which drunkenness was framed by medical doctors and psychiatrists in Santiago, Chile, and in Rio de Janeiro, Brazil, in the nineteenth century. The flows of scientific knowledge from select European countries, especially France and Germany, are traced, and the appropriation of different psychiatric traditions and the adjustments made to better suit local circumstances are examined. The comparative approach allows us to see how a psychiatric disease model came to be adopted within the context of two different industrialising societies in South America. The comparison between Brazil and Chile is particularly instructive as it also tells us that the flow from France and Germany of new theories about and socio-clinical approaches to the over-consumption of alcohol did not follow the same trajectory. There was no single or 'typical' South American style of dealing with alcohol-related issues before the transfer and integration of German and French medical practices into existing local methods. Nor was there one single blueprint for the implementation of new ideas and procedures. As the cases of Brazil and Chile show, specific Europe-bred ideas were not only absorbed at different periods over the course of the nineteenth century, but were also variedly modified, depending on the countries' different economic and institutional infrastructures and shifting socio-political ideologies as well as the strength of different medical sub-disciplines in the various rural and metropolitan areas in highly diverse cultural and socio-geographical localities. Nevertheless, in both countries the framing of alcoholism as a diagnostic category contributed to the pathologisation of alcohol consumption and the institutionalisation of psychiatry as a medical science and field of diagnostic competence and therapeutic intervention. By the end of the nineteenth century, 'alcoholism' was the most prevalent diagnostic category in psychiatric institutions in Chile and Brazil, subsequently underpinning intense campaigns of social hygiene.

In this chapter, the importance of professional networks and the role of individual doctors' agency employed at different institutions is highlighted within the wider contexts of transnational knowledge transfer and personal connections with local elites. The chapter also traces the nexus between Brazil's place in international trade networks and the flow of alcohol and resulting over-consumption. For the case of Chile, the persistence of traditional medical practices alongside the newly introduced (and locally modified) approaches from Central European countries is mapped. The chapter also discusses the importance of statistics in the configuration of the subject of alcohol over-consumption as a public health and socio-political problem, highlighting the epistemological role of the numerical dimension in the conceptualisation of a medical phenomenon.

Medical dissertations are important primary sources that lend themselves particularly well to an identification of the points in time when specific cutting-edge ideas became known among a new generation of medical practitioners in different localities. On account of the need for medical students to assess which medical theories and practices were considered as outdated or, conversely, as advanced, an analysis of medical dissertations, together with the subsequent publications of former medical students, helps us identify the points at which new ideas were received, modified and implemented and when the prominence of others was seen to have waned.

The colonial and post-colonial context

Chile and Brazil became independent from the Spanish and Portuguese respectively in 1818 and 1822 respectively. Before colonisation, alcoholic beverages were obtained by fermenting a variety of plant species, such as potatoes and corn. From the sixteenth century onwards, the Taíno word *chicha* was appropriated by the Spanish to designate all types of alcoholic beverages prepared by different groups of indigenous peoples.[1] The various forms of *chicha* were of great use in pre-Hispanic times and continued to be integrated into rituals and religious ceremonies even during the colonial period.[2] As the Chilean central zone, which is endowed with a Mediterranean climate, seemed to the Spaniards to be similar to the regions of Andalusia, they introduced the black grape for cultivation and produced a characteristic local wine. Among the indigenous people who populated Brazil, the main beverage was *caium*, made by fermenting sweet fruits such as yucca, pineapple and cajú, while people who were enslaved from Africa brought with them fermentation techniques, producing a concoction known as *pombe*, sorghum beer, and palm sap wines called *malafo*.[3]

The production of alcoholic drinks shaped Brazilian and Chilean society during Portuguese and Spanish colonial rule from 1500 to 1822 and from 1540 to 1818 respectively. In the Luso-Brazilian Empire, cane cultivation had shaped the economy and colonial society ever since the sugar trade dominated the transatlantic market in the mid-sixteenth century.[4] This stimulated the founding of sugar mills in the north-east, the massive exploitation of slave labour and the production of *cachaça* (alcohol distilled from fermented sugar cane).[5] Cane alcohol and Caribbean rum served as bargaining chips for the purchase of enslaved people in Africa, as international direct trade with Brazil was vetoed by the Portuguese monarchy, which in 1649 unsuccessfully tried to prohibit the manufacture of cachaça in Brazil and its export to Angola. The resistance generated to the measure is highlighted by Carneiro, not only in its economic dimension, but also in regard to the Brazilian liquor having become a symbol of national identity.[6] Del Pozo comments that at the beginning of the colonial period in Chile, in the sixteenth century, the cultivation of wine was one of the main bases of the consolidation of an agricultural economy.[7] By the nineteenth century, the Chilean winemaking enterprise was consolidated. Vineyards became a space for socialising for the local oligarchy as well as valuable assets, and, together with Catholicism, a symbol of identity and belonging for the families of the economic, political and institutional elite.[8]

From the 1870s onwards, Latin American societies experienced an accelerated process of modernisation. Rio de Janeiro and Santiago saw the arrival of thousands of migrants attracted by an incipient industrial development, a process that advanced further during the next century and transformed the urban landscape completely.[9] In Chile, this process was driven by the extension of its territories following the Pacific War (1879–83), the annexation of the Araucanía (1884) and the consolidation of an export economy based on nitrates in the north of the country. The Brazilian Empire witnessed the abolition of slavery (1888) and the transition from monarchy to republic (1889).[10] The profound changes and the emergence of new urban social actors increased social instability.[11] Medical doctors in the different countries began to base their status as experts on the scientific nature of their work. They also presented themselves as qualified to suggest ways of maintaining the desired social peace, while developing a utopia aimed at transforming the lifestyles of the population.[12]

During the early part of the nineteenth century, drunkenness was approached in medical writing mainly in relation to other issues such as food. With the establishment of medical teaching at the Imperial Academy of Medicine in Rio de Janeiro (AMRJ) and at Salvador de Bahia in 1839, and at the Faculty of Medicine in Santiago in 1843, the use of intoxicants was explored in medical dissertations and scientific publications. Valuable insights into the scientific thinking extant at the time can be derived from these dissertations, in which the students assessed and promulgated the prevalent professional views and the knowledge considered valuable within the medical tradition in which they were being trained. For example, a Brazilian dissertation written in 1839 explored the impact of food and drink on the morals of humankind. Its author, Alexandre de Rosario, argued that coffee- and tea-based drinks had modifying powers on the spinal-cerebral nervous system. These 'modifiers' could engender modifications in the brain and 'influence the character of our morals', while wine produced intoxication and the dullness of faculties.[13]

In regard to Brazil, Santos maintains that the construction of alcoholism as a pathological entity in the nineteenth century coincided with the medicalisation in capitalist societies of traditional behaviours, which was due to the need to prepare individuals for the demands of industrialisation and the consolidation of institution-based medical sciences.[14] Santos and Verani note that medical views about the use of alcohol are part of a process in which people's daily practices become scientifically inscribed.[15] The ways of life and customs of urban populations fuelled arguments about the use and abuse of alcohol. Fernández makes similar points for the case of Chile. He shows that lower-class drunkenness was represented via the figure of the poor and drunk man, a silhouette that projected a future of national degradation.[16]

The industrialisation process in Chile and Brazil also led to important changes in the availability of beverages and ways of drinking. Schivelbusch argues that the industrialisation of distillate production towards the late nineteenth century occasioned radical changes in traditional ways of drinking, just as the introduction of power looms had affected family economies at the end of the eighteenth century.[17] He claims that distillates were part of the generalised acceleration of change in modern times, together with rural exodus and experiences of displacement in hostile cities. Hard liquors maximised the effects of intoxicants and destroyed earlier forms of drinking and socialising, such as wine and beer consumption, causing heightened rates of alcohol abuse and the figure of the solitary alcoholic. In 1875 Ricardo Dávila Boza (1850–1937), a hygienist and medical inspector of the Consejo Superior de Higiene, pointed out that in Chile the most popular alcoholic drinks were *aguardiente* (strong distilled alcohol), *chicha*,[18] *chacolí* (wine)[19] and, in smaller quantities, beer.[20] Carvalho listed in his dissertation of 1880 the alcoholic liquids consumed in Brazil, namely the derivatives by distillation of sugar cane, beets and potatoes. He noted that distilled liquor was 'an extremely detestable liquid, and in our country the opium of the poor class in general, which is usually the cause of alcoholism'.[21]

Alcohol: nutrition, medicine and poison

In Chile and Brazil wine was still found within the available medical arsenal until the late nineteenth century. Following the understanding of the forerunners of laboratory science – the German Justus von Liebig and the Irish physician Robert Todd – that alcohol was fuel for the body, it was recommended to treat a wide range of conditions.[22] Quoting von Liebig, the Chilean Salvador

Feliú's dissertation on liver problems of 1879 suggested that alcohol was a form of nutrition and was burned in the 'bodily economy' in a way analogous to what happens with sugar and fats.[23] A year later in Brazil, Carvalho, citing Todd, expounded a similar view that alcohol was 'a food, a fuel for hematosis, a stimulant of the nervous system and at the same time a sedative, moderator of temperature, which fights and prevents delirium and brings a peaceful and beneficial sleep'.[24] Carvalho added that alcohol medication had precise indications, which depended on a practical and intelligent judgement.[25]

In Chile, in his 1873 medical dissertation F. Grohuert wrote about Todd's treatment of acute pneumonia with alcohol used as an antipyretic, in particular the recommendation of high doses of cognac, port and wine, to reduce pulse rate and temperature.[26] Grohuert, however, considered alcohol to be stimulating rather than antipyretic. Grohuert's thesis was written at a time of radical transformation in therapeutics and testifies to a certain eclecticism, in which approaches such as hydrotherapy and bloodletting were employed alongside emergent science-based medicine. Although he maintained that in cases of alcohol-related pneumonia bloodletting was contraindicated, he still recommended it, in combination with tartar, for phlegmasia, acute pulmonary oedema and cerebral congestion.[27] For alcohol-induced delusions, Grohuert recommended cold baths on account of their calming effect on the nervous system and, above all, chloral hydrate (a sedative).[28] Another Chilean medical student, Clotario Salamanca, explored a few years later the link between alcoholism and degeneration, and observed that wine was used for dyspepsia and to lower the pulse and temperature in fever, especially in pneumonia; as a palliative in consumption (tuberculosis) by moderating heat, sweat and vomiting; as a prophylactic in the cure of cholera; and as a disinfectant for wounds and ulcers and, with similar properties to iodine, for serous cavities.[29]

In Brazil, T. Carvalho published his dissertation in 1880 on ethyl alcohol, which he considered to have a 'very important role as one of the most beneficial medication agents'.[30] He noted the physiological impact of alcohol on the digestive tract, nutrition, urinary secretions, blood, circulation and breathing, and on body temperature. The idea of vapour flows inside the human body served to explain the absorption by the lungs of alcohol, reduced to the state of vapour.[31] In 1883 another doctor even recommended the use of alcohol to control agitation and delirium, suggesting that 'if, alongside the symptoms of pneumonia or any other acute discomfort, nervous phenomena were revealed by agitation, insomnia and delirium, alcohol will again be indicated for excellent results'.[32]

Until the end of the nineteenth century, the medical value assigned to alcohol was ambiguous. This is expressed in *Elementos de higiene* (Treatise on Hygiene) by the new director of the Institute of Hygiene in Chile, Federico Puga Borne, published in 1892.[33] The chapter on food includes the notion of 'nervous foods' (*alimento nervino*), defined by the Italian doctor Paolo Mantegazza as a group of nutrients that encompassed alcohol and products such as yerba mate (South American holly), coca leaf, coffee, tobacco and sugar cane.[34] Referring to the medical value of alcohol, Puga commented that:

> In our civilisation, where there are so many artificial things, the artificial stimulant of alcoholic drinks cannot be condemned at all. The moderate use of this liquid, especially in the form of fermented drinks, undeniably encourages the vigour of men, both of the manual and intellectual worker. This drink causes pleasant sensations, makes bad foods more attractive, raises strength momentarily, awakens joy and even makes you forget misery and grief.[35]

However, Puga warned that while alcohol in low doses was a nutritious drink, large doses were 'absolutely toxic'.[36] This kind of view was prevalent in the literature at the time, yet it was not unopposed. In the same year a doctoral student in Chile ranked alcohol among toxic substances, next to lead and mercury. He suggested in his dissertation, entitled 'Alcoholismo y degeneración' (Alcohol and degeneration), that 'the excessive exclusivism of hygienists comes undone when one asks with avid curiosity about or attentively investigates the role that alcohol has come to play in human life'.[37] In a similar vein, a Brazilian doctoral student commented in 1884 that intoxication by alcohol resembled true poisoning,[38] and in Chile in 1898, Moises Loyns directly quoted Orfila and his treatise on poisons to describe death in cases of ingestion of large amounts of alcohol.[39]

Alcohol's effects on body and mind

Alongside the idea of alcohol as nutrition, the focus on liver cirrhosis constituted an early approach to inebriation within the context of the clinical-anatomical paradigm that was so prominent in early nineteenth-century somatic medicine. The path started in the research on liver cirrhosis marked the terms by which alcoholism was constructed as a medical pathology and organic disease in Chile and Brazil. Within this framework, many medical dissertations on alcoholism described the effect of alcohol first on the bodily systems (circulatory, respiratory and reproductive, and the liver, kidneys, lungs and heart) and then on the nervous system. Doctors strove to find organic lesions, mainly in the stomach and liver. In both Chile and Brazil the modification of organic structures due to excessive use of intoxicants became defined as part of a degenerative process.[40]

Nevertheless, in Chile, the miasmatic paradigm remained prominent in the understanding of liver cirrhosis until the mid-nineteenth century. José Juan Bruner (1825–1899), a doctor of German origin who settled in Chile after arriving in 1844 and one of the founders of the Sociedad Médica de Santiago, held that alcohol aggravated the living conditions of the masses and led to liver diseases.[41] He wrote:

> What contributes to a high degree to destroy the constitution of the masses, already sufficiently undermined by miasma, nudity, syphilis and poor nutrition, as we will see later, is undoubtedly the growing abuse of alcoholic beverages. The excessive frequency of liver diseases, the great part of which develops, as we have seen, from miasmatic intoxication of the blood, has fertile ground in the abuse of alcohol.[42]

In a similar vein, in 1873 the doctor Wenceslao Díaz stated that liver diseases were common in Chile because of the abundance of cases of dysentery, the dryness of the environment, which exaggerated pulmonary and skin evaporation, and the 'excesses of the regimen of alcoholic beverages'.[43]

Halfway between the miasmatic tradition and the physiology of the Frenchman and father of experimental medicine Claude Bernard (1813–1878), Salvador Feliú argued in 1879 in his medical dissertation on 'alcohol as a cause of liver disease' that the main organs affected by alcohol were the kidneys and lungs. The processing of alcohol by the kidneys was understood by Feliú within the frameworks of physiology, while the effects on the lungs were interpreted in terms of the miasmatic theory, thus explaining 'drunken pneumonia'. Feliú noted that alcohol

> is eliminated by the lung in equal quantity to the urine, yet it is very difficult to condense the vapours contained in the expiratory stream; its irritating action accounts for the pneumonia of drunkards, which possesses such a distinctive character.[44]

Feliú held that in the same way as the vapours attacked the lungs, alcohol reached the brain through the circulation of the blood, which produced the states typical of acute alcoholism.

In Brazil, three medical dissertations dedicated to Laënnec's 'atrophic cirrhosis' were published in 1882, agreeing that its aetiological origin was the excessive use of alcohol and that autopsies confirmed lesions in the liver.[45] These theses owed much to the professor of medicine João Torres Homem, who noted that both in Brazil and in Europe alcohol consumption was becoming widespread. Homem's clinical experience in Rio de Janeiro led him to suggest that alcohol-related bodily damage varied, depending on the social class of the drinker. He held that in the Brazilian well-off classes, lesions in the heart were more frequent, while among the working classes damage manifested itself in the liver. Although Homem vaguely considered malnutrition among the poor as a factor, he did not develop this aspect any further.[46]

The emergence of a disease paradigm

The first medical texts in Chile that framed alcohol abuse as a disease in itself were written in 1873. They predominantly referenced European publications and adopted new epistemic paradigms, methods of observation and scientific knowledge styles. To some extent they reflected what was at the time considered the state of the art in the medical field.[47] This was in contrast to Brazil, which lagged somewhat behind North American and European countries, as in Brazil chronic alcoholism was not conceptualised as a mental illness in line with the tradition of French alienism until 1883.[48] The francophone influence was also apparent in Chile, where the medical establishment had been made up of Spanish and French doctors since independence in 1818 and the Chilean government began to fund medical students' training in Europe, mainly in France, from 1874. On their return to Chile, the doctors adapted the European models to local circumstances.

Between 1873 and 1890, Chilean medical theses framed alcohol over-consumption as both a 'social evil' and a mental illness, distinguishing the latter's acute and chronic forms.[49] In Brazil, a comprehensive delimitation of the different mental conditions connected with chronic alcoholism emerged from 1883 onwards, and acute alcoholism was described as a morbid process that affected functional nervous activities such as motility and cognition and caused injuries to organs and tissues.[50] Azevedo commented that 'alcohol exerts on the brain an action in which intensity and duration are proportional to the amount absorbed and to the individual's susceptibility'.[51]

In Rio de Janeiro, the anatomical pathologist João Vicente Torres Homem presented a case of hemi-chorea, which, in the absence of rheumatism and other causes, he attributed to the abuse of alcoholic beverages.[52] In 1878 he published the first work on mental illnesses in Brazil, *Lições sobre as moléstias do sistema nervoso* (Lessons on Diseases of the Nervous System). Torres Homem's emphasis on research provided the impulse for laboratory investigations and the foundation of the physiology laboratory at the National Museum. Vimieiro comments that new ideals of science and of civilisation were being forged in Brazil, in the midst of modernisation processes that were driven by the coffee industry and in which scientists felt they had a role to play.[53] Medical reforms during the 1880s followed the German model, promoting laboratory disciplines, such as physiology and experimental therapeutics.[54] This trend was further enhanced when anatomical pathology and histochemical analysis sections were established in the Hospício Pedro II during the late 1880s.[55]

In Chile, laboratories were formed only from the 1880s onwards, although the San Vicente de Paul Hospital had been assigned to clinical-medical teaching since 1872. Chilean alienists were not involved in research on alcoholism, despite or perhaps because of the attention given to the subject by hygienists. Augusto Orrego Luco (1848–1933) is a case in point. He is regarded in the historiography of medicine as a prominent figure of Chilean psychiatry at the end of the nineteenth century.[56] After graduating in 1873 and working at the Casa de Orates (House for Madmen),[57] he studied for a year in Paris with the neurologist Jean-Martin Charcot. Upon his return to Chile, he was a devoted disseminator of the anatomical clinical model in his capacity as chair of mental diseases.[58] In 1884 Orrego Luco published *La cuestion social*, outlining the social problems that the elite attributed to the Chilean people. He argued in favour of state intervention to regulate the living and leisure spaces of the poor and referred to alcoholism as an eminent problem. However, he did not focus in his own scientific research on the very diagnostic category that at the time was responsible for the largest number of psychiatric patients. In his dissertation on hallucinations, he had described the behavioural effects of alcoholism, asserting that regardless of the moral habits or constitution of an individual, hallucinations were bound to follow frequent use of alcohol. He considered hallucinations identical, independent of the toxin that produced them or induced 'by an innate or acquired predisposition'.[59]

Adeodato García Valenzuela (1864–1936) is another example of a Chilean doctor who wrote important pamphlets on the 'alcohol problem', yet did not focus on it in his own research. Valenzuela was a professor of physiological and pathological chemistry and, from 1899, chief of the General Council of Temperance, which brought together various temperance associations.[60] In an article that was read at the Chilean Scientific Congress, held in 1896 in the city of Concepción, he built his arguments mainly on German sources and, unlike Luis Orrego Luco, only to a lesser extent on French sources, without presenting studies based on local cases or his own investigations. In 1898 García published a new work on alcoholism, which had received second place in a contest run by the Ministry of Finance that asked for proposals on how to deal with the use of intoxicants by Chileans. García suggested the suppression of alcohol consumption by means of the criminalisation of drunkenness and the creation of doctor-managed specialist asylums for drinkers. He also included a chapter on 'Alcohol bajo punto de vista químico, fisiolójico i médico' (Alcohol from a chemical, physiological and physician's point of view), which was based mainly on German sources, such as Kraepelin's studies on the influence of alcohol on memory. These interventions led to the prevalence of German theoretical models and approaches in Chilean medical thinking by the end of the nineteenth century.[61]

Although psychiatrists and hygienists in both Brazil and Chile used the subject of alcoholism as a means of promoting their status as experts and of expanding their areas of expertise throughout the nineteenth century, differences in the extent of institutional consolidation (or lack thereof) affected the focus of medical discourse in each country. In Brazil, where the Junta Central de Higiene was established in 1852, physicians had consolidated their decision-making power, at least within the limits of Rio de Janeiro and in large cities such as Bahia and São Paulo. In contrast, in Chile, the earlier lack of a centralised health institution, such as the Consejo Superior de Higiene, which was not established until 1892, meant that medical discourses on alcoholism emphasised its serious social consequences, instead of producing research based on the prevailing model of biomedical science and employing the new insights of anatomical pathology and physiology research. Chilean physicians saw this lack of institutional power and scientific focus as a problem, and many strongly emphasised the need to establish specialised medical institutions. However, although they engaged in research and published scientific texts, some of them, such as Augusto Orrego Luco and Federico Puga Borne, ended up opting for political careers as parliamentarians and diplomats.

In Brazil, medical alcohol discourses were based on hygiene theories from the 1880s. But within the context of consolidated spaces of medical expertise, and during the rise of science-based experimental medicine, research on alcohol emerged that approached alcoholism systematically and on the basis of contemporary cutting-edge theories and methodologies, such as anatomical pathology and descriptive symptomology. Thus a greater focus on the tightening of nosological delimitations and the enhancement of clinical psychiatric knowledge was evident among doctors in Rio de Janeiro.

As well as engaging with political power, medical professionals in Brazil were also embedded within a more consolidated scientific space than their colleagues in Chile.

The role of statistics

The Hospicio Nacional de Alienados (HNA) in Brazil and the Casa de Orates in Chile were both opened in 1852. By the end of the nineteenth century, they were well-established medical spaces.[62] The establishment of chairs of mental and nervous diseases in 1881 was an important step towards the consolidation of psychiatry as a medical specialisation in both countries. For doctors in training, mental hospitals provided the opportunity to contrast the theories gleaned from European treatises with their own observations and scientific practices, and to expand the continued influence of Western modes of thinking. The opening of Observation Pavilions in 1893 in the HNA in Rio de Janeiro and, two years later, in the Casa de Orates in Santiago allowed doctors to develop their expertise. Medical internships, too, helped transform hospitals into loci of specialist learning and teaching.[63] In the 1890s psychiatrists took an increasing interest in alcohol-related conditions and developed their careers in this field within the context of particular institutions, mainly nursing homes and medical schools. The first systematic work on alcoholism in Chile was carried out by Manuel Segundo Beca (1863–1919), who began his career in internal medicine at the Casa de Orates in Santiago, devoting his dissertation to the statistical analysis of diagnostic practice at the institution.[64] In 1892 he focused on alcoholism, publishing several articles in which he combined the criminology of Lombroso and French positivism.[65]

In Brazil, Marcio Nery (1865–1911) stands out. After graduating from the faculty of medicine in Rio de Janeiro, he worked at the HNA from 1890. Following the French model, Nery was one of the people in charge of the Clinic of Psychiatry and Nervous Diseases, which was based in the Observation Pavilion. In 1893 he published articles on epileptic phenomena caused by alcohol and on the treatment of alcoholism.[66] He noted:

> … especially in the less affluent classes, which constitute the majority of the patients at the Hospício Nacional de Alienados, alcoholism is the most important aetiological factor. A toxic substance that slowly undermines the body, alcohol in its multiple forms, and taken in both small and large libations, stands accused of [producing the] largest contingent of madmen and heart patients in hospitals.[67]

Nery and Beca developed similar career trajectories focusing on alcoholism. Both were concerned with tightening the diagnostic category, recording observations, testing treatments and producing the first statistics based on data from the institutions in the respective two countries' major cities.

The production of statistics on mental illnesses in general and, subsequently, on alcoholism in particular helped establish psychiatry as an important medical field in Chile and Brazil. The creation of data from mental hospital statistics allowed doctors to substantiate their own wider social importance, as they could show that they were tackling a problem that occupied the attention of the authorities. At the same time, the institutions provided spaces for professional advancement. In regard to knowledge construction, research anchored in institutional numbers and graphics constituted a stepping stone towards the objectification of mental illness. Following the positivist tradition in science, diseases became circumscribed in terms of numerical magnitude. The counting of population and disease groups and their numerical representation constituted the foundation for population and disease management and control.[68] As Golonski has argued, statistical inventories and the production of positive knowledge tend to correspond to the rationality of a political and social governance that aims to manage phenomena such as alcoholism.[69] The presentation of reality in figures corresponded to an epistemological ideal that had permeated European scientific thought since the end of the eighteenth century. The precision and measurability of social phenomena were strongly grounded in mathematical models as forms of the ideal type of science.[70] The drive for exact quantification did not, as T. Porter has argued, arise from an inherent condition of scientific practices, but was part of a strategy of de-personalisation that assigned objectivity to representations, which thus could enjoy epistemological authority.[71] The epistemological role of statistics has also been addressed in Nina S. Studer's chapter in this volume on the understanding of alcoholism by French colonial psychiatrists in Algeria (see Chapter 8).

Manuel Beca performed the first statistical analysis related to alcoholism in Chile at the Casa de Orates in Santiago in 1884. Among the 486 patients resident that year, diagnoses of alcohol-related intoxication (dementia and alcoholic mania) did not surpass 7 per cent, in contrast to other diseases such as mania (47.75 per cent) and dementia (27.56 per cent).[72] By 1890/91, when the new diagnostic categories of 'acute alcoholism' and 'chronic alcoholism' were in use, alcohol was reported as the main cause of hospitalisation for 57 per cent of men.[73] In a later article, Beca established a link between alcoholism and criminality based on the diagnosis of thirty-six alcoholics among fifty-five prison inmates admitted to the Casa de Orates between 1883 and 1892.[74]

The alcohol statistics also had a political dimension. The conversion of the complex problem of drunkenness into seemingly clear-cut numbers allowed psychiatrists to isolate the phenomenon and visualise it in graphics, making it easier to plan interventions. The numerical data thus enabled psychiatrists to present their work as part of objective knowledge, establish a dialogue with the political powers that be, and channel and access the distribution of state resources for the implementation of policy measures.

In the wake of Beca's work in Chile, the first statistical report commissioned by the government was concerned with alcoholism. The aim was to base the implementation of public policy measures on actual figures gleaned from institutional and population surveys. The French engineer Francisco de Bèze was employed to produce the first official study, entitled *El alcoholismo, estudio y estadística* (Alcoholism, Research and Statistics), an investigation that was based on data collected by public institutions in 1895.[75] The report established the per capita consumption of *aguardiente* or distilled liquor (which apparently amounted to 60 litres per year); a significant annual expenditure on spirits; arrest rates for drunkenness (4.67 per cent of the population); the proportion of inmates in prisons who offended while intoxicated (12,013 people, equivalent to 40.79 per cent of the prison population); and hospitalisation in the Casa de Orates for alcoholism (57.11 per cent of men and 14.7 per cent of women).[76] The figures highlighted the extent of the alcohol problem, but Bèze did not suggest any medical measures to contain it. Instead, he proposed punitive actions such as forced patient work and confinement of 'incorrigible drunkards' in agricultural penal colonies.[77]

In Brazil, more comprehensive statistical data were collated in 1910 by the medical student Duque Estrada, who calculated that, between 1899 and 1909, 2,007 of the 8,228 people at the HNA were admitted because of alcoholism, representing 24.42 per cent of the total.[78] Similarly, that same year the psychiatrist Henrique Roxo, who, along with Marcio Nery, was in charge of the Clinic of Psychiatry and Nervous Diseases at the Imperial Academy of Medicine in Rio de Janeiro, compiled the first official statistics of the diagnoses assigned to patients in the HNA Observation Pavilion between 1895 and 1900, showing that 31 per cent of the patients (1,257 people) were assigned the diagnosis 'alcoholic psychosis' as the main cause for admission.[79]

In 1914 Hermeto Lima provided a wide range of statistical data in his dissertation, arguing that alcoholism was a cause of crime and of intellectual degeneration.[80] He included photographs of bars in the city and representations of alcoholics as well as a diagram that showed the numbers of people imprisoned for different crimes, deaths and hospitalisations due to the use of intoxicants. The diagram revealed that in Rio de Janeiro alone alcoholism was implicated in 6,000 of 7,500 cases of prisoners; 4,000 of the 5,000 people awaiting conviction; 2,700 of 4,100 deaths from tuberculosis; 1,200 of 1,900 suicides (between 1908 and 1912); and 1,200 of 1,500 hospital admissions.[81]

From *delirium tremens* to psychosis

A main challenge for doctors was to identify which organs were affected by alcohol consumption. Within the prevalent anatomical-clinical framework, the brain and hence the nervous system were seen to be implicated the most, leading to profound changes in drunken people's behaviour and mood. In regard to Brazil, Santos suggests that a 'whole array of enduring mental disorders' was seen to be 'produced by the prolonged intoxication of the nervous system by alcohol' and that 'this phenomenon was seen as a form of inflammation, often appearing under the term *neuritis*'.[82] In Chile, similar views were held, as is evidenced by a dissertation from 1873: 'There is a form of *delirium tremens* that closely resembles the frenzy of madness; in this case there is always an actual inflammation of the brain.'[83]

The concept of *delirium tremens* was well represented in Chile from the 1860s onwards. Dr Wenceslao Díaz pointed out that *delirium tremens* had 'become very common because of the excesses [caused by the consumption of] alcoholic beverages'.[84] A decade later, A. Zenteno offered in his dissertation a complete systematisation of *delirium tremens*, which he described as a transitory and nervous pathological state. He noted that this state was characterised by disturbances in brain and nervous functions, such as insomnia, delirium and hallucinations, and was accompanied by tremors and a tendency to collapse, which disappeared after a prolonged sleep. He suggested that for the phenomena 'to be truly *delirium tremens* they must be preceded by excessive abuse of spirits'.[85] The Chilean doctor also referred to the presence of visual, tactile or auditory hallucinations and noted that, although the patient might initially be aware of the non-reality of these phenomena, as the disease progressed, hallucinations tended to overcome judgement to the point that 'the drunkard believes in the reality of the visions that float before his eyes'.[86] Zenteno also highlighted the resemblance of alcohol-induced delirium episodes to delusional states caused by intoxication from other substances, such as opium, coffee, belladonna, lead and mercury.

Delirium tremens presented a new condition for psychiatry, which became further circumscribed in 1869 following John Hughling Jackson's conceptualisation of the tremors observed in the morbid process of *delirium tremens* as discharges similar to the seizures of epilepsy. At this stage, the alcoholic came to embody two of the most significant contemporary signs of mental disease: delusion and seizures. Santos and Verani argue that once psychiatry began to align symptoms of excessive drunkenness to madness, doctors also started to identify mania, melancholy, paranoid ideas, persecutory hallucinations, auditory and visual hallucinations, disorientation and mental confusion in cases of alcoholic intoxication.[87] Between the 1870s and the 1890s, both Brazilian and Chilean doctors increasingly began to talk about 'alcoholism', a new diagnostic category coined in Europe. Clinical attention shifted towards behaviours that then came to stand as symptoms for either acute or chronic versions of one specific condition.

An analysis of medical journals and dissertations in Chile attests to the continued influence of the French school of alienism until the early twentieth century. This influence was also present in Brazil, but from the 1880s onwards doctors there were particularly interested in identifying the physiological localisation of the sources of the behavioural alterations observed in alcoholics, and in mapping a systematic delimitation of different pathological conditions. For example, in 1883 Antonio de Azevedo argued that '*delirium tremens* is an acute epiphenomenon of chronic intoxication' by alcohol, distinguishing it from lipemanic insanity, another mental illness caused by alcoholism.[88] Brazilian physicians located *delirium tremens* in the encephalon, as affirmed by Loureiro in 1884, who noted that 'the cephalo-spinal nervous system is the theatre of disorders produced by alcohol abuse'.[89] This enabled them to explain delirium as located in the brain as well as the discharge of tremors through the nerves and spinal marrow. As Loureiro put it: 'the delirium is the tremor of the encephalon, just as tremors are the delirium of the marrow'.[90]

In 1890 the term 'toxic psychoses' appeared in Brazil to encompass delusions caused by alcohol and other intoxicating substances. The notion of psychoses was coined by the Austrian physician, poet and philosopher Ernst von Feuchtersleben in 1845 to label cases of extreme mental problems arising from a brain dysfunction that nonetheless presented no underlying pathological changes.[91] Later, psychosis was mobilised as a synonym for mental disorders *per se* and contrasted with neurosis.[92] The notion appears in Jeronymo de Moraes's dissertation, 'Psicoses de origem tóxica' (Psychoses of toxic origin), a systematisation of the different alterations caused by substances such as alcohol, morphine and cocaine. He argued that the challenge was to 'define what the essential primitive disorder is' for each form of psychosis.[93] Alcohol-related conditions and psychosis became progressively entangled in Brazilian psychiatry. This was not so in Chile. The different ways in which *delirium tremens* was framed by Brazilian and Chilean doctors puts into sharp relief how knowledge transfer from European countries to Latin America was not a uniform process but characterised by local adaptations and innovations.

Degeneration and dipsomania

Since the 1880s, one particular phrase has been widely quoted in scientific writing in both Brazil and Chile: 'A drop of sperm from an alcoholic contains a whole neuropathic family.' It was coined by the French alienist Jean-Martin Charcot and provides, in a nutshell, the emerging framework for alcoholism in Latin American psychiatric science. This framework appropriates the theory of degeneration, according to which mental illnesses were hereditarily transmissible forms of degeneration.[94] Originally developed in 1857 by the French alienist Benedict Morel (1809–1873), the theory was developed further by his fellow Frenchmen Valentin Magnan (1835–1916) and his disciple Paul Legrain (1860–1939), who used experiments with absinthe on animals to investigate the assumed morbid process to which the degenerate body was seen to succumb irreversibly.[95] The theory of degeneration opened the way for French medicine to adopt a strongly biologicist view on alcoholism, leaving environmental and social conditions second.[96] In contrast to developments in Chile and Brazil, an initial distance to and, from the 1890s, absorption of Morel's and Magnan's theories has been explored by Ricardo Campos in this volume in regard to the Spanish context (see Chapter 2).

As early as 1879, the Chilean physician Clotario Salamanca recognised the medicinal uses of alcohol, while at the same time suggesting that the dipsomaniac was an alcoholic and the product by inheritance of the vice of the parents, who in turn would have epileptic, insane, deaf-dumb, cretin and suicidal children, as well as bandits and murderers.[97] In Brazil, Emilio Loureiro announced in 1884 that 'all mental discomforts can be caused by the abuse of spirits'. He added that 'if we consult the annals of human teratology, we will see that the greatest physical and intellectual monstrosities appeared in alcoholics'.[98]

Although the ideas of Magnan had been referenced in earlier Latin American publications, it was only from the 1890s that dissertations in Chile and Brazil adopted his framework of degeneration in relation to alcohol.[99] In 1892 the medical journal *Brazil médico* published Magnan's book of 1874 *De l'alcoolisme, des diverses formes de délire alcoolique et de leur traitement* (On Alcoholism: The Various Forms of Alcoholic Delirium and their Treatment) with the new title 'Da dipsomania' (On dipsomania).[100] To judge from the wide range of dissertations published from the 1890s onwards, degeneration became the core concept for the framing of alcoholism in Brazil until the first decades of the twentieth century.[101] In Chile, Beca, for example, configured the notion of 'dipsomania' as a disease that could produce other diseases and 'hereditary psychological degeneration' in alcoholics' offspring.[102] He regarded it less as a special mental illness than as a syndrome of spontaneous appearance in individuals predisposed through heredity, presenting as mental obsessions and impulses, such as the wide range of manias of the time, for example kleptomania and nymphomania. In both countries, alcholism was also discussed in combination with other pathological phenomena like cirrhosis and alcoholic pneumonia (conveying lingering miasmatic ideas[103]), as well as epilepsy,[104] neuroses[105] and hysteria.[106]

The description of alcoholism was also linked with and compared to general paralysis of the insane (GPI). In 1879, for example, the Chilean Salamanca suggested that 'the general evil of the lower classes of modern nations is the immoderate and excessive abuse of alcoholic drinks, causing dementia and general paralysis'.[107] In a similar vein, in 1900 the Brazilian Jonathas Pedrosa suggested that morbid inheritance was a neuropathic state that could affect the entire organism or a specific organ. He argued that 'both in chronic alcoholism and progressive general paralysis, lesions of the brain and spinal cord are palpable', and listed symptoms such as frequent peripheral lesions, the gradual disorganisation of intelligence, and a drastic dissolution of cognitive ability.[108]

Conclusion

From the second half of the nineteenth century onwards, doctors in Brazil and Chile conceptualised alcohol over-consumption and its morbid forms by appropriating the theoretical and epistemic models of European science. Previously, the nutritional qualities of the various types of alcohol were widely promulgated, but discarded once liver cirrhosis became understood in an anatomo-clinical vein as a consequence of excessive alcohol consumption. As Santos, Santos and Verani, and Leyton and Fernández have pointed out, in both Chile and Brazil the emergence of over-drinking as a medical problem occurred within the context of industrialisation. Furthermore, in both countries alienists had established psychiatry as a scientific discipline and consolidated its practice and working spaces. Medicine came to offer prescriptions for social problems on the basis of psychiatry's scientific authority. In Chile, late nineteenth-century medical discourses had a hygienicist emphasis, which lent itself to the objectification of social problems as diseases. This allowed physicians to assume new competences in urban spaces while it also strengthened the institutionalisation of their profession. Similarly, in Brazil, around the same time as the establishment of the Republic in 1888, doctors began to develop their own theories, independent of those promulgated by European scientists. However, in neither country did the epistemological model mobilised to interpret the use of intoxicating beverages escape the Western medical framework. The link between excessive alcohol consumption and madness was seen to be *delirium tremens*, characterised by the delusions of chronic alcoholics in its advanced stage. Here the alcoholic's body became the focal point of two old concerns of nineteenth-century psychiatry, namely delirium and seizures. Over the years, the concept of *delirium tremens* evolved into the notion of alcoholic psychosis.

Although psychiatric communities in both countries shared certain paradigms and theoretical models in regard to alcohol, they also emphasised different focus points. In Brazil, doctors privileged the production of anatomo-clinical knowledge, whereas doctors in Chile focused on the compilation of statistical databases on alcoholism. While Chilean doctors gathered separate sets of detailed statistics on alcoholism from 1892 onwards, in Brazil such figures were presented alongside other diagnostic categories. These differences can be accounted for by the effort on the part of the Chilean medical profession to consolidate its spaces of competence, as the collation of statistics regarding alcoholism allowed them to encourage interest from the authorities in their work. In contrast, in Brazil psychiatrists had gained wide-ranging social and political legitimisation earlier on.

By the beginning of the twentieth century, the excessive use of alcoholic beverages was framed as a form of mental alienation in both Brazil and Chile. The definition of alcohol abuse as a psychiatric diagnostic category was initially informed by the French anatomo-clinical model and subsequently by the theory of degeneration and German organicism. The connection between over-drinking and mental illness was established during an era when large asylums were established for what were considered incurable chronic patients. These institutions became spaces *par excellence* for the professional performance of psychiatry. By the 1920s, patients suffering from alcohol-related problems constituted the largest number among hospital inmates.

As this chapter shows, the use of a comparative perspective has enabled us to identify the similarities and differences in two South American countries' psychiatric responses to the over-consumption of alcohol. The transnational focus highlighted the extent to which German and French medical theories and practices were transferred to, or re-fashioned in, Chile and Brazil, and brought into sharp relief differences in the ways in which alcoholism emerged as a disease category within very different socio-cultural, economic, political and institutional localities. At the same time, a Euro-centric analytical gaze was avoided by means of a close reading of medical dissertations that mapped the development of new, locally bred ideas and practices alongside those imported from other regions. Medical dissertations clearly constitute an invaluable primary source base for a history of knowledge transfer and knowledge production.

Notes

1 A. Bauer, *Goods, Power, History: Latin America's Material Culture* (New York: Cambridge University Press, 2001), 97.
2 Ibid., 98.
3 H. Carneiro, 'O corpo sedento: bebidas na história do Brasil', in M. del Priore and M. Amantino (eds), *História do corpo no Brasil* (São Paulo: Editora da Unesp, 2011), 131–56.
4 H. Carneiro, *Filtros, mezinhas e triacas. As drogas no mundo moderno* (São Paulo: Editora Xamã, 1994), 74.
5 Ibid.
6 H. Carneiro, *Comida e sociedade: uma história da alimentação* (São Paulo: Editora Campus, 2003), 74.
7 J. Del Pozo, *Historia del vino chileno* (Santiago: Lom Ediciones, 2014), 23.
8 Ibid., 79.
9 For an analysis of the economic development of Latin America at the time see J. Scobie, 'The growth of Latin America cities, 1870–1930', in L. Bethell (ed.), *The Cambridge History of Latin America*, vol. 4: *c. 1870 to 1930* (Cambridge: Cambridge University Press, 1986), 233–65.
10 For an analysis of the economic development of Brazil in the period see W. Dean, 'The Brazilian economy, 1870–1930', in Bethell (ed.), *The Cambridge History of Latin America*, vol. 5: *c. 1870 to 1930* (Cambridge: Cambridge University Press, 1986), 685–724.
11 In Chile colonial haciendas and agricultural labourers emerged towards the end of the nineteenth century. In Brazil identities were strongly determined by the social relations forged during slavery in the *ingenio azucarero* (sugar mills). For Brazil, see G. Freyre, *The Masters and the Slaves: A Study in the Development of Brazilian Civilization* (Berkeley: University of California Press, 1986). For Chile, see G. Salazar, *Labradores, peones y proletarios: formación y crisis de la sociedad popular chilena del siglo XIX* (Santiago: LOM Ediciones, 2000).
12 R. Campos Marín, *Alcoholismo, medicina y sociedad en España (1876–1923)* (Madrid: CSIC, 1997), 40.
13 A. Rosario, 'Dissertação sobre a influencia dos alimentos e bebidas sobre o moral do homem' (thesis, Faculdade de Medicina do Rio de Janeiro, 1839), 2. Translations are by the author except where otherwise stated.
14 F. Santos, 'Moderação e excesso; uso e abuso: os saberes médicos acerca das bebidas alcoólicas', *Clio – Revista de pesquisa histórica*, 24, no. 2 (2006), 105.

15 F. Santos and A.C. Verani, 'Alcoolismo e medicina psiquiátrica no Brasil do início do século XX', *Historia ciências saude – Manguinhos*, 17, no. 2 (2010), 400–20, at 406.

16 M. Fernández, 'Las puntas de un mismo lazo: discurso y representación social del bebedor inmoderado en Chile, 1870–1930', in Marcos Fernández Labbé et. al. (eds), *Alcohol y trabajo. El alcohol y la formación de las identidades laborales en Chile, siglos XIX–XX* (Osorno: Colección Investigadores, Editorial Universidad de Los Lagos, 2008), 91–119, at94; M. Fernández, 'Alcoholismo, herencia y degeneración en el discurso médico chileno. 1870–1930', in R. Gaune and M. Lara (eds), *Historias de racismo y discriminación en Chile* (Santiago: Uqbar Editores, 2009), 17–40; and M. Fernández, 'Fuera de sí: cuerpo, ebriedad y conciencia en Chile, 1870–1940', in A. Góngora and R. Sagredo (eds), *Fragmentos para una historia del cuerpo en Chile* (Santiago: Taurus, 2010), 285–327, at 285.

17 W. Schivelbusch, *Tastes of Paradise: A Social History of Spices, Stimulants, and Intoxicants* (New York: Pantheon Books, 1992), 153–4.

18 In pre-colonial Chile, *chicha* was made mainly of corn, but with the arrival of the Spaniards its production diversified into fruits such as apples, pears and grapes. The various types of *chicha* reflect its popular and artisan character, and accompanied the social and cultural life of the peoples of South America from pre-Columbian times. See P. Lacoste et al., 'Historia de la chicha de uva: un producto típico en Chile', *Idesia*, 33, no. 2 (2015), 89.

19 *Chacolí* is a variety of popular wine produced from the province of Huasco in the northern and central zones of Chile and was consumed at the end of harvest festivities, carnivals and national holidays, especially in the nineteenth century. Subsequently, consumption declined because of the wine industry's contempt for local varieties and artisanal methods of production. See P. Lacoste, A. Castro, F. Briones, F. Cussen, N. Soto, B. Rendón, F. Mujica, P. Aguilera, C. Cofré, E. Núñez and M. Adunka, 'Vinos típicos de Chile: ascenso y declinación del chacolí (1810–2015)', *Idesia*, 33, no. 3 (2015), 97.

20 See E. Laval, 'El Doctor Ricardo Dávila Boza: pionero de la infectología chilena. Higienista y salubrista', *Revista chilena de infectología*, 25, no. 6 (2008), 475–82. A list of the most popular liquors in Chile is given in R. Dávila Boza, 'Apuntes sobre el movimiento interno de la poblacion en Chile i sobre las principales circunstancias que tienen sobre él una notable influencia', *Anales de la Universidad de Chile*, 47 (1875), 546.

21 T. Carvalho, 'Dos alcoólicos: sua ação fisiológica e terapêutica' (thesis, Faculdade de Medicina do Rio de Janeiro, 1880), 34.

22 In the 1840s, the chemist Justus von Liebig (1803–1873) analysed the effects of alcohol on the body, concluding that it was a food. Some of these ideas were expressed in the book *Chimie organique appliquée à la physiologie et à la pathologie* (Paris, 1842). Robert Bentley Todd (1809–1860) was an Irish-born physician who is best known for describing the condition *postictal paralysis*, now known as Todd's palsy, in his Lumleian Lectures in 1849. He wrote *Cyclopedia of Anatomy and Physiology* (1835–59).

23 S. Feliú, 'El alcohol considerado como causas de las afecciones hepáticas' (thesis, Facultad de Medicina y Farmacia, Universidad de Chile, 1879), 371.

24 Carvalho, 'Dos alcoólicos' (1880), 28.

25 Ibid.

26 F. Grohuert, 'Del tratamiento de la neumonia aguda' (thesis, Facultad de Medicina i Farmacia, Universidad de Chile, 1873), 121.

27 Ibid., 126–7.

28 Ibid., 130–1.

29 C. Salamanca, 'Efectos del alcool' (thesis, Facultad de Medicina i Farmacia, Universidad de Chile, 1879), 360.

30 Carvalho, 'Dos alcoólicos' (1880), p. 4.

31 Ibid., 10.

32 M. Carneiro, 'Acção phisiologica e therapeutica dos alcoolicos' (thesis, Faculdade de Medicina do Rio de Janeiro, 1883), p. 85.

33 Federico Puga Borne (1855–1935) was a hygienist and director of the Institute of Hygiene, professor of legal medicine in the Faculty of Medicine of the University of Chile and later president of the Scientific Society of Chile and a deputy in the Chilean parliament. The Institute of Hygiene was the first specifically scientific health institution founded in Chile. Under the direction of Puga Borne, departments of hygiene and statistics, and chemistry and bacteriology were established. In 1896 a department for the production of sera and vaccines called the Institute of Animal Vaccine was added. See M.A. Illanes, *En el nombre del pueblo, del Estado y de la ciencia. Historia social de la salud pública, Chile 1880–1973* (Santiago: Impresión La Unión, 1993), 90.

34 Paolo Mantegazza (1831–1910) was an Italian neurologist, physiologist and anthropologist who in the late nineteenth century travelled through northern Argentina, where he came to know about the use of mate and other products of the region. Back in Italy, he investigated the anaesthetic effects of cocaine in humans. In 1858 he published

in Italy *Sulle virtù igieniche e medicinali della coca e sugli alimenti nervosi in generale.*

35 F. Puga Borne, *Elementos de higiene* (Santiago: Imprenta Gutenberg, 1891), 495.

36 Ibid., 492.

37 L. Vergara, 'Alcoholismo y degeneración', *Revista médica de Chile*, 20 (1892), 81.

38 E. Loureiro, 'Do alcoolismo chronico e suas consequencias' (thesis, Faculdade de Medicina do Rio de Janeiro, 1884).

39 M. Loyns, 'Alcoholismo inveterado como causa de dejeneracion hereditaria' (thesis, Facultad de Medicina i Farmacia, Universidad de Chile, 1898), 18.

40 For Chile, see W. Díaz, 'Geografía médica de Chile. Enfermedades reinantes en Chile', *Anales de la Universidad de Chile*, 47, no. 1 (1875), 13–40; Feliú, 'El alcohol considerado como causas' (1879); A. Tirado, 'Perturbaciones visuales en las cirrosis del hígado' (thesis, Facultad de Medicina i Farmacia, Universidad de Chile, 1886); A. Del Río, 'Contribución al estudio de la etiología y anatomía patológica de los abscesos al hígado', *Revista médica de Chile*, 18 (1890), 249–305. For Brazil, see M.J. Cruz, 'Cirrhose hepathica' (thesis, Faculdade de Medicina do Rio de Janeiro, 1882); L. Lage, 'Cirrhose hepatica' (thesis, Faculdade de Medicina do Rio de Janeiro, 1882); F. Martins, 'Cirrhose hepatica' (thesis, Faculdade de Medicina do Rio de Janeiro, 1882).

41 José Juan Bruner's interest was in natural history. He developed the Universidad de Chile's teaching in embryology and histology. In 1869 he was one of the founders of the Sociedad Médica de Santiago. See A. Orrego Luco, *Recuerdos de la Escuela* (Buenos Aires: Editorial Francisco de Aguirre, 1976). His contribution to psychiatry is investigated in Jaime Santander, Pablo Santander and Juan Enrique Berner, 'José Juan Bruner (1825–1899): una estrella fugaz en la historia de la psiquiatría chilena', *Revista médica de Chile*, 140, no. 11 (2012), 1495–500.

42 J. Bruner, 'Fragmentos de una hijiene pública en Santiago. Discursos de incorporación de don Juan Bruner en la Facultad de Medicina', *Anales de la Universidad de Chile*, 15, no. 1 (1857), 306.

43 The text was presented at the Congress of Geographical Sciences in Paris by Wenceslao Díaz (1834–1895), who was one of the founding academics of the Faculty of Medicine and one of the generation of professionals who stressed the importance of medical geography in explaining morbid phenomena. He became president of the

Protomedicato, the main institution for the control of medical practice at the time. See R. Diaz, *Una vida al servicio de la ciencia. El profesor doctor don Wenceslao Díaz, 1834–1895* (Santiago: Publicaciones de la Universidad de Chile, 1945).

44 Feliú, 'El alcohol considerado como causas' (1879), 371.

45 Cruz, 'Cirrhose hepathica' (1882); Lage, 'Cirrhose hepatica' (1882); Martins, 'Cirrhose hepatica' (1882). During the nineteenth century, autopsies were relatively uncommon in both Chile and Brazil. In Chile, post mortems were sporadically carried out in the field of legal medicine between 1860 and 1880 and more regularly following the introduction of a new medical curriculum in 1889, the opening in 1900 of the Casa de Orates Pathological Anatomy Laboratory, run by Dr Carlos Ugarte, and the appointment of the German pathologist Max Westenhoefer as professor of pathological anatomy between 1908 and 1911. See R. Cruz-Coke, *Historia de la medicina chilena* (Santiago: Andres Bello, 1995), 490–3. Arturo Ulloa, who worked for two years as an assistant at the Casa de Orates, noted that 'only the Casa de Orates contemplated in its regulations the performance of autopsies on all the deceased'. See A. Ulloa, *Estudio estadístico sobre mil doscientas autopsias i mui especialmente sobre la tuberculosis en Santiago* (Santiago: Imprenta y Encuadernación Universitaria, 1905), 10. In Rio de Janeiro, pathological anatomy practices were institutionalised only after 1907, when the first professor of pathological anatomy and physiology, Raul Leitao da Cunha, took office. See F. Duarte, K. Madi, L. Chimelli, H. Pinto de Moraes and C. Basílio de Oliveira, 'História da anatomia patológica nas Faculdades de Medicina do Rio de Janeiro', in M. de Franco and F. Soares, *História da patologia no Brasil* (São Paulo: Sociedade Brasileira de Patologia, 2001), 120. In 1902 the psychiatrist Juliano Moreira noted the absence of laboratories in mental hospitals, particularly in Bahia. See J. Moreira, 'Da necessidade da fundação de laboratorios nos hospitaes', *Gazeta médica da Bahia*, 33, no. 33 (1902), 439–50. In São Paulo it was not until the 1930s that pathological anatomy gained momentum with the appointment of the Italian physician Alfonso Bovero (A. Talamoni and C. Bertolli, 'A anatomia e o ensino de anatomia no Brasil: a escola boveriana', *História, ciências, saúde –Manguinhos*, 21, no. 4 (2014), 1301–22.

46 João Vicente Torres Homem (1837–1887) was the son of the doctor Joaquim Vicente Torres Homen, who studied in Paris and introduced Laënnec's auscultation method in Brazil. João Vicente studied at the Faculty of Medicine of Rio de Janeiro, specialising in internal medicine from 1861. In 1869 he published *Elementos de clinica medica*

and from 1882 his *Lições de clinica medica: feitas na Faculdade de Medicina do Rio de Janeiro (1867–1881)*. See L.O. Ferreira, 'João Vicente Torres Homem: Descrição da Carreira Médica no. Século XIX', *PHYSIS – Revista de saúde coletiva*, 4, no. 1 (1994), 57–78, and P. Nava, *Capítulos da história da medicina no Brasil* (São Paulo: Ateliê Editorial, 2004).

47 A. Zenteno, 'Alcoholismo' (thesis, Facultad de Medicina, Universidad de Chile, 1873) and V. Dagnino, 'El alcoholismo en Chile' (thesis, Facultad de Medicina i Farmacia, Universidad de Chile, 1887).

48 G. Bella, 'Do alcoolismo chronico e suas consequencias' (thesis, Faculdade de Medicina do Rio de Janeiro, 1883); J. Braga, 'Do alcoolismo chronico e suas consequencias' (thesis, Faculdade de Medicina do Rio de Janeiro, 1883); C.A. Azevedo, 'Do alcoolismo chronico e suas consequencias' (thesis, Faculdade de Medicina do Rio de Janeiro, 1883); and Loureiro, 'Do alcoolismo chronico' (1884).

49 Zenteno, 'Alcoholismo' (1873); Salamanca, 'Efectos del alcool' (1879).

50 Azevedo, 'Do alcoolismo chronico' (1883), Loureiro, 'Do alcoolismo chronico' (1884).

51 Azevedo, 'Do alcoolismo chronico' (1883), 1.

52 Loureiro, 'Do alcoolismo chronico' (1884), 23.

53 A. Vimieiro, 'Uma Ciência Moderna e Imperial: a fisiologia brasileira no final do século XIX (1880–1889)' (these Programa de Pós-Graduação em História, Faculdade de Filosofia e Ciências Humanas da Universidade Federal de Minas Gerais, Belo Horizonte, 2009), 74.

54 F.C. Edler, 'O debate em torno da medicina experimental no segundo reinado', *História, ciências, saúde – Manguinhos*, 3, no. 2 (1996), 284–99.

55 J. Moreira, 'Notícia sobre a evolução da assistência a alienados do Brasil', *Arquivos brasileiros de psiquiatria, neurologia e ciências afins*, 1, no. 1 (1903), 52–98.

56 Cruz-Coke, *Historia de la medicina chilena*; M.A. Illanes, *En el nombre del pueblo, del Estado y de la ciencia. Historia social de la salud pública, Chile 1880–1973* (Santiago: Impresión La Unión, 1993); M. Sánchez, 'La teoría de la degeneración en Chile (1892–1915)', *Historia*, 47, no. 2 (2014), 375–400; C. Leyton, 'El Gobierno de las poblaciones: Augusto Orrego Luco y la cuestión social en Chile', *Asclepio*, 72, no. 1 (2020), 297–313.

57 The Casa de Orates de Nuestra Señora de Los Ángeles was the institution opened by the Chilean government in 1852 to house people labelled as mentally ill. It was opened in the Yungay neighbourhood,

adjacent to the centre of the capital, and from its early years housed a high population of patients, with serious overcrowding problems. By the first half of the twentieth century, the House of Orates included a *manicomio* (asylum), intended for the insane considered dangerous; a psychiatric hospital and a temperance asylum for drinkers (*asilo de temperancia*). In 1928 its name was changed to Manicomio Nacional (National Asylum).

58 Augusto Orrego also cultivated political journalism, being editor of the newspapers *El Ferrocarril* and *El Mercurio*, while developing an institutional and political career and becoming director of the Faculty of Medicine (1871), president of the Chilean Medical Society (1895), deputy to the Liberal Party, president of the Chamber of Deputies (1886–88) and minister in two governments, holding the positions of Minister of the Interior (1897) and Minister of Justice and Public Instruction in 1898 and 1915. See P. Camus, 'Filantropía. Medicina y locura: la Casa de Orates de Santiago 1852–1894', *Historia*, 27 (1993), 109; C. Araya, 'Mujeres, médicos y enfermedad mental en la segunda mitad del siglo XIX', in A. Stuven and J. Fermandois (eds), *Historia de las mujeres en Chile*, vol. 1 (Santiago: Taurus, 2010), 453; E. Escobar, 'Las publicaciones psiquiátricas nacionales y sus autores en 150 años de la especialidad: los primeros cincuenta años (1852–1902)', *Revista chilena de neuro-psiquiatría*, 52, no. 4 (2014), 278.

59 A. Orrego, 'Causas indirectas de la alucinación mental', *Revista médica de Chile*, 2, nos 11–12 (1873), 441.

60 Adeodato García Valenzuela was trained in medicine and received a scholarship to specialise in physiological and pathological chemistry in Germany in 1891. Upon his return, he was appointed professor of physiological and pathological chemistry (1894). He also held the chair of chemistry in subjects affiliated to medicine, pharmacy and dentistry. Like Orrego, he wrote an essay titled 'La cuestion social' in 1907. See L. Corona, 'Recuerdos del profesor Adeodato García Valenzuela (1864–1936)', *Revista médica de Chile*, 95, no. 11 (1967), 154–9.

61 In A. García Valenzuela, *El alcohol i las bebidas espirituosas. Su reforma legal y social* (Santiago: Imprenta, Litografía i Encuadernación Barcelona, 1898), 104.

62 With the foundation of the Republic in 1889, the name of Hospicio Pedro II was changed to Hospicio Nacional de Alienados. The Academia Imperial de Medicina is now called Facultad de Medicina (FMRJ).

63 A.T. Venancio, 'Ciência psiquiátrica e política assistencial: a criação do Instituto de Psiquiatria da Universidade do Brasil', *História, ciências, saúde – Manguinhos*, 10, no. 3 (2003), 888.
64 M.S. Beca, 'Algo sobre las enfermedades mentales en Chile: recopilacion de la estadística de la Casa de Orates, desde su fundación en 1852 hasta la fecha' (thesis, Facultad de Medicina, Universidad de Chile, 1885). After publishing his statistics on mental illness in Chile, Beca specialised in criminology and anthropometric measurements. He was director of the Sociedad Médica de Santiago and editor of *Revista médica de Chile*. From 1903 he contributed to the development of anthropometric identification and dactyloscopy (fingerprinting) for the police of Santiago. In his book *Antropolojia I antropometria criminal. Estado de la cuestión* (1898) he developed the concepts of criminal predisposition and of the function of medicine as a therapeutic aid.
65 M.S. Beca, 'El alcoholismo', *Revista médica de Chile*, 20 (1892), 296–310; M.S. Beca, 'Una de las causas del alcoholismo crónico', *Revista médica de Chile*, 20 (1892), 361–9; M.S. Beca, 'Alcoholismo y criminalidad', *Revista médica de Chile*, 20 (1892), 442–50.
66 M. Nery, 'Fenômenos de índole epilética determinadas pelas bebidas alcoólica', *Brazil médico*, 7 (1893), 29–31; M. Nery, 'A loucura alcoólica e seu tratamento', *Brazil médico*, 7 (1893), 2–3.
67 Nery, 'A loucura alcoólica' (1893), 2.
68 Once the Office of Statistics and the Census Law were created in Chile in 1843, systematic population censuses were carried out every decade, which were made possible because of the small size of the Chilean population, mainly residents near cities and towns. In Brazil, although there was interest in carrying out a census in 1851, the first one meeting the standards of a modern state was not completed until 1872.
69 J. Golinski, *Making Natural Knowledge: Constructivism and the History of Science* (Chicago and London: University of Chicago Press, 2005).
70 Ibid., 72.
71 T. Porter, *Trust in Numbers: The Pursuit of Objectivity in Science and Public Life* (Princeton: Princeton University Press, 1995), 74.
72 Beca, 'Algo sobre las enfermedades mentales en Chile' (1885), 340.
73 Beca, 'El alcoholismo'.
74 Beca, 'Alcoholismo y criminalidad', 447.
75 The hiring of Francisco Béze can be understood in light of his relationship with Freemasonry and their sponsorship of positivism, in addition to his presentation of himself to the government of Chile as

an engineer and of French origin, within a context of shortages of professionals. The statistics on alcoholism were dedicated to the Minister of Justice and Public Instruction, Domingo Amunategui Rivera, also a Freemason. Between 1909 and 1911, Béze was director of the Chilean Statistics Office.

76 F. Bèze, *El alcoholismo, estudio y estadística* (Santiago: Imprenta, Litografía y Encuadernación La Ilustración, 1897), 12, 13. Other reports of statistical studies carried out in Chile by Bèze were *El suicidio en Chile* (1899) and *El capital y el trabajo* (1896).

77 Bèze, *El alcoholismo*, 6.

78 D. Estrada, 'Ethio-pathogenia do delirio alcoolico (contribuição ao seu estudo)' (thesis, Faculdade de Medicina do Rio de Janeiro, 1910), 87.

79 Henrique Roxo (1877–1969) received a doctorate in medicine from the FMRJ. He developed research on cerebral syphilis (1899), hysteria in men (1903), epilepsies (1905) and other topics. In 1921 he became a professor at the Psychiatric Clinic, and he published a *Manual of Psychiatry* in 1925. Between 1938 and 1946, he was the first director of the Institute of Psychiatry of the Universidade do Brasil. He had an important role in the institutionalisation process of Brazilian psychiatry. See A. Venancio, 'Os alienados no Brasil segundo Henrique Roxo: ciência psiquiátrica no Brasil no início do século XX', *Culturas psi*, 0 (2012), 19–44, at 30; H. Roxo, 'Causas de reinternação de alienados no Hospício Nacional', *Archivos Brasileiros de psychiatria, neurologia e medicina legal*, 6, nos 1–2 (1908), 403–15; H. Roxo, *Manual de psychiatria* (Rio de Janeiro: Livraria Francisco Alves, 1925), 257.

80 H. Lima, 'O alcoolismo no Rio de Janeiro' (thesis, faculdade de Medicina do Rio de Janeiro, 1914), 65.

81 Ibid.

82 Santos and Verani, 'Alcoolismo e medicina psiquiátrica', 403.

83 A. Zenteno, 'Alcoholismo' (thesis, Facultad de Medicina, Universidad de Chile, 1873). *Delirium tremens* was the term used to connect the effects of alcohol with madness. Thomas Sutton described it in 1813 as a delirium with tremors that occurred during abstinence after a prolonged intake of alcohol. Subsequent understandings of alcohol over-consumption built on this, and by 1890 alcohol delirium became seen as a form of alcohol psychosis. Thus *delirium tremens* was a central element that paved psychiatry's entry into the field of alcohol-related disorders. In nineteenth-century psychiatry, 'delirium' was an equivocal term as it designated both a global disorder of psychological life and states of mental confusion or delusional ideas. In the case

of *delirium tremens*, it referred to delusional states. Berrios argues that until 1855 mental alienation was considered a distinctive process in the French tradition, whose central expression was delusion. See G.E. Berrios and F. Fuentenebro, *Delirio: historia, clínica, metateoría* (Madrid: Editorial Trotta, 1996).

84 In 1863 the same doctor had already referred to *delirium tremens*. In a summary of the history of diseases in the country, the Chilean doctor Wenceslao Díaz responded to the paper 'De l'étar du Chili considéré sous le point de vue hygiénique et médical' published by the doctor Francisco Julio Lafargue, professor of anatomy between 1841 and 1850, and in *Bulletin de l'Académie nationale de médicine*, 17 (1851), 189–210. Lafargue had deplored what he called the 'debased existence' of Chilean peasants and asserted, among other things, that the upper classes indulged in drunkenness and gluttony. Díaz criticised Lafargue's conclusions, saying that his observations were based on exaggeration and prejudice. See W. Díaz, 'Documentos relativos a la historia de las enfermedades en Chile. Comunicacion de don Wenceslao Diaz a la Facultad de Medicina en su sesion del 10 de junio de 1863', *Anales de la Universidad de Chile*, 23 (1863), 737.

85 Zenteno, 'Alcoholismo' (1873), 19.

86 Ibid., 21.

87 Santos and Verani, 'Alcoolismo e medicina psiquiátrica', 403.

88 Azevedo, 'Do alcoolismo chronico' (1883), 15.

89 Loureiro, 'Do alcoolismo chronico' (1884), 19.

90 Ibid.

91 J. Gach, 'Biological psychiatry in the nineteenth and twentieth centuries', in E.R. Wallace and J. Gach, *History of Psychiatry and Medical Psychology: With an Epilogue on Psychiatry and the Mind–Body Relation* (New York: Springer, 2008), 390.

92 P. Pichot, *Un siglo de psiquiatría* (Madrid: Triacastela, 2010), 65.

93 J. Moraes, 'Psicoses de origem tóxica' (thesis, Faculdade de Medicina do Rio de Janeiro, 1890), 8.

94 On the theory of degeneration in Chile see Sánchez, 'La teoría de la degeneración'. For Brazil see O. Serpa, 'O degenerado', *História, ciências, saúde – Manguinhos*, 17, no. 2 (2010), 447–73.

95 See M.J. Eadie, 'Absinthe, epileptic seizures and Valentin Magnan', *Journal of the Royal College of Physicians of Edinburgh*, 39, no. 1 (2009), 73–8.

96 Campos, *Alcoholismo, medicina y sociedad*, 57.

97 Salamanca, 'Efectos del alcool' (1879), 303.

98 Loureiro, 'Do alcoolismo chronico' (1884), 23.

99 Vergara, 'Alcoholismo y degeneración'; Loyns, 'Alcoholismo inveterado' (1898); A. Sanhueza, 'Alcoholismo hereditario' (thesis, Facultad de Medicina I Farmacia, Universidad de Chile, 1898).

100 V. Magnan, 'Da dipsomania', *Brazil médico*, 4 (1892), 68–9. The use of the term *dipsomania* in Portuguese instead of the French original's *alcoolisme* is intriguing, as the former goes back to the Germanic tradition, namely Christoph W. Hufeland (1762–1836) in the early nineteenth century.

101 J. Nova, 'Capacidade civil dos alcoolistas' (thesis, Faculdade de Medicina do Rio de Janeiro, 1894); J. Pedrosa, 'Do alcoolismo como causa da degeneração' (thesis, Faculdade de Medicina do Rio de Janeiro, 1900); A. Bandeira, 'Gangrena social' (thesis, Faculdade de Medicina do Rio de Janeiro, 1904); M. Lima, 'Alcoolismo hereditario' (thesis, Faculdade de Medicina do Rio de Janeiro, 1904).

102 Beca, 'Alcoholismo y criminalidad'.

103 Feliú, 'El alcohol considerado como causas' (1879); Grohuert, 'Del tratamiento de la neumonia aguda' (1873).

104 G. Velis, 'Anotaciones sobre la epilepsia (esencial y jacksoniana)', *Revista médica de Chile*, 24 (1896), 201–32; Sanhueza, 'Alcoholismo hereditario' (1898); Loyns, 'Alcoholismo inveterado' (1898), Pedrosa, 'Do alcoolismo como causa da degeneração' (1900).

105 Loureiro, 'Do alcoolismo chronico' (1884).

106 Loyns, 'Alcoholismo inveterado' (1898); Pedrosa, 'Do alcoolismo como causa da degeneração' (1900).

107 Salamanca, 'Efectos del alcool' (1879), 302.

108 Pedrosa, 'Do alcoolismo como causa da degeneração' (1900), 27.

4

'White man's kava' in Fiji: entangling alcohol, race and insanity, *c.* 1874–1970

Jacqueline Leckie

When Fiji's Acting Governor, Juxton Barton, addressed the *Bose Levu Vakaturaga* (Great Council of Chiefs) on 18 September 1936, he appealed to them to control alcohol abuse among indigenous Fijians.

> There was nothing so degrading before man and God, than a drunkard, and there was no more potent poison to a native race than alcohol. It breeds diseases, crime and insanity; it ruins both the body and the mind; it separates husband from wife; and it inevitably means that sickly children are brought into the world.[1]

Barton expressed his concern despite the existence of legislation that prohibited the majority of indigenous Fijians from having access to alcohol and of customary and religious strictures against alcohol consumption. It seems that Europeans imbibed and abused alcohol to a far greater extent than other ethnic groups in Fiji, but Barton's speech points to the complex dynamics of alcohol and race.[2] Alcohol's effect upon health was among the consequences that Barton listed. This chapter explores the entanglement of local and global flows of alcohol from Europe, the USA and other colonies to Fiji — not just the transfer of the commodity — but also the discourses and practices that were medicalised, moralised, racialised, gendered and politicised.[3] At its most extreme, medical discourse focused in particular on 'alcohol insanity', while the clamour of moral, racial and gendered discourses became entangled with contesting calls over liberalisation versus prohibition of alcohol. These discourses were imbued with race, reflecting the assumptions about degeneracy, entitlement and civilisation that were directed at Fiji's plural indigenous and immigrant communities. The intersections of race and imperialism and debates about alcohol and its relationship to mental and other illnesses in Fiji resonate with Simon Heap's chapter on Nigeria in this book (see Chapter 5).

Fijians, along with other peoples in the Pacific Islands, had no alcoholic substances before their contact with outsiders.[4] European voyages in the Pacific, led by the Spanish during the sixteenth century, may have been predated by visits from island Asia. As Mac Marshall and Leslie Marshall have suggested, it is possible that from such early interaction Pacific peoples learned how to make

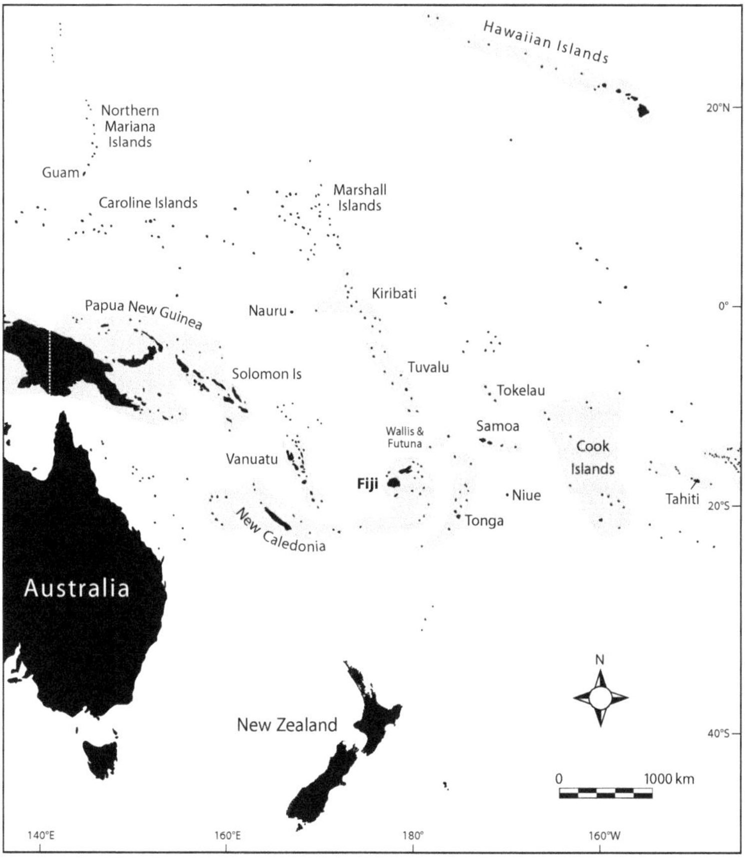

Figure 4.1 Map of the South Pacific

alcoholic beverages, including fermenting toddy from coconut palms to produce an intoxicating drink.[5] By the nineteenth century, alcohol had become a powerful trading commodity and hence was widely known among indigenous communities. As European colonialism unfolded, varying responses and meanings were attached to alcohol by indigenous people and Europeans. Many indigenous Pacific Islanders consumed kava, a drink prepared from the kava root (*piper methysticum*). This substance is not alcoholic but is sedative, and was used for centuries for ceremonial, social and spiritual purposes (as depicted in Figure 4.2). In Fiji kava is known as *yaqona*.[6] Not surprisingly, in some Pacific societies alcohol was initially referred to as 'White man's kava',[7] and in Fiji as *yaqona ni valagi* (referring to the English) or *yaqona ni kaivalagi* (referring to someone from outside Fiji, usually European).[8] *Mateni*, a Fijian term now used for being drunk on alcohol, once applied only to *yaqona*.[9] The connection made between kava and alcohol was not just one of terminology. Alcohol and kava were sometimes mixed together. They also became associated in legal, moralistic, racial, gendered and medical debates. Fijians called alcohol 'white man's kava', while some white men condemned kava along with other

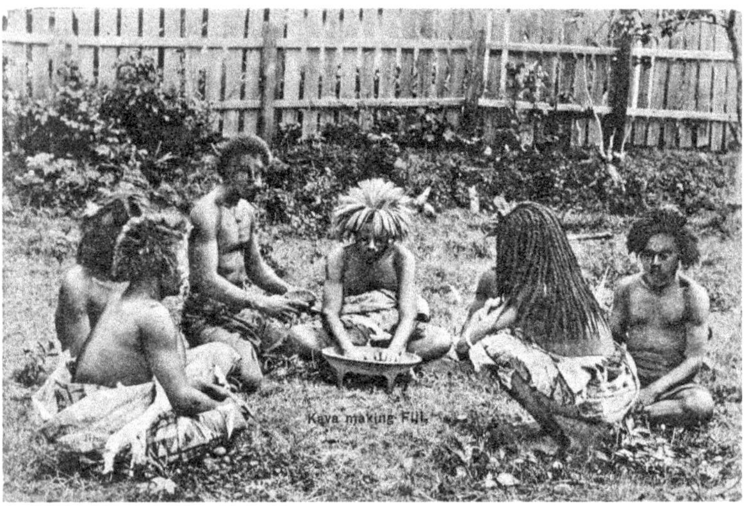

Figure 4.2 Postcard of 'Kava making Fiji', early 1900s

substances. For example, in 1862 Reverend Joseph Waterhouse's doctrine on teetotalism for Wesleyans in Fiji included kava, described as the 'opium' of Fiji. He was unsuccessful: 'In addition to ardent spirits the *yaqona* or kava root, is the curse of Fiji. For 12 years I have preached moderation, but in vain. With the Fijian of the present day it is all or none, – stupefaction, or sense.'[10] In 1871, after the Wesleyans' Fiji District Meeting, a ban on intoxicating liquor (except for medicinal and sacramental purposes) was introduced.[11] The alcohol ban appears to have been unpopular and was flouted. The number of expulsions from the church for intoxication equalled those for all other causes, and church membership in Fiji's eastern circuit declined from 3,598 to 2,808 in 1874. In some parts of Fiji, notably Rotuma, the missionary ban on intoxicating substances extended to kava. This restriction lasted only until 1873.

Barton's speech was directed at the Great Council of Chiefs, ostensibly representative of *iTaukei* (indigenous Fijians). However, colonial Fiji was ethnically complex. The 1936 census showed that Indo-Fijians made up 43 per cent of Fiji's population.[12] The roots of this community lay with the *girmitiyas*, indentured labourers who were shipped from India between 1879 and 1920 to work in Fiji, mainly for Europeans, in the sugar and copra industries.[13] Between 1865 and 1911, indentured labourers also originated from the Solomon Islands, the New Hebrides (Vanuatu), Tokelau, New Guinea, and the Gilbert and Ellice Islands (Kiribati and Tuvalu). Only a small proportion of Indians in Fiji were 'free' immigrants from Gujarat and Punjab. Other communities in Fiji included small numbers of migrants from China and other Pacific Islands.

Europeans were at the apex of the colonial hierarchy. They were also multi-ethnic in origin, being drawn from various regions in England, Scotland, Ireland, Australia, New Zealand, the USA and Europe. Some were born in Fiji, and represented diverse classes and interest groups such as planters, traders, missionaries, artisans and public servants. But in effect, 'European' was a racial category that equated to whiteness and white privilege and power. There were also the descendants of European men and indigenous Fijians and other Pacific Islanders – variously known throughout Fiji's history as part-Europeans, part-Fijians, half-castes and mixed-race – and, by the late twentieth century, more commonly as Kailoma.[14] Unlike non-Europeans, many Kailoma were granted access to alcohol. This potent beverage was a powerful marker of racialised and gendered boundaries; the regulations to enforce these were also part of the extension of control and order within a changing colonial society.

Regulation and race

By the late nineteenth century, almost all colonies within the Pacific Islands and the British white settler colonies of Australia, New Zealand and Canada had regulated indigenous and much of non-European access to alcohol, on the basis of common assumptions about race, civilisation and alcohol.[15] Although alcoholism and drunkenness were considered to be negative consequences of white people's advanced civilisation, and indicative of moral failing and degeneracy, drinking was also seen as an entitlement of race. Throughout the Pacific indigenous people were prohibited from buying and consuming alcohol. Fiji's policy was influenced by the negative impact alcohol was seen to have had on indigenous peoples in New Zealand and Australia. Its restrictive legislation was in large part derived from New South Wales legislation, which had banned alcohol for indigenous Australians. A few years after Fiji's cession to Britain in 1874, legislation was introduced that made it an offence to supply intoxicating liquor to natives or Polynesian immigrants. 'Native' did not just equate to indigenous Fijians but, as defined in the 1911 Liquor Ordinance, included Indians if they were indigenous Pacific Islanders or members of 'an aboriginal race of India'.[16] Those with a parent or grandparent indigenous to the Pacific or India were also considered to be natives. However, Pacific and Indian men who could trace European ancestry through their fathers' descent were entitled to possess and drink alcohol.[17] Heavy fines could be imposed on those who supplied alcohol to 'natives', while the latter could be fined up to £5 or imprisoned for up to one month if possessing or drinking liquor. This policy, which was in place until the 1950s, reinforced assumed connections between race, crime and alcohol. Court records in 1924 revealed a 'continual stream of offenders, mainly natives and Indians'.[18] 'Natives' caught with almost any quantity of alcohol could be prosecuted and criminalised. There were three exceptions, the first of which was the consumption of hop beer in native saloons. Legislation in 1917 formalised the licensing of saloons that could sell hop beer containing under 2 per cent proof spirit.[19] Fijians and Indians may have learned how to manufacture hop beer when they worked in European households or through socialising and working with Kailoma.[20] Further legislation in 1928 tightened the manufacturing and licensing of places that could sell hop beer, but this failed to control the illegal brewing of beer over 11 per cent proof.[21] In the hop beer saloons established throughout Fiji, 'the potency of the liquid sold and its harmful effects were legend'.[22]

Second, an elite minority of 'natives' – 'men of rank, who can be trusted with a permit' – were exempted from the 1911 liquor restrictions.[23] Non-indentured Indians of good character who had resided in Fiji for more than a year could apply for restricted permits, but policy stipulated that full permits were to be issued only to Indians in exceptional circumstances. Colonial officials were directed to use their discretion when issuing full or restricted liquor permits to 'half caste natives' of European descent. The most common (and less prestigious) liquor permits allowed holders to drink beer at hotel bars; a smaller number of holders could consume spirits, and a very restricted minority were permitted to purchase bottled liquor. Chinese, like Europeans, were not prohibited from access to liquor, ostensibly because they were 'reputed to have little tendency to become intoxicated having strong heads for liquor'.[24] Concern that Chinese storekeepers allegedly supplied liquor to prohibited persons led to Chinese, but not Japanese, being classified as 'natives' and requiring a liquor permit under the 1929 Liquor Ordinance. The Chinese government and consulate in Australia strongly objected to this amendment and the regulation was soon lifted.[25]

Medical reasons were the third exception to the 1911 Liquor Ordinance – but as will be expanded on later in this chapter, this was an area of considerable ambiguity. A doctor could prescribe quantities of alcohol to a patient of any ethnicity. This became a loophole through which some alcoholics obtained liquor. At the same time the ordinance enabled anyone, including Europeans, of 'confirmed intemperate habit' to be prohibited from consuming alcohol. This order was publicly posted and presumably referred to those who were considered alcoholics or of persistent danger to themselves or others.

The gendered boundaries of access to alcohol were far less complicated than those pertaining to race or status. Although some indigenous women had high status, generally men's authority was dominant in the domestic and public spheres. The colonial state and Christian churches reinforced traditional gender hierarchies and constraints on women's activities.[26] Until 1969, all non-European women were prohibited from purchasing alcohol. However, from 1962 European women were allowed to obtain alcohol permits. In the early twentieth century, even the serving of alcohol and kava by women had provoked an outcry. During the nineteenth century several European barmaids had worked in the boisterous hotels in Fiji's first capital, Levuka, but by 1933 there were only three barmaids in Fiji.[27] Similarly, the operation of kava saloons by Fijian women led to moral concerns during the late 1920s and 1930s, with claims that such 'dens' were also meeting places for sexual assignations and prostitution.[28] However, some colonial officials suggested that women had a moderating influence on men's behaviour in the saloons.[29] Women's access to alcohol was one of the most contentious issues when the 1911 ordinance was replaced by the Liquor Ordinance of 1962. By then, the race issue had become less prominent, with all men in Fiji aged over eighteen years allowed to buy and drink liquor.[30]

Transferring temperance and prohibition

The introduction and subsequent gradual lifting of liquor restrictions spanned the whole period of British colonial rule in Fiji, from 1874 to 1970. During the nineteenth century, most indigenous Fijians embraced Christianity, abandoning, or being forced to reject, their prior 'polytheistic cosmology.'[31] Some pockets of pre-Christian indigenous Fijian spiritual beliefs persisted, although many of the practices associated with these beliefs were outlawed.[32] Colonial Fiji was a strongly religious society, embracing Christian, Hindu and Islamic faiths. All of these religions taught abstention from or moderation of alcohol consumption. International discourses on liquor prohibition and temperance, especially those prevalent in the USA, New Zealand and Australia, resonated also in Fiji, where sharply contesting views over alcohol consumption and legislation developed. The resulting debates became entangled with ideas on racial difference prevalent at the time.

Ideas on temperance and prohibition flowed into Fiji through transcolonial church links and temperance movements during the late nineteenth century and the first half of the twentieth. When *HMS Pearl* docked in Fiji during 1874 – the year Fiji was declared a British colony – those on board included members of the International Order of Good Templars. Three lodges were eventually established, and during the 1880s the lodge in Suva housed the Freemasons' Lodge of Fiji. The Fiji Templars were part of the Grand Lodge of New South Wales and Fiji, with Reverend Arthur Small of the Methodist Mission and G.A.F.W. Beauclerc (the Deputy Grand Chief Templar) as property trustees.[33] Earlier visitors to Fiji had included George Grant, a temperance evangelist from New Zealand, in 1896.[34] During the heyday of prohibition in the USA, advocates toured the Pacific Islands. For example, Reverend J. Dawson of the World's League Against Alcoholism visited Fiji and Samoa in 1924.[35] Soon after, in 1925, the Fiji League Against Alcoholism was founded, and it was succeeded by the Fiji Social Service Alliance in 1931. The league and allied bodies ardently lobbied government against any potential liberalisation of Fiji's liquor policy.

In 1927 the league tried to publish temperance propaganda in the official Fijian vernacular newspaper *Na Mata*. However, the Secretary of Native Affairs objected to the transfer of foreign prohibition discourse to Fiji. The intended material told a story from South Africa: 'Khama: The Chief Who Worked Wonders'.[36] The Secretary of Native Affairs argued that the story was not applicable to Fijian culture and objected to the view that prohibition should embrace all classes.[37] Officials at the time wished to retain the privilege of access to alcohol for elite Fijians.

Nevertheless, international visitors set on pushing the prohibition message continued to arrive. Foreign Christian missionaries warned of the evils of alcohol when they proselytised Indo-Fijians. In 1924, for example, Reverend A.W. McMillan was sent from

New Zealand as Field Secretary of the Young Men's Christian Association. He was a founder of the Indian Reform League and secretary of the Indian League Against Alcoholism, which was concerned about the effect of alcohol on the Indian community.[38]

In a similar vein, Reverend Frank Lade, President of the Methodist Church of Australia, applauded the successes of prohibition in the USA when he addressed a meeting at Suva's town hall in 1931.[39] International prohibition propaganda flowed freely into Fiji and drew upon examples from the USA and other colonies such as South Africa, India and those in the Pacific.[40] In 1962 the Pacific Christian Literature Society and the Stanmore Missionary Press in Sydney published tracts on 'Danger in the Pacific', warning that 'Strong Drink will spoil you' and lead to fighting, swearing, competition, stealing, bad debts, murder, cursing, evil thoughts, sickness and arguments.[41]

The prohibition lobby in Fiji used its strongest argument against alcohol by invoking racial considerations, especially when government sought to amend the 1911 Liquor Ordinance. The Methodist missionary and President of the Fiji Social Service Alliance, G.H. Findlay, argued in 1932 that Fiji's liquor laws did not work well in a 'mixed community', because they aggravated issues of race.[42] This had 'the additional bad effect of making the native think of liquor as a privilege of the superior races, which, in certain circumstances, he might obtain'.[43] An impressive line-up of groups that advocated prohibition presented a petition to Fiji's Governor and the Secretary of State for the Colonies in early 1932. These bodies included the Fiji Social Service Alliance, the Methodist Mission, St Andrew's Presbyterian Church, the London Missionary Society in Fiji, the Fiji Mission of Seventh Day Adventists, the European and Indian branches of the Women's Christian Temperance Union, the Young Fijian Society, the Indian Reform League, the Arya Samaj, the Sikh Gurdwara Committee and the Fiji Muslim League.[44] This multifaceted coalition was united by the common purpose of abstinence from alcohol, but it also reflected emergent politicised criticism of racial discrimination in Fiji, especially among Indo-Fijians. As the Fiji Social Service Alliance put it in its recommendations to the select committee on the amendment of the liquor ordinance:

> The system of certificates of exemption under the present ordinance tends to create the impression that the use of liquor is evidence of social prestige to be sought after. Racial discrimination prohibiting the large majority and granting privilege to the small minority may be regarded as suggestive of partiality in the government of British subjects and tending to engender racial antipathy.[45]

A poison to the 'native race'

The speech of the Acting Governor, Juxton Barton, to the Great Council of Chiefs in 1936 reflected the operation of indirect rule – the alliance between Europeans and the chiefly elite – in maintaining the colonial state in Fiji. This alliance was based upon the doctrine of the paramountcy of Fijian interests and its dependence upon the British Crown's protection.[46] Charles Turner, Secretary of the Fiji Social Service Alliance, linked the government's 'duty of trusteeship towards native races for their training and education to a higher moral and education level' with the liquor question.[47] Government's duty towards indigenous Fijians was expected to prevail over the interests of a small minority entitled to liquor who had financial interests in the liquor business. The small minority included the Fijian elite, who were accorded special privileges, including access to alcohol. The state expected chiefs to enforce prohibition in villages even when these chiefs were allowed to consume the very substance that was banned. Although many, though not all, chiefs were teetotal for religious and cultural reasons, Barton disapproved of alcohol consumption among Fijian chiefs, just as missionaries had during the nineteenth century. In 1870 the Levuka missionary Joseph Nettleton observed an 'increase in drunkenness' and chiefs 'boldly' imbibing their 'drams'.[48] The Wesleyan missionary Frederick Langham expelled several church members on the island of Bau because of their alcohol consumption. 'The rage for English liquors both among members and nonmembers, chiefs and people is something appalling.'[49] The paramount chief Ratu Seru Epenisa Cakobau was reprimanded by Langham for his drinking habits. During the 1880s, annual gatherings of the Great Council of Chiefs were described by European observers as 'a saturnalia of drunken debauchery, riotous extravagance, and rampant, profligacy'.[50] Ratu Rabici's alcohol consumption was so persistent that in 1878 he was suspended from his post of Roko Tui Rewa and banned from visiting Suva for a year in 1891. He was also forced to retire from his official post.[51] During the early twentieth century, an outspoken temperance campaigner, Beauclerc, demanded that chiefs – many whom he called 'drunken sots' – be denied alcohol permits. That privilege had:

> the effect of demoralising and abasing the highest and most intelligent class of the coloured community. If the chiefs are to be allowed to become a degraded class, unfitted to work for the elevation or even the preservation of the people, what hope is there of preventing the whole native race from falling into as low a state as the aborigines of Australia, and eventually dying out, as those are dying out?[52]

The plummeting population of indigenous Fijians was also given as a reason for prohibiting indigenous access to alcohol. In 1907 Reverend F. Stubbs attributed falling Fijian population numbers to the 'evil' illegal supply of liquor to Fijians.[53] The decline in population (and also the 'sickly children' Barton had mentioned) had a longer history and was associated with introduced and infectious diseases, such as measles, influenza and dysentery, rather than the impact of alcohol.[54]

Beauclerc's comments and European preconceptions that alcohol abased the most intelligent class in the colony seemed to be confirmed twenty-four years later with the tragic circumstances surrounding the death in 1935 of the Fijian native medical practitioner Mesulame Taveta.[55] He had been posted to the British and French Condominium of the New Hebrides, where he was treated with disdain by the French doctors and the British administrators. Taveta began drinking heavily and, although forbidden to consume alcohol, continued to binge-drink. He contracted malaria and blackwater fever but was refused admission to the nearest hospital because the doctor misdiagnosed this, assuming that his delirium was due to drunkenness. Taveta died soon after, not from alcohol poisoning, but because of European medical preconceptions about alcohol and indigenous Pacific Islanders. His former tutor Dr Thomas Clunie had asserted in 1932 that 'few natives lifted out of their natural sphere escape death from alcoholic poisoning'.[56] Dr Sylvester Lambert, the Rockefeller Foundation's International Health Division's Pacific representative in 1934, also stated that alcohol had a toxic effect on Pacific Islanders, as they supposedly lacked Europeans' 'acquired immunity'.[57] Or as Barton had put it: liquor was a poison to the 'native race'.

One reason why liquor could be so toxic was that much of what was consumed was unregulated, illicitly brewed or distilled, with dubious additives to increase potency and keep costs down. Restrictive policies and high import duties encouraged illicit brewing but also inflated the price of commercially manufactured alcohol. During the 1920s regular supplies of whisky flowed into the rural districts and sold at sixteen shillings a bottle:[58] hardly affordable for the majority of indigenous Fijians and Indo-Fijians who had a subsistence or small farming livelihood, or for unskilled wage-earners, who earned around two shillings a day.[59] Illegal alcohol included home brew usually made of hops, sugar and yeast, and spirits distilled from ingredients such as molasses, rice, pineapple or raisins (often known as 'Raisin Jack').[60] Methylated spirits ('metho') was among the toxic concoctions that was sometimes added, and was sometimes even mixed with *yaqona*, a practice reputably favoured by southern Indians in Fiji. American servicemen stationed in Fiji during World War II taught Fijians how to make 'Black Jack', an alcoholic drink containing boot polish.[61] In 1957 an article in the *Pacific Islands Monthly* reported that 'Kava, laced with 'metho' and 'Black Jack', provide cheap horrible concoctions, but [are] well in the reach of the average Fijian who wants to become 'blind' drunk.'[62] Other names for home brews used in the 1940s included *tevoro* (devil), *siviyara* (plough), *kaukamea* (iron) and Fiji Airways.[63] Police raids in Macuata Province in 1940 seized liquor distilled by Indo-Fijians that, when tested, was shown to have proof spirit levels ranging from 25 to 109 per cent.[64] By the 1960s some Fijians in the Nakelo, Bau, Rewa and Noco *tikinas* (districts) became intoxicated by soaking a cloth in methylated spirits, tying it to their wrist and then inhaling alternate breaths of meths and cigarette smoke.[65]

While its effects were not usually as enduring as the 'alcoholic insanity' that pushed a very small number of drinkers into Fiji's

Public Mental Asylum, alcohol, especially illicit brews, could lead to temporary mental problems. In 1948 Kailoma and Fijians brewed a concoction mixture of hops, brasso, vanilla, raisins and 'coconut spey' on the island of Taveuni.[66] The District Officer claimed that 'two glasses are enough to put the drinker into a raving condition'.[67] Police reported Gilbert and Ellice Islanders in Fiji becoming 'fighting drunk' through drinking fermented toddy.[68] Fermented toddy apparently could sometimes drive the drinker 'almost crazy'.[69] In 1938 the Macuata District Commissioner R.N. Caldwell reported that a Fijian had run 'amok', burning an Indian's house and threatening other Indians with an axe, while under the influence of an 'Indian made spirit'.[70] Even hop beer, when brewed to a high level of potency, was said to make 'natives' drunk and, 'in many cases, very violently ill'. In 1924 an employer thought that one of his Indian staff would die, while one of his Fijian workers 'was silly for days'.[71]

Racial stereotypes about the impact of alcohol on non-Europeans were common in Fiji and were used to justify restrictions and prohibition. Even when alcohol was legally available to non-Europeans, Europeans perpetuated the stereotype: 'It is well known that the Fijian "just cannot hold his liquor" … the most amiable of South Sea Islanders – except, when, "under the influence", he becomes a quarrelsome pest.'[72] One medical doctor observed that alcohol 'made the usually gentle, polite' Taveta 'aggressive and insubordinate'.[73] Prohibitionists in Fiji, such as McMillan, also cited international temperance literature to prove that there were 'points of resemblance' with conditions in South Africa and in Fiji, concluding that 'Natives can't be moderate drinkers.'[74] When Reverend Anare Raiwalui declared in 1962 that 'Liquor is public enemy no. 1', he noted that he knew of 'Fijians whose careers had been marred by the influences of liquor'.[75]

'Liquor Drives Fijians Mad'

This eye-catching headline from the popular regional journal *Pacific Islands Monthly* fed into racial stereotypes about indigenous Fijians and alcohol.[76] The media also reflected colloquial discourse, whereby 'madness' referred to a temporary state or behaviour that was bizarre or contrary to racialised preconceptions. The journal editor Robert Robson, reporting on Fijian troops stationed in Malaya during the 1955 emergency, said that liquor 'maddens' Fijians: 'Very wisely, the officers keep their Fijians away from all alcohol', as it 'destroys their great good-humour and invariable courtesy'.[77]

Barton did warn the Fijian chiefs that alcohol could cause insanity. Popular and medical discourse stating that alcohol was an important cause of insanity was transferred to the Pacific from Europe, Australasia and the USA. In 1915 a Samoan newspaper cited an article from the American *Everybody's Magazine*: 'it is a universally accepted belief that alcohol is an important factor in producing insanity'.[78] Alcoholic insanity was also a recognised diagnosis within mental asylums,[79] including the Public Lunatic Asylum in Suva.[80] Alcoholic insanity and alcoholism have been ambiguously located in Western psychiatry. They were considered both causative and symptomatic of moral failing. According to degeneration theory, which was favoured by many Western doctors during the late nineteenth century, 'racial weakening' could be accounted for by behaviours such as alcohol consumption and masturbation.[81] It was believed that such weakening could lead to hereditary mental illness, linked to physical and intellectual disabilities. This is possibly why Barton warned the Great Council of Chiefs that the abuse of alcohol brought sickly children into the world.[82]

Yet doctors' notes from Fiji's asylum were generally devoid of moral judgement about alcohol and tended to describe alcoholism as an organic condition that had disturbing consequences for the patients and their families. The asylum record of what became St Giles Psychiatric Hospital in the 1960s show that alcohol abuse between 1884 and 1964 was never as prominent in the aetiology and nosology of mental disorders as it was in other regions under British control, such as colonial New Zealand and Australia.[83] Alcoholic insanity was also often confused with general paralysis of the insane (GPI) because of similar symptoms of mental restlessness, confusion, facial and bodily tremors and grandiose delusions.[84] This connection was problematic in Fiji, where the majority of patients diagnosed with general paralysis of the insane were indigenous Fijians who showed no evidence of alcohol abuse.[85]

Asylum records in Fiji also belie media and popular discourse that highlighted any links between indigenous Fijians, liquor and certifiable insanity. Governor Sir John Thurston noted that Ratu Alifereti Ravulo was sent to the lunatic asylum following alcohol abuse during what was referred to by him as the 'X'mas orgies' of 1888,[86] but there is no record of Ravulo's admission.[87] Between the asylum's opening in 1884 and 1964, only two indigenous Fijians were admitted to St Giles with alcohol given as a cause of their illness. One, a young native medical practitioner, was reported in 1946 to have drunk methylated spirits. He was disciplined but then became acutely depressed and refused to work. He was re-diagnosed with manic depression and never practised medicine again.[88] The other, a fifty-five-year-old Fijian foreman, was diagnosed with senile dementia in 1953. His condition was said to have been caused by financial worry and alcohol. He died in St Giles in 1961.[89]

Just one Indo-Fijian was diagnosed with alcoholism (along with violent mania and melancholia) and admitted to the asylum before World War II.[90] This gradually changed after the war when more Indo-Fijians were admitted. Like indigenous Fijians, the majority of Indo-Fijians were not entitled to buy alcohol. Many chose to abstain from consuming liquor, for cultural, religious and economic reasons. But kava was legal and enthusiastically imbibed by many Indo-Fijians. Kava did not induce insanity, although a male Indo-Fijian mental hospital patient with manic depression was labelled a 'yagona addict' in 1953, while another, with schizophrenia, was described as a heavy *yaqona* user.[91]

Women rarely drank kava, so it is surprising that it was reported in 1888 that villager Mele's excessive *yaqona* drinking made her abstain from eating, causing her to succumb to insanity.[92] Another female patient, diagnosed with manic depression, was said to have drunk *yaqona* 'all day'.[93] Only two European and one Chinese woman had alcohol listed as a cause for their condition on admission to St Giles during the colonial era, in 1956, 1959 and 1937 respectively. More female patients, especially Europeans and Kailoma, bore and suffered from the impact of their husbands' alcohol abuse. In 1948 Molly, a Kailoma, was in despair about her European husband, who was a 'compulsory alcoholic'. This was echoed in other accounts of the social and mental effects of alcohol within families in Fiji.[94]

There is however evidence that alcohol abuse among Europeans was more widespread outside the confines of medical institutions. Drunkenness in Pacific port towns, such as Levuka, was legendary during the nineteenth century,[95] and alcohol dependence seems to have been common among planters and early colonial administrators.[96] Reports of 'heavy drinking' and the large consumption of spirits by Europeans in Fiji persisted in later decades.[97] The alcohol problem in Fiji was a problem for the very race that was entitled to drink (for instance at Navua Hotel, depicted in Figure 4.3). Those admitted to the asylum for 'alcoholic insanity' before World War II were almost exclusively male Europeans. This ethnic predominance, however, did not reflect the asylum's overall ethnic makeup. Europeans never formed more than 15 per cent of patients and, after 1914, around 5 per cent. Europeans also comprised only 2.57 per cent of Fiji's population in 1911. From around 1905, Indo-Fijians made up the highest percentage of admissions, with Fijians never constituting more than 40 per cent of admissions until the 1970s.[98] In 1901 Indians made up 14 per cent and

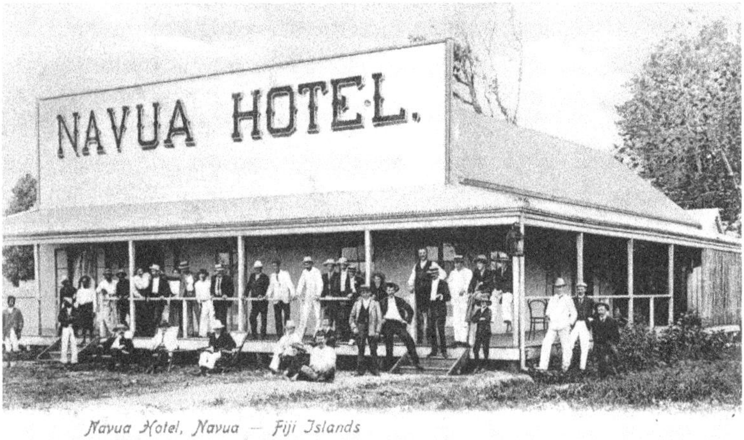

Figure 4.3 Postcard of Navua Hotel, Fiji Islands, 1900–1920

Fijians 79 per cent of Fiji's population; these respective percentages changed to 50.5 and 43 by 1966.

Michael, a European civil servant, was diagnosed as an 'alcoholic maniac' in 1910.[99] He had attempted suicide by drinking potentially lethal perchloride of mercury, and during his transfer to the asylum he had tried to jump off a cliff. Michael spent four months in the asylum, where he was under constant supervision and sometimes confined to a straitjacket. He was delusional, violent, anorexic and manic. He heard voices that directed him to commit murder, and he believed that his presence on earth damned a million people a day. Michael's severe depression resurfaced, and there were further suicide attempts. Michael saw his madness as a moral struggle between God and the devil. The devil won through driving him to drink, and also to chronic masturbation. Probably because of this moral failing, he urged the medical superintendent to cut out or open his genitalia, presumably to stop him masturbating.

Michael regarded alcohol as the source of his moral failing, although the causes of his severe mental condition were likely to have been more complex. Alcohol abuse often coexisted with other mental conditions, and doctors sometimes prioritised alcohol as a cause of a patient's illness. Conversely, the role of alcohol consumption within the aetiology of mental disorders could be underestimated because patients might hide the true extent of their alcohol consumption patterns and abuse – especially within cultures where the consumption of liquor was considered immoral, shameful or illegal. Mani, an Indian storekeeper, had six admissions between 1934 and 1962.[100] He was initially diagnosed with dementia, then with mania, and only on his fourth admission was his disorder listed as 'alcoholic psychosis'. The debilitating impact of alcohol abuse on physical and mental health is also often cumulative and may be evident only after several years of alcohol addiction. Some of the patients admitted with alcohol-related conditions were also very ill physically. In 1902 a European patient admitted with 'alcoholic insanity' died from thrombosis in the brain, dementia and exhaustion, all thought to have been directly related to his alcohol abuse.[101] He had been a baker and continued to believe he was still baking loaves every morning during his time in the asylum. He was also convinced that people were trying to cut off his head.

The asylum was sometimes a space to 'dry out' the alcoholic fever and madness that gripped some travellers and crew, either on board ships or within Pacific ports. Alcohol abuse was a problem for workers on Pacific steamships and was partly exacerbated by working conditions, boredom and depression.[102] A European fireman on the *SS Atua* was admitted with 'alcoholic insanity' in 1911 for two days after throwing himself overboard and trying to assault officers and crew.[103] The sudden cessation of alcohol could have lethal consequences for alcoholics. In 1907 a European veterinarian, 'temporarily depressed in mind', sailed from New Zealand to Fiji on the *Moura*.[104] After he was denied alcohol, he went into *delirium tremens*. He was refused urgent medical treatment at Suva's main hospital and instead sent to the asylum, where he soon died. Thomas, a former sailor from Ireland who had settled in Noumea in New Caledonia, was diagnosed with alcoholic insanity and spent eight years in Suva's asylum.[105] His mental condition had deteriorated after his wife's death, and in 1882 he stowed away in the coal bunkers of the *PS Thistle*. He was discovered when the ship docked in Fiji and was declared insane. Thomas was initially placed under restraint in a police cell and then drifted into prison as a vagrant, remaining until he was committed to the asylum after it was founded in 1884. On his discharge, the medical superintendent predicted that Thomas would slide back into alcoholism in Suva. He was shipped back to Noumea, considered 'a more civilised & larger port', on the condition that he was not given any liquor during the voyage.

Small amounts of alcohol were administered to patients of all ethnicities within the mental asylum. Under section 77 of the 1911 Liquor Ordinance, registered medical practitioners could prescribe liquor. Within the asylum, whisky was sometimes given as a stimulant, or combined with milk and egg and passed through a nose-tube for patients who, like Michael, had 'wasted away' or refused food or drink.[106] On 13 January 1907, for example, a long-term female European patient who became very weak and vomited frequently was given a special daily diet of three ounces of whisky, one pint of beef tea, two pints of milk, bread and butter, tea and rice pudding. It is unclear whether alcohol was given in small doses to hospitalised alcoholics, but samples of the permits issued outside the asylum suggest that some doctors enabled a steady supply of alcohol to be given to patients who probably suffered from alcohol dependency. For example, one medical doctor, Dr Miller, wrote in 1916 that 'a patient of mine is suffering from a chronic disease and is in need of a bottle of good whisky per fortnight'.[107] There is no record of what this illness was. Until 1918, prescriptions could be issued for one bottle of spirits per week, fortnight or month, for a duration of six months, and then renewed.

After 1918 doctors could only supply a medical certificate for procurement of a liquor permit, which the patient (unless bed-ridden or hospitalised) used to apply for a permit through the district commissioner and the inspector general of constabulary.[108] For example, during the 1920s and 1930s, Prasad consulted doctors several times for acute alcoholism.[109] For many years he had been able to obtain a liquor permit on medical grounds, but eventually the District Medical Officer of Lautoka, Dr Philip Harper, persuaded Prasad to surrender the certificate. Several years later Prasad persuaded Dr F. Roth Carrick to recommend a dose of one bottle of beer a day, but clearly Prasad obtained more liquor through other means, as he nearly killed himself through drink on several occasions. In 1935 Carrick managed to get Prasad to again hand in his liquor permit when he suffered 'a fit of remorse and a bad headache'. Harper had often seen Prasad and his son drunk and advised against issuing further permits.[110]

Reasons given in applications for liquor permits on medical grounds included rheumatism, debility, chronic cough and bronchitis. The Nadroga District Medical Officer recommended that an Indo-Fijian patient be allowed one bottle of spirits per month because he needed stimulants: 'I can think of no stimulant to compare with the judicious exhibitive of alcohol.'[111] An Indo-Fijian storekeeper on Taveuni was able to obtain a liquor permit to purchase four bottles of whisky and eight bottles of beer per month because his doctor said that liquor was of great value to him during his frequent attacks of *waqaqa* (infection and fever from filariasis).[112] This was contrary to the Governor's view in 1934 that there was no value in alcohol for treating medical conditions: 'There are medicines which in practically every case are quite as efficacious as alcohol, and Fijians and Indians who can afford alcohol can afford to buy medicines.'[113] The Governor ruled that henceforth no liquor permits were to be issued on medical grounds except on a recommendation by the Chief Medical Officer to the Colonial Secretary.

Change of brewing in the colony

The patterns of reported alcohol abuse changed after World War II, when Indo-Fijians rather than Europeans were noted in St Giles' records with alcohol-related mental disorders. One reason for this was that more Indo-Fijians, and more people in all other ethnic communities, now had access to alcohol – both illicitly and legally. The war had been a catalyst in the growth of the informal liquor industry, from which some Indo-Fijians profited, as well as allowing easier access to alcohol. The total number of liquor permit holders increased from 7,542 in 1947 to 20,088 in 1953.[114] Of these, 14,815 were Indians, and 5,473 were Fijians and others.[115] More liberal attitudes among Indo-Fijian communities towards the consumption of alcohol also changed after World War II, but many Hindus and Muslims, as well as *iTaukei*, were still teetotal. The class structure of Indo-Fijian communities was also shifting, with a growing middle class enjoying a slightly higher disposable income. The majority of Indo-Fijians admitted with alcoholism to St Giles before the 1960s were storekeepers (seven, and also one Chinese storekeeper), who probably stocked liquor. Contrary to stereotypes in Western countries of the homeless as alcoholics, none of the destitute or homeless people admitted to St Giles during the colonial period appear to have had serious alcohol problems.

Outside the mental hospital, both the pro- and anti-liquor lobbies remained vocal, but in Fiji medical reasons were never prominent in demands to further restrict access to alcohol. Instead the race issue came to the fore as the liquor question became politicised. By the late 1940s, political divisions over prohibition were sharply drawn between Indian politicians – notably the Arya Samaj leader Vishnu Deo and A.D. Patel.[116] Deo advocated total prohibition while Patel considered that restrictions on alcohol should be lifted for all ethnic communities. Patel's stance was supported by most of the Indian advisory committees to government. It was argued that prohibition in fact promoted the manufacture and consumption of illicit liquor and methylated spirits. Both Patel and Deo saw the liquor laws as racially discriminatory: alcohol was a signifier and concrete expression of racialised lines in Fiji. Patel saw the permit system as paternalistic. Deo's and the Samajists' views were informed by the situation in India, where teetotalism was a key symbol of nationalism and anti-colonialism.[117]

Alcohol remained an important ingredient within the state's paternalistic protection of indigenous Fijians.[118] In 1947 the government proposed lifting liquor restrictions for Indo-Fijians but keeping those for indigenous Fijians, thus 'establishing racial equality while protecting the Fijians'.[119] This proposal was strongly opposed by most Fijian and European members of the Legislative Council, and the ensuing select committee failed to reach a decision.[120] It was commerce and industry, not patronising racial considerations, that brought a considerable change to Fiji's liquor laws and the legal availability of alcohol in 1958. In the same year as Carlton Brewery began brewing Fiji Bitter, restrictions on the consumption of beer in licensed bars were lifted for all males aged over eighteen. However, the prohibitionists did not give up. In 1962, when government proposed removing the permits required by Fijians to purchase spirits, and the restrictions on women's access to alcohol,[121] Reverend Doug Fullerton of the Methodist church claimed that he had support from many Fijians in villages for the view that everyone, including Europeans, should have to apply for a permit if they wanted to drink.[122]

Debates about alcohol became again entangled with issues of race during the 1960s amid talks about universal franchise and Fiji's impending independence from Britain. Fullerton, Europeans and many Fijians argued that Fijians needed more time to learn how to make responsible decisions about drinking and the alcohol legislation[123] – a well-established paternalistic and protectionist stance, which was also echoed in views about franchise and political independence. Furthermore, one section of Fijian society remained deprived of equal rights in terms of suffrage and access to alcohol: Indian women. According to the official report of the liquor committee in 1962, almost everyone in Fiji agreed that Indian women should not consume alcohol.[124] Restrictions on the buying and drinking of liquor by Indian women were not lifted until 1969 – the same year they attained the right to vote, and one year before Fiji's independence from Britain. Even then, women (excepting barmaids) were prohibited from entering public bars for several more years.

Conclusion

It has been argued in this chapter that the global flow of alcohol and alcohol discourse across cultures was embedded in assumptions of race and gender. Conceptions of alcoholic insanity were transferred from Europe, North America and British colonies to become entangled with Fiji's plural cultures. As the historian Brij Lal states: 'Maintaining strict separation of the races was an essential component of the colonisers' desire to control the colonised … colonial rule was premised on the ideology of inequality.'[125] The power dynamics between coloniser and colonised are integral to understanding past patterns of access to and consumption of alcohol in Fiji. Alcohol symbolised racial and gendered separation and hierarchy. But 'alcoholic insanity' revealed the cracks in this logic. While legal access to alcohol was an entitlement of race, those suffering from 'alcoholic insanity' before World War II were almost exclusively Europeans. Yet popular discourse linked native races, alcohol and madness, and thus justified exclusion and protection.

Elite Fijians, such as Taveta, were pivotal in the maintenance of racialised lines. Colonialism in Fiji worked through co-option of and cooperation with the indigenous elite, as Barton so clearly reminded the Great Council of Chiefs in 1936. Fijians like Taveta had their behaviour and drinking scrutinised, and the hegemonic discourse that 'natives' cannot hold their liquor lingered for many decades. Europeans such as Michael let the side down, and his punishment was evident in his insanity. Colonial Fiji certainly had an alcohol problem but it also had a race problem, full of contradictions.

The 1960s were a decade of unprecedented change in Fiji – not least in regard to alcohol.[126] Access was no longer an entitlement of race (although gendered boundaries remained), but access and desire were influenced by money, product commodification and advertising. 'Alcoholic insanity' was no longer a medical term and was replaced by 'substance abuse', which, in Fiji, as in many other countries, included psychiatric concern about cannabis use. In post-colonial Fiji white man's kava has been legally available to all adults and is firmly entangled with local cultures. As in the colonial era, a strong anti-alcohol lobby persists, fuelled by religion and sometimes entangled with indigenous nationalism. Kava is consumed by people of all communities in Fiji – albeit predominately by men. It is now also exported globally, but more than ever has become a symbol of Fijian culture and pride.

Notes

1 Colonial Paper (CP) 36/36, 'Report of the proceedings of the Council of Chiefs, held at Mbau on 16th September 1936, and following days.' All archival sources, unless stated, are from the Colonial Secretariat Office (CSO) files, National Archives of Fiji, Suva.

2 Evidence of European alcohol consumption in Fiji during the nineteenth century is based on contemporary accounts such as those quoted in D. Scarr, *Viceroy of the Pacific: The Majesty of Colour: A Life of Sir John Bates Thurston* (Canberra: Australian National University Development Studies Centre, 1980), 188. A minute by Fiji's Inspector General of Constabulary, 22 October 1909, stated that the consumption of liquor by the white population was greater than that of any Australasian colonies, but that it was difficult to obtain precise figures. CSO 8133/1909. It is not clear how true this statement was. Figures for Fiji for convictions of drunkenness and being under the influence of alcohol reported higher numbers for Europeans and people of mixed race in a minute in 1910, in F40/15, 'Native liquor trade – control of'.

3 I sincerely thank Mac Marshall and Judy Bennett for advice and information, Waltraud Ernst for feedback, Opeta Alefaio and staff of the National Archives of Fiji, and the Stout Research Centre of New Zealand Studies, Victoria University of Wellington and the University of Newcastle for support.

4 For an overview of alcohol and drugs in the Pacific Islands see E.M. Lemert, 'Forms and pathology of drinking in three Polynesian societies', *American Anthropologist*, 66, no. 2 (1964), 361–74; M. Marshall, 'A review and appraisal of alcohol and kava studies in Oceania', in M.W. Everett, J.O. Waddell and D.B. Heath

(eds), *Cross-Cultural Approaches to the Study of Alcohol: An Interdisciplinary Perspective* (The Hague and Paris: De Gruyter, Mouton 1976), 103–18; M. Marshall, 'A Pacific haze. Alcohol and drugs in Oceania', in V.S. Lockwood, T.G. Harding and B.J. Wallace (eds), *Contemporary Pacific Societies: Studies in Development and Change* (Englewood Cliffs, NJ: Prentice Hall, 1993), 260–72; M. Marshall, 'Pacific islands', in Jack S. Blocker, Jr, David M. Fahey and Ian R. Tyrrell (eds), *Alcohol and Temperance in Modern History: An International Encyclopaedia*, vol. 2 (Santa Barbara, Denver and Oxford: ABC-CLIO, 2003), 472–4; M. Marshall, 'Market highs: alcohol, drugs and the global economy in Oceania', in V. Lockwood (ed.), *Globalization and Culture Change in the Pacific Islands* (Upper Saddle River, NJ: Pearson, 2004), 200–21.

5 M. Marshall and L.B. Marshall, 'Opening Pandora's bottle: reconstructing Micronesians' early contacts with alcoholic beverages', *Journal of the Polynesian Society*, 84, no.4 (1975), 441–66.

6 See S. Aporosa, 'Yaqona (kava) and education in Fiji: investigating "cultural complexities" from a post-development perspective' (PhD dissertation, Massey University, 2012), 177–84.

7 Marshall, 'A Pacific haze', 264.

8 C. Toren, *Mind, Materiality and History: Explorations in Fijian Ethnography* (London: Routledge, 1999), 134.

9 R. Gatty, *Fijian–English Dictionary: With Notes on Fijian Culture and Natural History* (Suva: Southeast Asia Program, Cornell University, 2010), 166. Elsewhere in the Pacific, in Tahiti, alcohol was called *ava no Beretania* (British kava), while Chuukese adopted the Pohnpeian word for kava (*sakau*) to refer to alcohol. In the Cook Islands, kava can mean both the *piper methysticum* and liquor. Imported alcohol is *kava papa'ā* while home brew, and also traditional kava, is *kava Māori*. Alcohol in Samoa is known as *ava malosi* (strong kava).

10 N. Gunson, 'On the incidence of alcoholism and intemperance in early Pacific missions', *Journal of Pacific History*, 1, no.1 (1966), 60. Although these effects are not common, kava can induce intoxication ('grog doped') and hangovers (*lomoloma ca*). Aporosa, 'Yaqona (Kava) and Education in Fiji', 177–84.

11 Gunson, 'On the incidence of alcoholism', 60–1; A. Thornley, *Exodus of the I Taukei: The Wesleyan Church in Fiji, 1848–74* (Suva: University of the South Pacific, Institute of Pacific Studies, 2002), 484–5.

12 Fiji Bureau of Statistics, '1.2A census population of Fiji by ethnicity' (Suva, 2012), www.statsfiji.gov.fj (accessed 19 December 2019).

13 See K.L. Gillion, *Fiji's Indian Migrants: A History to the End of Indenture in 1920* (Melbourne: Oxford University Press, 1962); K.L. Gillion, *The Fiji Indians: Challenge to European Dominance, 1920–1946* (Canberra: Australian National University Press, 1977); B.V. Lal, *Girmitiyas: The Origins of the Fiji Indians* (Canberra: Journal of Pacific History, 1983); J. Leckie, '"Race has nothing to do with anything": Indians in Fiji', in R. Starrs (ed.), *Nations under Siege: Globalization and Nationalism in Asia* (New York: Palgrave Macmillan, 2002), 243–68.

14 See L. de Bruce, 'Histories of diversity: Kailoma testimonies and "part-European" tales from colonial Fiji (1920–1970)', *Journal of Intercultural Studies*, 28, no. 1 (2007), 113–27.

15 Marshall, 'Pacific islands', 473; Marshall, 'A Pacific haze', 264; S. Saggers and D. Gray, *Dealing with Alcohol: Indigenous Usage in Australia, New Zealand and Canada* (Cambridge: Cambridge University Press, 1998), 45–67.

16 'An ordinance to consolidate and amend the law relating to the sale of spirituous liquors', 17/1911. Part II referred to liquor prohibition. In Fiji, the term 'aboriginal Indian' referred to any Indian, whether tribal, caste Hindu or Muslim.

17 Provided they had the qualifications to be registered as an elector of the Legislative Council. Ordinance 17/1911, Part II, subsection 72.

18 'A campaign commenced', *New Zealand Herald*, 27 May 1924, p. 5, https://paperspast.natlib.govt.nz/newspapers/NZH19240527.2.39 (accessed 5 July 2021).

19 Licence Ordinance 9/1917. On hop beer saloons see Minute Paper (MP) 4142/24.

20 According to F40/5, 'Liquor and hop ban. Illicit distillation and brewing'. Memorandum from Acting Inspector-General (AIG) to Colonial Secretary (CS)', 11 July 1932.

21 F40/5, 'Memorandum on sly-grog traffic' from AIG, 28 September 1936.

22 F40/5, 'Memorandum from AIG to CS', 11 July 1932.

23 MP 6079/09. Saggers and Gray, *Dealing with Alcohol*, p. 49, refer to exemptions on alcohol restrictions for Australian aboriginals and the colonial French and Belgian concept of *évolué* or *assimile*, permitting the rights of full civic status if an indigenous subject could prove that they were civilised.

24 MP 3508/28, 'Memorandum from CS to Governor on question of instituting prohibition for Chinese residents', 1 August 1928.

25 B.N.K. Ali, *Chinese in Fiji* (Suva: University of the South Pacific,

Institute of Pacific Studies, 2002), 80–1; MP 5341/28, 'Bill to amend Liquor Ordinance 1911, 1928'; MP 461/29, 'Petition of Chinese residents with reference to the liquor bill'.

26 However, on women's agency see J. Leckie, 'The complexities of women's agency in Fiji', in B. Yeoh, P. Teo and S. Huang (eds), *Gender Politics in the Asia-Pacific Region* (London: Routledge, 2002), 156–80.

27 J. Young, 'Evanescent ascendancy: the planter community in Fiji', in J.W. Davidson and D. Scarr (eds), *Pacific Islands Portraits* (Canberra: Australian National University Press, 1976), 154; F40/1/pt. 1, Minute by AIG, 13 January 1933.

28 F40/5, 'Memorandum on sly-grog traffic' by AIG, 28 September 1936; MP 4668/24, 'Memorandum by Ratu Joni Mataitini and 36 others re. suspension of prohibition of Fijian women serving in yagona saloons'; petition by *c.* 31 Indians (probably Indian Reform League), organised by Methodist Missionary Society of Australasia (Fiji District).

29 MP 4668/24, 'Memorandum on Suva kava saloons'.

30 Restrictions on the consumption of beer were lifted in 1958.

31 J. Ryle, 'Roots of land and church: the Christian state debate in Fiji', *International Journal for the Study of the Christian Church*, 5, no. 1 (2005), 62.

32 See M. Kaplan, *Neither Cargo nor Cult: Ritual Politics and the Colonial Imagination in Fiji* (Durham, NC: Duke University Press, 1995).

33 E.H. Cherrington, *Standard Encyclopaedia of the Alcohol Problem: 1877–1950*, vol. 3 (Westerville, OH: American Issue Publishing Company, 1926), 987.

34 Ibid., 1131.

35 'A campaign commenced'.

36 Prohibition Paper no. 3 MP C7/27, 'Fiji League Against Alcoholism requests publication in "Na Mata" of pamphlet on prohibition', 8 March 1927.

37 MP C7/27, 'Fiji League Against Alcoholism requests publication in 'Na Mata' of pamphlet on prohibition', 8 March 1927.

38 Gillion, *The Fiji Indians*, 105. The Indian Reform League appealed to Indian Christians and 'modern-minded Indians', many who were government clerks and interpreters.

39 F40/1/pt. 1, *Fiji Times* (*FT*), 6 November 1931.

40 On international developments, see Johan Edman, 'Transnational nationalism and idealistic science: the alcohol question between the wars', *Social History of Medicine*, 29, no. 3 (2016), 590–610.

41 F60/6–2, 1962, reprint from *Pacific Island World*, 10, no. 3 (December 1958).
42 'Liquor laws and mixed races: Fijian system aggravates racial feeling', *The Advertiser* (Adelaide), 6 May 1932, 16. See K. Close-Barry, *A Mission Divided: Race, Culture and Colonialism in Fiji's Methodist Mission* (Canberra: ANU Press, 2015) on the complexities of race and Methodism in Fiji, DOI: http://doi.org/10.22459/MD.12.2015).
43 'Liquor laws and mixed races', 16.
44 F40/1, pt. 1, 8 January 1932, 'Deputation from Fiji Social Service Alliance to Governor', 24 January 1932.
45 F40/1/pt. 1, 'Recommendations to the select committee appointed to consider the amendment of the Liquor Ordinance from the Fiji Social Services Alliance', 1932.
46 S. Durutalo, The Paramountcy of Fijian Interest and the Politicization of Ethnicity (Suva: USP Sociological Society, 1986).
47 F40/1, pt. 1, 24 January 1932.
48 Cited in Thornley, *Exodus of the I Taukei*, 483.
49 Ibid.
50 'Fiji', *New Zealand Herald*, 11 September 1883, p. 6.
51 D. Scarr, *Viceroy of the Pacific: The Majesty of Colour: A Life of Sir John Bates Thurston* (Canberra: Australian National University Development Studies Centre, 1980), 44, 202–3.
52 MP 8133/09, Beauclerc to Governor, 21 April 1911.
53 'The future of Fiji', *New Zealand Herald*, 7 February 1907, p. 7, https://paperspast.natlib.govt.nz/newspapers/NZH19070207.2.97 (accessed 5 September 2021). See B.V. Lal, *Broken Waves: A History of the Fiji Islands in the Twentieth Century* (Honolulu: University of Hawai'i Press, 1992), 18.
54 See V. Lukere, 'Mothers of the Taukei: Fijian women and "the decrease of the race"' (PhD dissertation, Australian National University, 1997), https://openresearch-repository.anu.edu.au/handle/1885/10978 (accessed 5 February 2022).
55 A. Stuart, 2006. 'Contradictions and complexities in an indigenous medical service', *Journal of Pacific History*, 41, no.2 (2006), 125–43.
56 Cited in ibid., 139.
57 Ibid.
58 'A campaign commenced'.
59 Fiji Government, *Commission to Inquire into the Cost of Living*, Legislative Council Paper, CP 46/20 (Suva: Government Printer, 1928). Compare those Fijian and Indian wages with those of other workers within the Colonial Sugar Refinery Company; white artisans

earned 12–15 shillings a day; clerks earned £12–25 a month, while a manager received £300–400, plus housing, per year. W.A. Chapple, *Fiji: Its Problems and Resources* (Auckland: Whitcombe & Tombs, 1921), 161.

60 F40/5, 'Memorandum on sly-grog traffic' by AIG, 28 September 1936.

61 'Liquor drives Fijians mad', *Pacific Islands Monthly* (*PIM*), 1 November 1957, p. 22.

62 Ibid.

63 Pennefather, Advisor on Native Affairs, in CSO F40/10/1. Cited in Lal, *Broken Waves*, 114.

64 F40/5, 'Police extract from Labasa monthly report for November 1940', 27 December 1940. Note: a level of about 120 proof is considered the maximum.

65 District Commissioner, Central, 1 July 1962 to CS, F60/6–2.

66 It is not clear what the meaning of 'spey' is here. The Spey is a river in Scotland, and an area famous for the production of whisky. Probably 'coconut spey' refers to fermented toddy, which quickly attracts wild yeast, needed to make alcoholic drink. Fermented toddy was made from juice collected from the coconut flower and the cut stalk was secured to a bottle that the liquid flowed into. The stem of the coconut flower is very sweet and also adds sugar. Judy Bennett, personal communication, 15 January 2020; F40/5, 'Memorandum on sly-grog traffic'.

67 F40/5, CF 23/3, pt. 6, confidential report of District Officer, Northern Taveuni, March 1948.

68 F40/5, 'Memorandum on sly-grog traffic'.

69 Frank Coffee, *Forty Years on the Pacific* (New York and Sydney, Australia: Oceanic Publishing Company, 1920), referring to the Line Islands in Kiribati, https://en.wikisource.org/wiki/Forty_Years_On_The_Pacific/Kava_and_Toddy (accessed 5 February 2022). Fresh toddy is a highly nutritious drink but if left to ferment can become alcoholic.

70 MP 407/38, 'Quarterly report on Indian affairs', letter to CS, 6 July 1938.

71 MP 4142/24, 'Memorandum from District Inspector Eastern to Inspector General of Constabulary', 29 October 1924.

72 'Liquor drives Fijians mad'.

73 Cited in Stuart, 'Contradictions and complexities', 138.

74 MP 4809/26, 'Deputation to wait upon His Excellency in regard to the administration of the Liquor Ordinance'.

75 'Letter to the editor', *FT*, 16 June 1962.

76 'Liquor drives Fijians mad', 22.
77 'How Fijians hunt and kill in Malayan jungles: R.W. Robson in Singapore June 2', *PIM*, 1 July 1955, 72–3.
78 'Insanity and prohibition', *Samoanische Zeitung*, 6 February 1915. The original author, Dr E.H. Williams, found that insanity was worse in states with prohibition.
79 G. Davis, *'The Cruel Madness of Love': Sex, Syphilis and Psychiatry in Scotland, 1880–1930* (Amsterdam: Rodopi, 2008), 108–9, discusses alcoholic insanity. See also 'Types of alcoholic insanity', *The Lancet*, 28 January 1905, p. 244.
80 See J. Leckie, 'Modernity and the management of madness in colonial Fiji', *Paideuma*, 50 (2004), 551–74; J. Leckie, *Colonizing Madness: Asylum and Community in Fiji* (Honolulu: University of Hawai'i Press, 2020).
81 G.E Berrios, *The History of Mental Symptoms: Descriptive Psychopathology since the Nineteenth Century* (Cambridge: Cambridge University Press, 1996), 428–9.
82 CP 36/36.
83 See, for example, C. Coleborne, *Insanity, Identity and Empire: Immigrants and Institutional Confinement in Australia and New Zealand, 1873–1910* (Manchester: Manchester University Press, 2015), 120.
84 Davis, *'The Cruel Madness of Love'*. See also E.J Engstrom and I. Crozier, 'Race, alcohol and general paralysis: Emil Kraepelin's comparative psychiatry and his trips to Java (1904) and North America (1925)', *History of Psychiatry*, 29, no. 3, 263–81.
85 J. Leckie, 'Missing or misdiagnosed? General paralysis of the insane, yaws, and syphilis in Fiji, 1884–1940', *Journal of Pacific History* (2020), 37–57.
86 Cited in Scarr, *Viceroy of the Pacific*, 203.
87 My research at St Giles Psychiatric Hospital in Suva, Fiji, examined admission certificates between 1884 and 1964 and the relevant Mental Hospital Register. Tables generated from this and other data are indicative of general patterns and, because of gaps and some inconsistencies in the data, do not represent precise statistical validity. See Leckie, *Colonizing Madness*.
88 Patient Number (PN) 1478. A PN refers to the number of the admission certificate to St Giles. Pseudonyms are used unless referring to individuals in the public domain.
89 PN 1953.
90 PN 1189, first admitted in 1936, but it was only on his second

admission in 1941 (PN 1300) that a toxic reaction to excessive alcohol consumption was recorded.

91 PN 1248; PN 1787; PN 2136.

92 PN 45.

93 PN 1248.

94 PN 1537. See also e.g. O. Scott, *Deep beyond the Reef: A True Story of Madness and Murder in the South Pacific* (Auckland: Penguin, 2004) concerning his family in Fiji.

95 See C. Ralston, *Grass Huts and Warehouses: A Study of Five Pacific Beach Communities of the Nineteenth Century* (Honolulu: University of Hawai'i Press, 1978); Scarr, *Viceroy of the Pacific*, 188–9.

96 J. Young, 'Evanescent ascendancy: the planter community in Fiji', in Davison and Scarr (eds), *Pacific Islands Portraits*, 147–75; Scarr, *Viceroy of the Pacific*, 188.

97 'A campaign commenced'.

98 For more discussion of admission rates see Leckie, *Colonizing Madness*. Population statistics from Fiji Bureau of Statistics, Key Statistics, June 2012, '1.2A census population of Fiji by ethnicity', https://www.google.com/url?sa=t&rct=j&q=&esrc=s&source=web&cd=1&ved=2ahUKEwjFk_uC_p3mAhX663MBHcDEAcYQFjAAegQIBRAC&url=http%3A%2F%2Fcatalog.ihsn.org%2Findex.php%2Fcatalog%2F3602%2Fdownload%2F50136&usg=AOvVaw3MhJds4hzD1H2J7GAadptS (accessed 5 December 2019).

99 PN 329.

100 PN 1062; PN 1065; PN 1883; PN 1943; PN 2159; PN 2650.

101 PN 192.

102 See Frances Steele, *Oceania under Steam: Sea Transport and the Cultures of Colonialism, c. 1870–1914* (Manchester: Manchester University Press, 2011), 84–8.

103 PN 344.

104 'Inhumanity in Fiji', *Feilding Star*, 11 April 1907, p. 2.

105 PN 7.

106 Information from case books, 2 December 1903 to 1953, St Giles Hospital, Suva. These are not detailed individual cases.

107 MP 1266/16.

108 MP 2733/18, April 1918.

109 Various letters on F40/12. Prasad is a pseudonym.

110 F40/12, 'Liquor permits – issue of on medical grounds', District Medical Officer, Lautoka to District Commissioner, Lautoka, 3 August 1935.

111 F40/12, memo from District Medical Officer, Nadroga to Chief Medical Officer, 28 September 1934.

112 F40/12, memo to District Officer, Taveuni, 8 August 1942.
113 F40/12, Circular MD 5/3, from Acting Chief Medical Officer to District Medical Officers, 17 September 1936.
114 'Fiji, too, has its liquor troubles', *PIM*, 1 July 1954, p. 164.
115 Ibid.
116 B.V. Lal, *Vision for Change: A. D. Patel and the Politics of Fiji* (Canberra: National Centre for Development Studies, Australian National University, 1997), 108–9; Patel to Governor, Fiji, 25 February 1949, cited in CP 16/49, 'Report of the Select Committee on the Liquor Bill', 1947.
117 For example, H. Fischer-Tiné and J. Tschurenev (eds), *A History of Alcohol and Drugs in Modern South Asia: Intoxicating Affairs* (London: Routledge, 2014), especially R.E. Colvard, '"Drunkards beware!": Prohibition and nationalist politics in the 1930s', 173–200.
118 See Durutalo, *The Paramountcy of Fijian Interest.*
119 See 'Fiji's racial-liquor problem', *PIM*, 1 June 1954, p. 115.
120 CP 16/49.
121 F60/6–2, 'Liquor Ordinance'.
122 *FT*, 9 June 1962. Fullerton's claims of widespread support were disputed by some district officers. For example, the district officer of Ba/Tavua wrote to the CS on 26 June 1962 that 'the claims of the Rev. Fullerton to report Fijian opinion are justified only in that the majority of Fiji are Methodists and that he speaks for the Methodist Church to which most Fijians are loyal.' F 40/6–2, 'Liquor Committee's report, 1962'.
123 *FT*, 23 June 1962.
124 See for example *FT*, 26 May 1962, 18 June 1962; F 40/6–2.
125 B.V. Lal, 'The passage out', in K.R. Howe, R.C. Kiste and B.V. Lal (eds), *Tides of History: The Pacific Islands in the Twentieth Century* (Honolulu: University of Hawai'i Press), p. 445.
126 Lal, *Broken Waves*, 164.

5

'In the hot and trying climate of Nigeria the European has a much stronger temptation to indulge in alcohol than the native': drunkenness in Nigeria, *c.* 1880–1940

Simon Heap

Alcohol consumption among indigenous people in pre-colonial and colonial Nigeria was a multifaceted affair, mixing concerns on personal, communal and ritual levels throughout the life cycle of the individual within wider contexts: naming ceremonies, entertaining guests at weddings, chieftaincy instalments, funeral obsequies and pouring libations to the ancestors. There existed a variety of alcohol drinks, such as palm wine and fermented grain beers, but pre-colonial Nigerians did not distil spirits. It was not until the Atlantic slave trade, which encouraged the purchase of slaves with rum and whisky, that a taste for European-style imported liquor was fostered. The more potent imported alcohol symbolised a stronger spiritual strength and became a socially prestigious commodity. There were also economic uses for liquor: as a transitional currency and powerful catalyst for trade. When the slave trade ended, the liquor trade continued, reaching large volumes in the second half of the nineteenth century.[1]

While British colonial officials and traders tended to favour European-style alcohol, indigenous communities consumed traditional brews and palm wines, as well as imported liquors. This chapter first discusses the impact of European alcohol imports on Nigerian communities, in particular in the southern regions, focusing on colonial debates on the merits of the wider availability of strong alcohol and its impact on African and European races.

It then maps the controversial assertion by the Church Missionary Society (CMS) Bishop of Western Equatorial Africa that three-quarters of Europeans in the country died as a result of drinking imported spirits. This detailed case study reveals how the arguments for and against alcohol consumption were heightened, leading a few years later to an inquiry into the impact of the liquor trade on Nigeria which revealed more evidence on both sides of the debate. The chapter then examines the role of alcohol in the lifestyles of expatriates in the country, illustrated by cases of drunkenness, disorderly behaviour and death.

'A Rum and Gin Civilisation'

The demand for imported alcohol in Nigeria grew in tandem with the growth and expansion of British control over the territory from the 1860s onwards. While Northern Nigeria became an imported alcohol prohibition zone, liquor was the most significant import in terms of volume and value in the British colonies of Lagos, Oil Rivers Protectorate, Niger Coast Protectorate and Southern Nigeria, all of which were eventually integrated into the Southern Provinces of Nigeria in 1914. By that time, Nigeria imported over four million gallons annually of alcoholic beverages, chiefly German *Schnapps* and Dutch gin.[2]

Before colonial intervention in the 1860s, the southern areas of what became Nigeria had various types of palm wine, while the north's cereals provided the basic ingredient for various food-like brews fermented without yeast. Imported drinks did not displace local beverages; rather, they coexisted, complemented and competed with each other. Yet in the view of some colonial commentators, there was too much consumer choice. As the author of an article in the *Lagos Standard* noted in 1909, 'The African has his palm wine and corn beer. To him spirituous liquor is a superfluous and dangerous luxury. He does not want it, he needs it no more than a cat needs two tails.'[3] But there was no going back to older drinking habits as imported liquor spread inland through the new transport networks to an ever-growing number of Nigerians.

Of course, gin and rum had stronger intoxicating effects than palm wine or grain beer, a fact that critics of the liquor trade kept pointing out to their opponents. Describing concerns over rising palm wine consumption as 'very much like ignoring the camel and trembling at the gnat', critics of the liquor trade argued that the taste for alcohol was already in place in Nigeria and that the much more potent strength of imported spirits could wreak widespread drunkenness and destruction on the population in the near future.[4] Such concerns were mirrored in Fiji, as is highlighted in Jacqueline Leckie's chapter in this volume (see Chapter 4).

The import of strong liquor provoked fierce debate and concerns about whether the consumption of alcohol advanced development or mired it. The liquor trade was caught between two opposing colonial perspectives on economic development: on the one hand, the civilise-through-trade concept seeking to modernise Africans by enticing the population into the cash economy, and, on the other hand, the paternalist principle that Western civilisation had a duty to protect Africans from bad external economic and moral influences. Humanitarian concerns and economic interests became entangled. Critics of the liquor trade used temperance narratives to further their cause: drinking alcohol was bad, abstinence was good. Arguing that the imposition of 'a Rum and Gin Civilisation' would be 'a hydra that devours the natives' – halting useful commerce and hindering economic development – they agitated for prohibition and a complete restructuring of the colonial economy along alcohol-free lines.[5]

In the 1930s, a new practice swept through Nigeria: the distillation of illicit gin or *ogogoro*, a drink similar in strength to imported spirits.[6] *Ogogoro* made serious headway against the long-standing imported liquor trade, substituting non-Nigerian drinks with locally made ones. The effect of an unlimited supply of crude, over-proof alcohol on the population raised grave health concerns. As one inhabitant of Aba, Soku Madu, put it in 1932: the consumption of '8,000 gallons per day of this Dreadfull [sic] liquor … is very injurious and dangerous to the human health'.[7] Such anxieties provided a basis on which the colonial government could initially attack illicit gin. Colonial pronouncements were clear. People attending the Sabagreia court in the Niger Delta in February 1932 were told:

'this crude liquor has very bad effects making people go blind, become paralysed and incapable of producing children'.[8] An official circular distributed at Agbor in September 1932 listed illicit gin's noxious side-effects in the following shock phrases: 'it is a poison'; 'it causes a wild state of drunkenness leading to death or insanity'; and 'it can lead to loss of use of legs, wasting away, total blindness and impotence'.[9] But as the years passed and the anticipated public health disasters did not materialise, colonial officers re-examined their warnings and concluded in 1947 that illicit gin had no more long-term health risks than licit liquor.[10]

Debate over the physical conditions that drinking spirits could induce became a key battleground in the liquor trade debate in Nigeria. From the late nineteenth century onwards the concept of over-indulgence in alcohol as a disease emerged, soon overshadowing parallel works by anthropologists that underscored the socio-cultural dimensions of alcohol use and abuse. As the historian Akyeampong has noted in relation to Ghana and Western countries, alcohol abuse became medicalised, and treatment by medical professionals advocated as the only remedy.[11] However, the disease concept failed to resonate with the social and cultural realities of alcohol consumption among Nigerians.

Many members of the medical fraternity gave evidence to the 1909 Inquiry into the Liquor Trade Inquiry in Southern Nigeria, set up by the British government to lay to rest questions over the liquor trade once and for all. Apart from Dr John Randle, a Sierra Leonean in private practice in Lagos, all doctors giving evidence were British colonial officers. The large and influential CMS had two medical missionaries, Dr John Miller in the north and Dr Henry Drewitt near Onitsha in the south, but neither of them appeared before the committee, leaving it to their bishop, Herbert Tugwell, to be their sole witness.[12]

Dr Henry Strachan, Southern Nigeria's Principal Medical Officer, was sure that habitual drinkers suffered more health complaints than those who occasionally indulged in a 'burst' or single session of excessive drinking.[13] With seven years' experience of Nigeria, Dr Thomas Adam disagreed. He recalled a post mortem carried out by a colleague in the south-eastern town of Calabar on a soldier who he knew to have been particularly abstemious in his drinking.

Yet the examination revealed death by acute alcoholic poisoning, the result of drinking half a bottle of gin straight off.[14]

Drinking alcohol formed part of a wider debate. Back in the nineteenth and early twentieth centuries, scientists and physicians theorised on the concept of acclimatisation as an important issue in imperial settings.[15] What was the ability of European colonialists to survive and prosper in non-European environments? And how was alcohol, among other things, part of the intrinsic cultural needs of Europeans far from home?

Medical opinion did agree on one issue: moderation in drinking habits was the healthy watchword, and abstention by those able to do without alcohol was even better.[16] Against the convivial background of social drinking in rural areas, the solitary drinker presented an unusual phenomenon among Nigerians and was viewed with disquiet by all. In urban areas, social relations formed over drink, as opportunities for drinking presented themselves in the bars and clubs of Nigeria's burgeoning towns and cities.

For the critics of the liquor trade, the prospect of wholesale physical degeneration of the entire African race loomed. In 1895 a Nigerian listed in the *Lagos Weekly Record* newspaper the unhealthy state of those countrymen who drank too much alcohol:

> It has been noticed, and proved as unalterable fact, that amongst the tribes that drink gin very excessively the following diseases are prevalent, Indigestion, Stricture, Diabetes, Nervous disorders, Bright's disease of the Kidneys resulting in apoplexy, convulsions or dropsy.[17]

The majority view among medical doctors at the 1909 Liquor Trade Inquiry was that there were no inherent differences in the physiological effects of alcohol on the two races. However, given the contemporary belief that the average Nigerian was probably physically stronger than the average European, some observers concluded that indigenous people could take more alcohol without ill effects. For example, on the basis of his long experience in Yorubaland, Principal Medical Officer Henry Strachan argued that Nigerians were less susceptible than Europeans to the action of alcohol.[18] That said, Strachan was struck by 'the paucity of evidence of chronic alcoholic poisoning'.[19] Hesketh Bell, a leading colonial official, claimed that 'a coloured man, without "turning a hair", can take a "shot" of rum or gin which would put a European into an almost helpless condition'.[20] Indeed, one missionary of the Holy Ghost Society compared the ability of Nigerians to take more alcohol to their ability to eat strongly spiced foods, which outsiders found too peppery for their constitution.[21]

There were also opposing views. Dr Oguntola Sapara, who ran the Ereko Dispensary in Lagos, with over 7,538 and 8,319 outpatients in 1907 and 1908 respectively, stated that, while health problems related to alcohol were on the increase, the dispensary still had only about ten cases on its record books of stomach inflammation due to various initial causes but aggravated by alcohol.[22] Sapara believed that his countrymen were more prone than Europeans to the effects of strong spirits.[23]

Death from excessive alcohol consumption was expected by some European officials even among the seemingly strong and healthy. Captain Frederick Lugard met the chief of Shaki in Northern Yorubaland in 1897 and found him 'of magnificent physique and in the prime of life'.[24] But this was just his outward appearance; inside, his kidneys and other vital organs were 'a complete wreck from Lagos drink, and [he was] doomed to a premature death'.[25] According to Lugard, only timely medical attention by his travelling physician, Dr Guy Mottram, who diagnosed the problem, turned the chief into a more sober, healthy patient. However, further south in the city of Ibadan, another leading chief was reported to have succumbed to the effects of excessive drinking and died at a relatively early age in February 1899.[26] In a further case, a Wesleyan minister in Abeokuta saw two 'heathen townsmen' waste away from excessive drinking: one apparently exposed himself after a heavy drinking bout and caught pneumonia; the other lost his appetite and 'was practically kept alive for weeks on nothing but gin, but eventually he died'.[27]

Evidence of drink-related medical conditions is scarce and mostly anecdotal. In fact, some reports from medical institutions did not list any diseases linked with alcohol consumption, as was the case for the Warri hospital.[28] Similarly, the Abeokuta Dispensary, which treated about 200 patients a month, reported no cases of alcohol over consumption or conditions caused by heavy drinking in the ten months up to May 1909. It was merely noted that people came to see the resident physician, Dr Rupert Welply, with concerns about 'guinea worm, ulcers, abscesses, and fevers'.[29] In relation to the Lagos hospital it was noted that there were few admissions for 'acute alcoholic poisoning and delirium tremens' between 1899 and 1905, and that all ten of them were discharged and no deaths recorded.[30] Two of the cases admitted at Lagos in 1905 were Europeans. Overall, the number of patients diagnosed with alcohol-related conditions was negligible. In 1903 the records for all government hospitals in Southern Nigeria revealed only one case related to alcohol in a Nigerian.[31] Between 1906 and 1911, recorded numbers were low, as is evident in Table 5.1.

Are the low numbers evidence of actual trends, official neglect or the difficulty of identifying alcoholics within society? Could there have been some reluctance to identify alcohol consumption as a

Table 5.1 Cases of 'acute alcoholic poisoning and delirium tremens' treated in hospital, Western, Central and Eastern Provinces, Southern Nigeria, 1906–1911

Hospital	1906	1907	1908	1909	1910	1911
Broad Street, Lagos	0	1	2	4	1	0
Massey Street, Lagos	0	5	0	0	0	0
Ebute Metta, Lagos	0	0	1	1	0	0
Ibadan	0	0	0	1	1	0
Ondo	0	2	0	0	0	0
Western Province total	*0*	*8*	*3*	*6*	*2*	*0*
Warri	2	1	0	9	0	0
Forcados	0	0	3	0	0	0
Sapele	0	0	0	2	0	1
Benin City	0	0	0	0	0	1
Central Province total	*2*	*1*	*3*	*11*	*0*	*2*
Calabar	2	0	4	5	3	1
Bende	0	1	0	0	0	1
Bonny	0	0	0	1	0	1
Brass	0	0	0	0	1	1
Obudu	0	0	0	0	0	1
Eastern Province total	*2*	*1*	*4*	*6*	*4*	*5*
Grand total	*4*	*10*	*10*	*23*	*6*	*7*

Source: NAI, Southern Nigeria Annual Report on the Medical Department, 1906–11.

health problem, or was it merely doctors' unfamiliarity with the diagnoses of 'acute alcoholic poisoning and delirium tremens', or rather a belief in the sobriety of both Nigerians and Europeans that could account for the low figures? After all, this was at a time when the import of European liquor had increased to over three million gallons annually, and a large but unknown quantity of indigenous brews was reported to have been consumed. The collection and recording of official figures on alcoholic-related conditions within Nigerian and expatriate communities and among hospital patients might need to be questioned for their accuracy and comprehensiveness. As they stand, they paint a rather sober picture.

Expatriate officials were granted six months' leave after every twelve months' duty in the colonial service. While there is not much official evidence on the treatment of alcohol-related conditions, anecdotal accounts suggest that for Europeans the procedures of choice were hospitalisation and 'drying out', with severe cases simply invalided out of the colony and sent home.[32] For the indigenous population, health implied wellbeing of mind, body and spirit, and this was expressed in a person's ability to perform their social roles and responsibilities. The misuse of alcohol was a spiritual ailment, and treatment had to directly address the spiritual dimension.[33] Given these notions, it was in psychiatry that African and European understandings and treatments potentially overlapped. Psychiatric practice in colonial Nigeria confirmed that what came later to be known as 'alcoholism' was a spiritual illness. As Sadowsky has shown, Nigerians viewed mental disorders as spiritual ailments, and the treatment of alcoholics in mental asylums from 1906 onwards reinforced the association of alcohol-related conditions with spiritual causes.[34] Despite the lack of recorded evidence on the incidence and epidemiology of alcohol-related problems, one man was sure alcohol abuse was rife among Europeans.

Bishop Herbert Tugwell and the number of European deaths due to alcohol

In a letter to *The Times* newspaper of 27 March 1899, Bishop Tugwell, the chief protagonist in the anti-liquor trade argument, made a bold, eye-opening intervention in the debate on Europeans' copious alcohol consumption in West Africa:

> Of the deaths which occur amongst Europeans on the [west] coast probably 75 per cent are to be attributed to habits of drinking at all hours of the day and drunkenness, these habits being directly fostered and encouraged by the cheap rate at which spirits can be purchased.[35]

The Times had a considerable circulation in Lagos and according to colonial official Captain George Denton, Tugwell's statement provoked 'a great deal of ill-feeling in Lagos ... more harm in Lagos than I can describe'.[36] After all, despite imported liquor's significant role in the local economy as a profitable business for the wholesale selling of it to local retailers and as a desired barter item for the lucrative trading in local commodities such as cocoa and palm oil, European merchants were being directly attacked. At a special meeting under the auspices of the Lagos Chamber of Commerce, local traders voiced their upset at what they saw as yet another of the bishop's 'jumped at' conclusions. They decided to teach Tugwell a lesson.[37] Just before he boarded a ship heading back to London for the centenary celebrations of the CMS, the police, armed with a criminal summons for libel, arrested Tugwell. Soon after, the Acting Police Magistrate of Lagos heard the case of John Peacock, Secretary of the Lagos Chamber of Commerce, versus the Right Reverend Herbert Tugwell, CMS Bishop of Western Equatorial Africa. Sir William Geary appeared for the plaintiff, while the defendant chose to speak for himself.[38]

The prosecution's case rested on an analysis of the available data relating to European fatalities in the colony. According to the medical certificates for Europeans dying in Lagos, there was no basis for the claim that every three out of four deaths were alcohol-related. Between 1880 and 1892, there were 113 European fatalities: 89 residents and 24 visitors.[39] Of the former group, two were alcohol-related deaths: in 1886, the Engineer of Government Vessels, H. Crane, died aged thirty of what was recorded as 'acute alcoholism', while in the following year a foreman of works, James Thomas Murphy, died aged thirty-seven of 'excessive intemperance'.[40] Incidentally, in the year after the Tugwell debacle, the Registrar-General of Lagos recorded another European death from alcohol abuse: that of Thomas Pearce, aged forty-five, a storekeeper with the Lagos Government Railway, who died on 22 February 1900.[41]

Between 1892 and 1898, 106 European men and 17 European women died in Lagos. Only two deaths were related to drink: in 1892 one person died of 'delirium tremens', and two years later another of 'acute alcoholic poisoning'.[42] During the first five months of 1899, eight European residents of Lagos died, two of whom are known by name and drinking habits: Senior Survey Officer Corporal W. H. Pratt, a total abstainer who died of fever aged thirty-eight on 23 March, and the thirty-year-old District Commissioner G.H. Gill, a moderate drinker who died of dysentery two days later.[43]

The figures in Table 5.2 show that of 17 deaths recorded for 1893, 9 were due to 'climatic diseases' and one was a case of 'accidental drowning'. There is nothing in that year's statistics to substantiate Bishop Tugwell's statement. In 1894 19 of the 23 deaths were due to 'climatic causes', while 'alcohol poisoning' entered the list, but only in a single case. In that year, seven missionaries lost their lives; therefore, if Tugwell's claim was true, it would imply that at least two of the missionaries died from drink, as pointed out by the *Lagos Weekly Record*:

> It would leave room for the startling insinuation that Bishop TUGWELL's predecessor Bishop HILL died of drunkenness. This insinuation ... is made more conspicuous in the returns for 1895. Of the total of 16 deaths in that year, if we deduct the two from drowning and one unknown, and one infant, we have according to Bishop TUGWELL, 12 deaths due to drunkenness of whom five were missionaries.[44]

The newspaper condemned the way the bishop had 'ruthlessly blasted the reputation of the whole European population on the West coast'.[45] Apart from commercial considerations and some individuals taking umbrage, the prestige of the colonial rulers may have been seen to be at stake, too, as when, some forty years later, the colonial film censors banned Africans from seeing on the big screen 'drunken white men and women' and 'white people drinking cocktails'.[46] However, like other newspapers, the *Lagos Weekly*

Table 5.2 European deaths, Lagos, 1893–1903

Cause of death	1893	1894	1895	1896	1897	1898	1899	1900	1901	1902	1903
Fever	3	5	7	8	5	0	6	11	0	0	0
Malarial fever	0	0	0	0	0	2	4	0	6	4	6
Blackwater fever	1	1	0	0	2	0	1	6	0	0	0
Haemoglobinuric fever	4	0	0	0	0	0	2	0	4	5	2
Other fevers	1	8	0	2	1	0	0	0	0	0	0
Heart diseases	2	2	1	4	3	0	1	0	0	1	0
Hyperpyrexia	0	0	0	6	3	3	1	0	0	0	0
Exhaustion	0	0	1	3	1	1	0	0	0	0	0
Accidents	1	0	0	3	0	0	0	0	1	1	0
Dysentery	0	0	1	0	1	0	1	1	1	1	1
Hepatitis	0	1	1	0	0	0	0	0	0	0	0
Gastroenteritis	0	0	0	1	1	0	0	0	0	1	0
Phthisis/pneumonia	1	1	0	0	1	0	0	0	0	0	0
Syncope	0	0	0	0	1	1	0	0	1	0	0
Brain haemorrhage	0	0	0	0	1	0	1	0	1	0	0
Alcohol poisoning	0	1	0	0	0	0	0	1	0	1	0
Abscess of the liver	0	0	0	0	0	0	0	0	0	1	0
Others	4	3	2	1	3	0	1	0	1	1	2
Total deaths	*17*	*23*	*16*	*28*	*23*	*8*	*18*	*21*	*15*	*17*	*11*

Sources: NA, CO 147/94, Lagos General Abstract of Registration, 1893, p. 4; 'The libel action against Bishop Tugwell', *Lagos Weekly Record*, 24 June 1899, p. 2; *Lagos Registrar-General Annual Report* (Lagos: Government Printer, 1899), 105; NAI, CSO 1/1/35, *Lagos Registrar-General Annual Report* (Lagos: Government Printer, 1900), 89; *Annual Report of the Principal Registrar of Vital Statistics* (Lagos: Government Printer, 1901), 34; *Lagos Medical Annual Report* (Lagos: Government Printer, 1901), 43; *Lagos Medical Annual Report* (Lagos: Government Printer, 1902), 27–8; *Lagos Medical Annual Report* (Lagos: Government Printer, 1903), 74–5.

Record soon came to treat the libel action as trivial and absurd, as Tugwell had not brought any particular individual into disrepute.[47] Indeed, events quickly turned Tugwell into a martyr to the cause of temperance and prohibition. Offers of help, both moral and financial as well as legal, came Tugwell's way. A Defence Fund was initiated. Back in London, Dr Charles Battersby, the Secretary of the Native Races and Liquor Traffic United Committee (NRLTUC), a CMS-led pressure group seeking alcohol prohibition in Africa and throughout the world, stepped in to defend Tugwell:

> It is impossible to deny that the drinking habits of the Europeans who work on the West African coast constitute a gigantic evil ... with the recklessness with which men indulge in decoctions of gin and bitters, commonly known as cocktails. They swallow them before meals to create appetite; they drink them whenever they meet together; and not to offer a guest a cocktail is considered the grossest form of hospitality. The result is that the habit grows upon them till it utterly enslaves them.[48]

Yet Tugwell's editorial in his own CMS magazine, *Niger and Yoruba Notes*, tried to downplay the whole affair, and other observers quibbled about the figures calculated on both sides of the argument:

> The Bishop will be writted for slander directly ... surely the slandered are those who are dead, which makes their action even more difficult; or rather '75 per cent of dead Europeans versus Bishop of Western Equatorial Africa'. Even '75 per cent of Europeans likely to die someday', would not look much better.[49]

In fact, another editorial by Tugwell in July 1899 stated that his opening salvo's initial words could only be taken to refer to 7.5 per cent, not 75 per cent, of the European community.[50] Later that year, Tugwell switched tack, believing that the liquor trade aggravated still further Lagos's already high death rate.[51] In fact, even with a figure ten times less than first stated, Tugwell's calculations totalled a higher number than the official records (as collated in Table 5.3). During the 1890s, the death rate peaked at 66.3 per thousand Lagosians, or 6.63 per cent. In the next decade, the rate stabilised at the mid- to low 40s, a rate comparable to that of the early 1890s. While it is acknowledged that such rates depended on the accurate

Table 5.3 Death rate among Lagos population of Europeans and Nigerians, 1893–1908

Year	Death rate per 1,000	Year	Death rate per 1,000
1893	41.0	1901	43.7
1894	45.0	1902	42.4
1895	53.0	1903	43.7
1896	52.0	1904	45.6
1897	59.0	1905	48.2
1898	58.0	1906	41.9
1899	66.3	1907	42.0
1900	60.0	1908	44.7

Sources: NRLTUC, *Native Races and the Drink Question* (London: NRLTUC, 1903), 2, 6–7; Dr Robert Laurie in *Report of the Committee of Inquiry into the Liquor Trade in Southern Nigeria*, Part II: *Minutes of Evidence*, Cd 4907 (1909), Questions 15960–80, pp. 394–5.

counting of all deaths and the total number of people in Lagos, the differences could be best explained by improvements in public sanitation, not diminishing consumption of alcohol.[52]

Wider questions about the freedom of speech and the seeming callous persecution of an individual's idiosyncratic views caused the Lagos government deep unease and embarrassment. It did not want to have a martyr to liquor prohibition on its hands.[53] Interest in the case both in Nigeria and abroad became intense. The colonialists decided that the best course of action was to prevent the case from reaching the Lagos court: a *nolle prosequi* (a formal notice of abandonment by a plaintiff or prosecutor of all or part of a suit) was entered by the Queen's Advocate to quash the libel action against Bishop Tugwell.[54] Such a move probably resulted from the fresh arrival in Lagos of Chief Justice Sir T.C. Rayner, who 'put an end to this vexatious action, and thus to uphold the honour and prestige of our British Courts'.[55] However, freed from the *sub judice* of the court case, the *Lagos Weekly Record* went on the attack over Tugwell's initial pronouncement:

> If we attempt a critical examination of the statement ... we find ourselves confronted with one of two things – either a sober and serious statement affecting alike the missionary, the official and the trader, or

> a wild, inconsiderate and meaningless exaggeration of a sensational-monger. The communication ... if examined by this standard of accuracy and honesty falls lamentably below the mark ... intended more for the purpose of creating sensation than an honest and accurate exposure of an existing evil.[56]

Alcohol and the enervating effects of the Nigerian climate

There may have been some truth in Tugwell's claim, however, as expatriate deaths could well have been accelerated by over-indulgence in alcohol. The Acting Governor of Lagos, George Denton, suggested:

> Some ten per cent of the cases which come under care of certain medical men I have consulted believe great injury has been done to the constitution by an excessive use of stimulants. From this it must not be supposed that drunkenness is common in the place, as this is not so, but only that many of the young men are apt to be imprudent in a climate which from its enervating effects decidedly begets longing for support.[57]

For Europeans, the Nigerian climate was debilitating and, coupled with frequent bouts of ill-health, made their residence particularly wearing on both their mental and physical condition. The Liquor Trade Inquiry contended:

> It is obvious that in the hot and trying climate of Nigeria the European has a much stronger temptation to indulge in alcohol than the native, who is inured to the climate of his own country, and the European, as a rule, has more means and opportunity of procuring spirits.[58]

Added to these factors was a frugal social life, especially for colonial district officers in rural areas, with loneliness and depression painfully present.[59] Recourse to alcohol as a prophylactic to stave off the possibilities of ill-health, or as a tonic to lighten one's spirits, proved to be a favourite option for Europeans living and working in Nigeria.[60] Alcohol was considered a necessity of life in the tropics. In 1918 the Civil Service Association sought a licence to import 200 cases of whisky because the local Nigerian retail rate was fifty shillings a case more than the price of getting it directly from the Scottish manufacturer. As Governor-General Lugard pointed out, 'These exorbitant rates are not checked by the Food Controller as whisky is not a food item, but it is a necessary article in moderate quantities in this climate.'[61] Only missionaries, with their generally abstemious practices, did not follow the pattern of over-indulgence in alcohol.[62] Blaming the climate for Europeans' excessive drinking was questioned, with some pointing out that the climate was not unhealthy if you drank moderately. One local newspaper, the *Western Echo*, argued: 'The climate may be enervating but it is not so deleterious as some wish to make out if Europeans will but use the brandy bottle judiciously.'[63]

In medical emergencies, the medicine of choice tended to be the same for everyone. Alcohol was almost routinely administered in cases of debility. In one case, Dr John Tichburne gave six to eight ounces of spirits to patients suffering from typhoid.[64] Finding himself in the bush with a bad attack of malaria and without medicine, Dr Ernest Tipper resorted to imported gin to help him through his fever.[65] In 1929 J. Olu Johnson, transferring to Lokoja to work for John Holt and Company, got his doctor to issue a prescription to preserve his health en route, which included small doses of brandy.[66]

From 1892 the heads of each department in the colonial service had to ask staff four questions regarding their behaviour, one of which was, 'Has he been temperate in his habits?'[67] The view among prominent officials seems to have been that moderate or temperate habits were conducive to the health status of Europeans. The soon-to-be Governor of Lagos Sir William MacGregor, for example, wrote from his previous position in British New Guinea that 'in my experience people that are total abstainers in the Colony enjoy better health, and have a lower mortality than those that are not total abstainers'.[68] His French counterpart in Madagascar agreed, cautioning at the International Temperance Congress in Paris against imbibing too much alcohol, and, on one tour, he himself took only water – 'I never had a brighter idea in the whole of my existence.'[69] Indeed, an official government guidebook for British colonial officers who were to serve in West Africa had this advice (rendered in bold type): 'Heavy drinkers should not go to West

Africa, moderate drinkers should be very moderate there, and total abstainers should remain so.'[70] However, as the Under-Secretary of State for the Colonies had noted in 1903 in his correspondence with the High Commissioner of Northern Nigeria,

> It has frequently been proved that men of excellent reputation in this country have, while on the West Coast of Africa either from the absence of the social restraint to which they have been accustomed or from the solitude of their situation and temporary lack of occupation given way to drink.[71]

There is evidence of colonial officers being censured for over-consumption of alcohol. Apparently, medical doctors also over-indulged in drink. In 1898 Dr William Murphy, stationed in the Niger Coast Protectorate, was reported to have been 'strongly addicted to drinks and [had] on one or more occasions been unfit for duty'.[72] Murphy was sacked. In Northern Nigeria, a doctor named as Sanderson resigned his post in 1902 after appearing under the influence of alcohol at a dinner with other government officials and proceeding to get very drunk. It was noted that 'his conduct and language during dinner was disgraceful'.[73] In 1910 Dr A.B.S. Powell resigned his position in Southern Nigeria when he faced a charge of excessive alcoholic indulgence while on duty; he died a few days later.[74] In another case, a colonial committee of inquiry in 1910 investigated Dr Stuart Snell, stationed at Ogoja in Southern Nigeria, following allegations that he had been frequently intoxicated. While it was established that he had occasionally over-indulged in liquor, the committee decided that this had not interfered with his work and so dismissed the case.[75]

There was a debate about the number of train drivers in the Railway Department who had reportedly succumbed to the lure of the bottle. The author of a letter to the editor of the *Lagos Standard* in July 1901 mused on one such employee: 'Poor fellow, but for the comfort he gets from the obedience of his engine his life would hardly be tolerable. He has to look after everything – guard, brakesmen, station-masters, passengers, wheels, axles, couplings and brakes.'[76] In early 1902 two railwaymen named Rodway and Smith, a driver and fitter respectively, were reported to have been caught working while in a drunken state.[77] The Lagos Governor labelled as 'scurrilous and false' the newspaper report that 'several of the drivers were not always strictly sober, with the result that the trains were very often late in arriving at Ebute Metta' railway station.[78] However, later that year, in October 1902, the railway platelayer foreman Buckley died from alcohol over-consumption at the age of thirty-seven.[79] And just a couple of years later, in 1905, the Railway Department dismissed an engine driver named Rolfe for severe intoxication, which had caused him to break up furniture and to become 'so violent that he had to be strapped to his bed'.[80] It also gave Henry Dyer, a permanent way inspector, an extra four months leave of absence to 'dry out' from his heavy drinking.[81]

More cases of excessive drinking were reported in subsequent years. In 1911 A.B. Healey, a sawmill foreman on the Baro–Kano line, was sacked after being found intoxicated on duty twice in a fortnight.[82] The clinical report of the death of a railway platelayer named Wilson in 1915 indicated a long personal history of intemperance: 'This man must have been drinking on the voyage out ... and ... as soon as he got to his station he started again, and finished himself off in a couple of days.'[83] In 1916 Rees Champion, a head guard on the Nigerian Railway, was sacked for being 'addicted to intemperance'.[84] Alcohol poisoning killed the platelayer William Butler in 1918.[85] One morning in September 1921, William Rothwell, the district station manager at Iddo on the Lagos mainland, was not at work. He was found drinking in his quarters with two other Europeans and, when asked if he was unwell, he replied, 'No, I'm on the booze today.'[86] Rothwell was suspended immediately. Fred Jones lost his driver's job in March 1922 for 'having given way to drink and therefore rendering himself unfit for the responsible duty of train working'.[87] Two years later, the locomotive driver Benjamin Gardner's pension was reduced by 20 per cent because he was found under the influence of alcohol while driving a train in the last year of his working life.[88]

Other branches of the Nigerian colonial service, such as the police, marine and customs departments, also had problems with drunken staff. James Owens, an assistant commissioner in the Southern Nigeria Police Force, had a five-year-long record of excessive drinking. Being described as a good officer, he was retained, but he was demoted to the bottom of the list for his rank without immediate prospects of salary increases.[89] The travelling commissioner Lieutenant Richard Morrisey resigned at the end of October 1904 after being found guilty of drunken behaviour.[90] William Coulter, a foreman carpenter with the Marine Department, died at Forcados in February 1914. His death from sun-stroke 'was not helped by four "stiff" whiskies and soda taken every evening after dinner'.[91] Thomas Broadhurst's long-standing alcohol habit finally forced him to seek medical help; he was sacked from the Customs Department in 1917.[92] William Langdon, the purser of the government steam yacht *Ivy*, was another case. He exhibited 'insomnia, nervous depression and a delusion that he was in danger of being murdered'.[93] In 1931 a police constable was arrested in Calabar. He was 'raving and manic drunk. He had to be kept in irons for 24 hours. It is conjectured that this could have only been the result of consuming locally distilled spirit.'[94]

In Northern Nigeria, where the government had imposed constraints on the sale of alcohol and alcohol consumption was more restricted among indigenous communities, Europeans' lifestyles tended to be sparser than in the south. Still, alcohol figured greatly. In 1902 Charles Russell, a temporary fitter, admitted that he had been on a week-long drinking binge.[95] Earlier that year, one colonial official, Thomas Robinson, did not even get to the region before being deemed unsuitable for taking up his position as postmaster because of his intemperate nature.[96] A clerk in Zaria's Treasury Department, F.B. Graham, tried the local native beer, soon became drunk and turned up for duty while still in that state.[97] Two Marine Department masters were dismissed for insobriety, having been in Northern Nigeria for only a month: P.W. Matthews was fired for frequent over-indulgence, while Ernest Cleave, on more than one occasion, took charge of his steamer 'in a muddled state'.[98] In 1927 an unnamed drunken colonial clerk was found lying at the side of a street in Zaria.[99]

A couple of acts of alcohol abuse were reported in the colonial records as having been aggravated by gross misconduct. One involved the curator in Southern Nigeria's Agricultural Department, John Williams, who was dismissed in 1909 for drunkenness and 'indecently assaulting his native [boy] servant'.[100] A secret despatch of 1919 revealed that the assistant district officer L.G. Grant 'resigned due to being constantly in a state of intoxication and of having committed indecent acts with natives at Ibadan'.[101]

How was life in West Africa perceived by fellow Europeans who passed through the colony or had retired from colonial service? In regard to the life of European traders who staffed the factories buying the hinterland's agricultural produce, for example, Mary Kingsley, the adventurer, considered it unremittingly bad:

> ... endless swamps made the person who lived among them think that nothing else but this sort of world, past, present, or future, can ever have existed; and that cities and mountains are but the memories of dreams. A more horrible life than a life in such a region for a man who never takes to it, it is impossible to conceive.[102]

But for Sir Alan Burns, a former colonial official, such isolation, without European wives and families, had some advantages for the expatriate male community:

> The 'Old Coaster' regarded them [white women] as intruders into what had been essentially a bachelor's paradise, where a man could dress as he pleased, drink as much as he liked, and be easy in his morals without causing scandal.[103]

Both views are given credence in the autobiography by Raymond Gore Clough, a Niger Delta trader of the 1910s and 1920s. He described in detail the life of the original 'Palm Oil Ruffians' and their descendants on the coast of Nigeria. He himself spent two tours working for 'a hard-living, hard-drinking palm oil ruffian called Hodgson'.[104] According to Gore Clough, alcohol figured prominently when he and his fellow traders and merchants met for supper, which was preceded by 'much more pink gin' or other beverages, as in the case of one Scotsman, John Willie, who apparently 'loved his whisky'.[105] On reaching the factory at Olomo, Gore Clough saw a gathering of the local agents on the veranda for their evening session of whisky: 'They moved slowly so as not to encourage the sweat; it was still very hot and humid. The drink was always whisky and soda taken in a long glass, the soda prepared in a contraption despatched from England.'[106] It is of course difficult to fathom whether the habits of hard drinking had been acquired back in Europe or had developed or exacerbated in the colony.

But it seems clear that alcohol was the European's consoler and comforter, the balm to a difficult existence.

As was the case in the military and navy, most European factories provided a daily ration of alcohol as part of their remuneration. Whisky and soda were common, some added a gin to the evening's supper, and others, like Miller Brothers, provided a £2 monthly wine allowance.[107] This system irked Bishop Tugwell when he visited a number of traders at a British factory who were drinking gin given to them free by their employer on a festive day: 'when intoxicated with it they were dancing about in a most horrible, disgusting, and disgraceful manner'.[108] In 1899 Dr Charles Battersby claimed that the African Association Trading Company would employ only teetotallers, having seen many of its alcohol-drinking clerks die from the climate and disease, resolved to.[109] However, for some, total abstention or moderation was difficult in the long run. One of the Niger Company's agents, John MacTaggart, was dismissed for alcoholic excesses. Apparently, he had been all right for the first year of his factory work, but 'then went to pieces and drank heavily, quarrelled with everybody, and left Igassa District in a state of chaos'.[110]

On the basis of cases of alcohol-related misconduct recorded in official correspondence, travellers' observations and autobiographies, it seems that local brews and imported liquor were central parts of the creature comforts enjoyed by European expatriates. Among Nigerians, alcohol had social as well as ceremonial functions, as when alcoholic spirits were used to libate the ground and waterways in honour of ancestral spirits. However, whether Nigerians drank excessively, leading to inebriation and 'alcoholic poisoning', is more problematic to ascertain. The evidence on drinking behaviours collected by the 1909 Liquor Trade Inquiry was, in its own words, 'conflicting'.[111] Evidence for the growing spread of excessive drinking among Nigerians was mainly given by eighteen (out of a total of 149) witnesses, all of whom belonged to the CMS. The Committee of Inquiry was not prepared to conclude that statements of eighteen representatives of a single missionary body should outweigh the bulk of other statements:

> The remaining 131 witnesses, drawn from all classes of the community, while admitting that individuals injured themselves by drink,

> were of opinion that the people as a whole were extraordinary sober and well able to exercise self-control in the matter of drink. They saw no signs that drunkenness was on the increase.[112]

The majority of witnesses agreed with the views of a succession of colonial governors. As the Southern Nigeria Governor Walter Egerton, for example, put it in 1909, 'the statements made that the inhabitants of the country are being ruined by drink are incorrect and contrary to the facts'.[113] In a similar vein, the Lagos administrator Captain Denton had claimed in 1899: 'A more fallacious idea cannot exist and it is a cruel shame to malign in this way a people whose temperate habits are an example to nearly every other race in the world.'[114] Nigeria's Inspector-General of Police Charles Johnstone compared the country very favourably in its absence of drunkenness with other places where he had served, England and India.[115] The head of the Forestry Department found the Nigerian population's sobriety comparable to that of the Burmese.[116] The Honourable Kitoye Ajasa, a noted lawyer and unofficial member of the Lagos Legislative Council, who went to the Lagos horse race meeting for ten consecutive years, said there were no arrests for drunkenness among the crowd made up of Europeans and Lagosians: 'I am sorry that I cannot say as much for England.'[117]

Conclusion

Nigeria's significant trade in imported liquor in the nineteenth and early twentieth centuries provoked passionate arguments about its impact on both indigenous and expatriate communities. At the time, patterns of drinking and addiction were drawn across time, between territories and between races. Yet the perceived and actual level of excessive alcohol consumption requires careful analysis in order not to tar whole sections of the population, indeed, whole races, with the brush of alcoholic degeneration. The exaggerated case put forward by Bishop Tugwell that the vast majority of deaths were drink-related and the fierce rebuttal by local traders showed how far beyond reasoned debate the discussions had reached. Though that episode produced little clarity as regards the impact of the liquor trade, the central role of alcohol in the lifestyles of many expatriates in the country can be illustrated by cases of drunkenness, disorderly behaviour, dismissal from employment and even death.

Notes

1 Simon Heap, 'The liquor trade and the Nigerian economy, 1880–1939' (PhD dissertation, University of Ibadan, 1995); Simon Heap, 'Before "Star": the import substitution of Western-style alcohol in Nigeria, 1870–1970', *African Economic History*, 24 (1996), 69–89; Simon Heap, '"We think prohibition is a farce": drinking in the alcohol-prohibited zone of colonial Northern Nigeria', *International Journal of African Historical Studies*, 31, no. 1 (1998), 23–51: Simon Heap, 'Transport and liquor in colonial Nigeria', *Journal of Transport History*, 21, no. 1 (2000), 28–53; Simon Heap, '"A bottle of gin is dangled before the nose of the natives": the economic uses of imported liquor in Southern Nigeria', *African Economic History*, 33 (2005), 67–84; Simon Heap, '"Those that are cooking the gins": the business of ogogoro in Nigeria during the 1930s', *Contemporary Drug Problems*, 35, no. 4 (2008), 573–609; Simon Heap, 'Liquor licences and spirit boycotts: the struggle to control liquor in Ibadan and Abeokuta, Southern Nigeria, 1908–9', *Social History of Alcohol and Drugs: An Interdisciplinary Studies Journal*, 25 (2011), 107–29.

2 Simon Heap, '"Living on the proceeds of a grog shop": liquor revenue in Nigeria', in D.F. Bryceson (ed.), *Alcohol in Africa: Mixing Business, Pleasure and Politics* (Westport, USA: Greenwood Publishing Group, 2002), 139–59.

3 'The liquor traffic question', *Lagos Standard*, 10 March 1909, p. 2.

4 'The report of the Liquor Traffic Commission', *Lagos Weekly Record*, 18 December 1909, pp. 2–3.

5 'Rum and gin', *Lagos Observer*, 17 April 1886, p. 2; 'The drink traffic and the natives', *Lagos Observer*, 7 May 1897, p. 2.

6 Heap, '"Those that are cooking the gins"'.

7 National Archives, Enugu (NAE), Aba District Office, ABADIST 14/1/169, S.T. Madu to C. J. Pleass, District Officer, Aba, 8 December 1932. For the gastro-intestinal symptoms in habitual *ogogoro* drinkers, see T.A. John, O. Onabanjo, R. Aiyedogbon and C.D. Aisa,

'Is "ogogoro" a potent ulcerogen?', *West African Journal of Pharmacology and Drug Research*, 9, supplement (1990), 65–9.

8 NAE, Brass District Office, BRASSDIST 10/1/80, E.N.C. Dickinson, Assistant District Officer, Brass, to Native Court, Sabagreia, 16 February 1932.

9 National Archives, Ibadan (NAI), Asaba Divisional Office, ASADIV 1/ AD.199, I.N. Hill, District Officer, Asaba, to J.M. Simpson, Assistant District Officer, Agbor, 22 September 1932.

10 NAE, Rivers Province Office, RIVPROF 2/1/17, A.T E. Marsh, Resident, Rivers Province, to F.B. Carr, Secretary, Eastern Provinces, 23 December 1947.

11 Emmanuel Akyeampong, 'Alcoholism in Ghana – a socio-cultural exploration', *Culture, Medicine and Psychiatry*, 19 (1995), 261–80.

12 Bishop Herbert Tugwell in *Report of the Committee of Inquiry into the Liquor Trade in Southern Nigeria*, Part II: *Minutes of Evidence*, Cd 4907 (1909), Questions 915–16, p. 26.

13 Dr Henry Strachan in *Minutes of Evidence*, Question 674, p. 17.

14 Dr Thomas Adam in *Minutes of Evidence*, Questions 2772, 2821–31, pp. 73–4.

15 Mark Harrison, 'A global perspective: refining the history of health, medicine and disease', *Bulletin of the History of Medicine*, 89, no. 4 (2015), 639–89; Michael A. Osborne, 'Acclimatizing the world: a history of the paradigmatic colonial science', in 'Nature and Empire: Science and the Colonial Enterprise', *Osiris*, 15 (2000), 135–51.

16 Strachan in *Minutes of Evidence*, Question 675, p. 17; Adam in *Minutes of Evidence*, Questions 2715–17, p. 71.

17 'The gin traffic controversy from an African point of view, by Abdul Mortaleb', *Lagos Weekly Record*, 27 July 1895, p. 2.

18 Strachan in *Minutes of Evidence*, Question 671, p. 17.

19 Strachan in *Minutes of Evidence*, Question 706, p. 18.

20 H.H. Bell, 'The liquor problem in West Africa', *Empire Review*, July 1929, p. 13. See also Adam in *Minutes of Evidence*, Question 2692, p. 76; Kitoyi Ajasa in *Minutes of Evidence*, Questions 2953–6, p. 77.

21 Reverend Father Shanahan in *Minutes of Evidence*, Question 4524, p. 117.

22 Dr Oguntola Sapara in *Minutes of Evidence*, Questions 5647–60, 5671–6, p. 142.

23 Sapara in *Minutes of Evidence*, Questions 5732–7, p. 143.

24 Frederick Lugard, 'Liquor traffic in Africa', *Nineteenth Century*, November 1897, pp. 770–1.

25 Frederick Lugard, 'Liquor traffic in Africa', *Nineteenth Century*, November 1897, pp. 770–1.
26 Herbert Tugwell, 'The liquor traffic in West Africa', letter to the editor, *The Times*, 27 March 1899, p. 10.
27 Reverend Abraham Walton in *Minutes of Evidence*, Questions 5932–6, p. 148.
28 Dr Edward Read in *Minutes of Evidence*, Questions 11703–8, p. 290.
29 Dr Rupert Welply in *Minutes of Evidence*, Questions 6033–5, p. 150.
30 *Lagos Blue Book of Statistics* (Lagos: Government Printer, 1899–1905).
31 *Southern Nigeria Annual Report* (Old Calabar: Government Printer, 1903), 47.
32 Staff lists, *Lagos Blue Book of Statistics* (1899–1905).
33 Akyeampong, 'Alcoholism in Ghana', 266–9.
34 Jonathan Sadowsky, *Imperial Bedlam: Institutions of Madness in Colonial Southwest Nigeria* (Berkeley: University of California Press, 1999).
35 Tugwell, 'The liquor traffic in West Africa', 10.
36 National Archives, Kew (NA), Colonial Office papers, CO 147/142, Captain George Denton, Administrator, Lagos, to Joseph Chamberlain, Secretary of State for the Colonies, London, 2 May 1899.
37 NA, CO 147/142, Denton to Chamberlain, 2 May 1899.
38 'Action for libel', *Gold Coast Aborigines*, 10 June 1899, p. 2. On informing the defendant that the case would be sent to the assizes, the magistrate bailed Tugwell with two sureties of £50 each.
39 *Payne's Lagos and West African Almanack and Diary for 1894* (London: J.S. Phillips, 1893), 55–9.
40 NA, CO 147/80, Denton to Lord Knutsford, Secretary of State for the Colonies, London, 22 May 1891.
41 NAI, CSO, 1/1/35, *Lagos Registrar-General Annual Report* (Lagos: Government Printer, 1900), 79.
42 'Action for libel', 2.
43 'Action for libel', 2; 'Death', *Lagos Government Gazette*, 25 March 1899, p. 184.
44 'The libel action against Bishop Tugwell', *Lagos Weekly Record*, 24 June 1899, p. 2. Capitals in original.
45 'The libel action against Bishop Tugwell', 2.
46 'Censored films for natives: no vamps, drink, or illicit love', *Lagos Daily News*, 5 December 1931, p. 3.

47 'The case of Bishop Tugwell', *Lagos Weekly Record*, 17 June 1899, p. 2; 'Editorial notes', *Niger and Yoruba Notes*, 5, no. 69 (June 1899), 87.
48 Charles Battersby, 'Bishop Tugwell's friends and the Lagos Chamber of Commerce', *Lagos Weekly Record*, 10 June 1899, p. 2.
49 'Editorial notes', *Niger and Yoruba Notes*, 5, no. 60 (June 1899), 87.
50 'Editorial notes', *Niger and Yoruba Notes*, 6, no. 61 (July 1899), 1.
51 'An African view of the liquor traffic question', *Niger and Yoruba Notes*, 6, no. 64 (October 1899), 31.
52 Native Races and Liquor Traffic United Committee (NRLTUC), *Native Races and the Drink Question*, 7.
53 'The case of Bishop Tugwell', *Lagos Weekly Record*, 17 June 1899, p. 2; 'Bishop Tugwell's Defence Fund', *Niger and Yoruba Notes*, 5, no. 60 (June 1899), 89.
54 'The libel action against Bishop Tugwell', 2; 'Junius', 'The Right Reverend Bishop Tugwell: a Christian or a pseudologist, letter to the editor', *Lagos Standard*, 10 July 1901, pp. 2–3.
55 'Editorial notes', *Niger and Yoruba Notes*, 6, no. 61 (July 1899), 1.
56 'The libel action against Bishop Tugwell', 2.
57 NA, CO 147/142, Denton to Chamberlain, 2 May 1899.
58 *Report of the Committee of Inquiry into the Liquor Trade in Southern Nigeria*, Part I: *Report*, Cd 4906 (1909), 18.
59 Joyce Cary, a former colonial officer in Northern Nigeria, later wrote of such experiences of Gollup in his novel *Mister Johnson* (London: Victor Gollancz).
60 W. Lauzun-Brown, 'Life and health in West Africa', *West Africa*, 10 September 1904, p. 238; 'Life and health in West Africa', *West Africa*, 17 September 1904, p. 258; 'Life and health in West Africa', *West Africa*, 24 September 1904, p. 287; Harry H. Johnston, 'Alcohol in Africa', *Nineteenth Century*, 70 (September 1911), 482, 493; *Report by the Honourable W.G.A. Ormsby-Gore, M.P., on his Visit to West Africa during the Year 1926*, Cmd 2744 (1926), 179.
61 NAI, CSO 1/32/39, Frederick Lugard to Walter Long, Secretary of State for the Colonies, 29 May 1918.
62 Dr John Tichbourne in *Minutes of Evidence*, Questions 4178–81, p. 109.
63 *Western Echo*, 16–23 December 1886, quoted in 'Editorial', *Lagos Observer*, 5 February 1887, p. 2.
64 Tichbourne in *Minutes of Evidence*, Questions 4200–1, p. 110; Johnston, 'Alcohol in Africa', 482.
65 Dr Ernest Tipper in *Minutes of Evidence*, Questions 5607–9, p. 139.

66 NAI, Commissioner of the Colony's Office, COMCOL 1/808, J. Olu Johnson, Agent, Messrs John Holt and Company, to G.H. Findlay, Acting Administrator of the Colony, Lagos, 26 June 1929.
67 NAI, CSO 1/22/2, Marquis of Ripon's circular despatch to All Governors, 10 September 1892, quoted in Earl of Crewe to James Thorburn, 18 January 1909.
68 *British New Guinea Annual Report* (Rabaul: Government Printer, 1897–98), 36, quoted in 'Europeans and alcohol', *Niger and Yoruba Notes*, 6, no. 62 (August 1899), 11.
69 'Europeans and alcohol in the Tropics, by General Gallieni, Governor of Madagascar, read at the International Temperance Congress, Paris', *Niger and Yoruba Notes*, 5, no. 60 (June 1899), 92–3.
70 *The West African Pocketbook – A Guide to Newly Appointed Government Officers*,' 2nd edn (London: HMSO, 1906), quoted in M. Crowder, *West Africa under Colonial Rule* (London: Hutchinson, 1968), 395.
71 NAI, CSO 1/28/3, William Mercer, Under-Secretary of State for the Colonies, London, to Lugard, High Commissioner, Northern Nigeria, 9 April 1903.
72 NA, Foreign Office, FO 2/180, A.C. Douglas, Acting District Commissioner, Opobo, 19 July 1898, quoted in H.L. Gallwey, Acting Commissioner and Consul-General, Niger Coast Protectorate, to Chamberlain, 13 October 1898.
73 NAI, CSO 1/27/2, D.K. McDowell, Principal Medical Officer, Northern Nigeria, to M.H.D. Beresford, Secretary to the Administration, Northern Nigeria, 9 April 1902.
74 NAI, CSO 1/21/7, John Thorburn, Acting Governor, Southern Nigeria, to Earl of Crewe, Secretary of State for the Colonies, London, 11 July 1910.
75 NAI, CSO 1/21/7, Thorburn to Crewe, 16 July 1910.
76 'Junius', 'The Right Reverend Bishop Tugwell', 2.
77 NAI, CSO 1/1/37, Sir William MacGregor to Joseph Chamberlain, 8 March 1902.
78 NAI, CSO 1/1/37, MacGregor, Governor, Lagos, to Chamberlain, 8 March 1902.
79 *Lagos Medical Annual Report* (Lagos: Government Printer, 1902), 28.
80 NAI, CSO 1/1/52, Thorburn, Administrator, Lagos, to Earl of Elgin, Secretary of State for the Colonies, London, 13 December 1905.
81 NAI, CSO 1/1/50, E.A. Speed, Administrator, Lagos, to Alfred Lyttelton, Secretary of State for the Colonies, London, 28 April 1905.

82 NAI, CSO 1/27/11, Charles Temple, Acting Governor, Northern Nigeria, to Harcourt, 3 July 1911.
83 National Archives, Kaduna (NAK), Secretary, Northern Provinces, SNP 8/2/81/1915, F.H. Waller, Acting General Manager, Nigerian Railway, to Donald Cameron, Central Secretary, Nigeria, 2 June 1915.
84 NAI, CSO 1/32/16, Lugard to A. Bonar Law, Secretary of State for the Colonies, London, 8 June 1915; NAI, CSO 1/32/26, A.G. Boyle, Deputy Governor, Nigeria, to Bonar Law, 21 October 1916.
85 NAI, CSO 1/32/37, Cameron, for Lugard in the Northern Provinces, to Long, London, 24 January 1918.
86 NAI, CSO 1/32/65, Report of the Committee of Executive Council Appointed to Enquire into the Charges against Mr W.B. Rothwell, District Station Manager, Nigerian Railway, 27 May 1922, pp. 1–2, 5.
87 NAI, CSO 1/32/64, Cameron, Governor's Deputy, Nigeria, to Winston Churchill, Secretary of State for the Colonies, London, 3 March 1922.
88 NAI, CSO 1/32/74, Cameron, Acting Governor, Nigeria, to James Thomas, Secretary of State for the Colonies, London, 6 June 1924.
89 NAI, CSO 1/21/5, Sir W. Egerton, Governor, Southern Nigeria, to Crewe, 3 September 1909.
90 NAI, CSO 1/15/5, Egerton, High Commissioner, Southern Nigeria, to Lyttelton, 26 August 1904.
91 NAI, CSO 1/32/2, Lugard, Governor-General, Nigeria, to Lewis Harcourt, Secretary of State for the Colonies, London, 25 February 1914.
92 NAE, Chief Secretary, Enugu, CSE 5/12/5, T.F. Burrowes, Comptroller of Customs, Nigeria, to Thomas Broadhurst, Wharfinger, Customs Department, Nigeria, 2 March 1917.
93 NAI, CSO 1/21/8, Egerton to Harcourt, 10 January 1911.
94 NAI, CSO 1/32/110, memorandum by G.H. Findlay, Resident, Calabar, 21 September 1931, p. 2.
95 NAI, CSO 1/27/2, Lugard to Chamberlain, 23 December 1902.
96 NAI, CSO 1/27/2, Lugard to Chamberlain, 15 March 1902.
97 NAK, SNP 6/3/83/1907, F.B. Graham, Clerk, Treasury, Zaria, to T.B. Phillips, Assistant Treasurer, Zaria, 5 June 1907.
98 NAK, SNP 6/5/53/1909, W. Wallace, Acting Governor, Northern Nigeria, to Crewe, 6 June 1909; NAK, SNP 6/1/78/1904, Lugard to Lyttelton, 2 September 1904.
99 NAK, Zaria Provincial Office, ZARPROF, FED 5/1/C.2475, C.A. Woodhouse, Acting Senior Resident, Zaria Province, to G.S. Browne, Secretary, Northern Provinces, Nigeria, 5 April 1927.

100 NAI, CSO 1/21/5, Egerton to Crewe, 18 October 1909.
101 NAI, CSO 1/36/5, Boyle, Acting Governor, Nigeria, to Viscount Milner, Secretary of State for the Colonies, 24 April 1919.
102 Mary Kingsley, *West African Studies* (London: MacMillan, 1899), 44.
103 Alan Burns, *Colonial Civil Servant* (London: Allen and Unwin, 1949), 42.
104 Raymond Gore Clough, *Oil Rivers Trader* (London: C. Hurst, 1972), 55.
105 Gore Clough, *Oil Rivers Trader*, 33, 48.
106 Gore Clough, *Oil Rivers Trader*, 46.
107 Frederick Pedler, *The Lion and the Unicorn in Africa* (London: Heinemann, 1974), 204, 208. Pedler refers to information from 1906 and 1913.
108 Bishop Herbert Tugwell, 'West African merchants and the liquor traffic', *Niger and Yoruba Notes*, 8, no. 96 (June 1902), 92.
109 Battersby, 'Bishop Tugwell's friends and the Lagos Chamber of Commerce', 2–3.
110 Bodleian Library, Oxford, Scarborough Papers, MSS.Afr.s.88, fols 479–80, J. Trigge, Agent, Niger Company, to Lord Scarborough, Chairman, Niger Company, 24 October 1903.
111 *Report of the Committee of Inquiry into the Liquor Trade*, Part I, 10.
112 *Report of the Committee of Inquiry into the Liquor Trade*, Part I, 11–12.
113 NA, CO 520/80, Egerton to Crewe, 23 July 1909.
114 NA, CO 147/142, Denton to Chamberlain, 2 May 1899.
115 Charles Johnstone in *Minutes of Evidence*, Question 422, p. 11.
116 Henry Thompson in *Minutes of Evidence*, Question 1778, p. 48.
117 Ajasa in *Minutes of Evidence*, Questions 1995–6, p. 78.

6

Alcohol, abstinence and rationalisation in Germany, *c.* 1870s–1910s

Jasmin Brötz

This chapter explores why the idea of abstinence received considerable attention among medical doctors and the public alike in Germany during the late nineteenth and early twentieth centuries. It focuses on the plural and at times ambiguous semantics of the terms 'alcoholism', 'addiction' and 'temperance'. The chapter maps how debates on alcohol were imbued with ideas about the irrationality of the 'masses', the nature of alcoholism as a process and the link between the body and the body politic, in other words between the health of individuals and the health of the nation. The varied impact of discourses of physical, mental and moral degeneration on medical views of alcohol consumption and on ideas pertaining to the creation of a 'New Man' is explored. In these discourses it became apparent that alcoholism contradicted the expectations of a rational society. It will be argued that increased interest in alcoholism was based on the idea of rationalisation as a society-changing process.[1] The anticipated realisation of reason was regarded as an unavoidable, almost natural process which, at the same time, encapsulated the potential for human action. Science offered such potential by promising to reduce alcoholism. It was feared that alcoholism would lead to inheritable degeneration, resulting in considerable economic loss to the wealth of the nation. Last but not least, alcohol was considered an obstacle to the global competition with other nations, especially during the period preceding World War I.

The chapter embraces previous research from social and cultural history on the scientification and medicalisation of alcoholism.[2] It also explores conceptual history perspectives by examining the semantics of the discourse on alcoholism, revealing recurrent elements in the debate.[3] These recurring themes require an assessment of continuities and ruptures, particularly in regard to earlier debates on alcohol. Temperance campaigns against hard liquor in early nineteenth-century Germany had focused on the miserable living conditions of the working classes and combined religious concerns with temperance values; drinking was conceived of as a sin. In the later decades of the century, the temperance movement was dominated by physicians and scientists. For them, 'alcoholism' was a disease. This view relied no longer on religious ethics, but on scientific explanations and statistics. Moreover, the alcohol problem became everyone's problem, because even small amounts of alcohol were perceived as causing devastating damage to the individual and therefore to public health. According to medical experts, alcohol in general ought to be avoided. The call for temperance turned more and more into a call for complete abstinence.

From the 1880s onwards, numerous abstinence associations were founded in Germany. Most popular were the Guttempler (1883), the Blaues Kreuz (1885) and the Kreuzbund (1896).[4] The Guttempler alone, which was based on the US association of the same name, had 50,000 members before World War I.[5] In 1883 the Deutscher Verein gegen den Mißbrauch geistiger Getränke (German Association against the Abuse of Spiritual Drinks), which was committed to moderation, was founded.[6] By the end of the century, the number of abstainers among members of temperance associations was three times as high as that of those favouring moderation. Popular support for these associations was in general relatively low.[7] However, these movements had a lasting influence on drinking culture in Germany; for example, while alcohol was not prohibited at the workplace, its consumption did become less common. During the 1880s, quantities of spirits consumed in factories lessened, and after 1900 the same could be said for beer.[8] From the 1880s, special coffee halls were opened, and in the 1890s, abstainers also considered producing other non-alcoholic beverages such as soda water and lemonade.[9] Furthermore, the naturopath Friedrich Eduard Bilz created a lemonade drink that has since 1907 been marketed worldwide under the name 'Sinalco'.[10]

The sources for this chapter mainly consist of popular scientific literature, such as public lectures, guidebooks and educational pamphlets. The social historian Heinrich Tappe uses similar sources in his comprehensive study of alcohol production, drinking behaviours and the abstinence movement in Germany. He attributes the emergence of abstinence associations to economic problems during the financial crisis of the 1870s, when social problems returned to the public eye. Although Tappe focuses on economic factors, he points out that social movements and cultural issues may have been influential as well.[11] In contrast, Hasso Spode pursues a cultural-historical approach in his history of alcohol in Germany. He shows that the rise of the abstinence movement was partly due to biopolitical factors and linked to ideas of 'racial hygiene'.[12] However, Spode interprets the debate on alcoholism with recourse to Max Weber's concept of rationalisation as part of modernisation.[13] Weber's work was contemporaneous with and underlay the views held by the main protagonists investigated in this chapter, and hence is considered a primary source rather than used as a theoretical framework for the chapter. In contrast to previous research, the conceptual history approach employed here sets out to reveal the connection between the alcohol problem on the one hand and the idea of rationalisation, as framed by Weber and others, on the other. It facilitates a better understanding of why the discussion about abstinence of the 1870s became prominent in the first place.

Alcohol as a problem of modern society

Although alcohol over-consumption had been considered as a threat to good health within German folklore and the Graeco-Roman and other medical traditions even before the rise of modernity, the transformation of 'drunkenness' from a sin to a disease in its own right occurred with the increased focus on the medicalisation of alcohol use and the 'discovery of addiction'.[14] In 1802 the German physician Christoph Wilhelm Hufeland described alcohol as a 'narcotic poison'.[15] In 1819 the German-Russian physician Constantin von Brühl-Cramer framed the term 'addiction to drink' (*Trunksucht*) as a new disease pattern that could be treated rather than being relegated to the realms of morals.[16] Translating Brühl-Cramer's concept, Hufeland subsequently coined the technical term 'dipsomania'.[17] Following the Swedish physician Magnus Huss's suggestion, the term 'alcoholismus chronicus' emerged in the mid-nineteenth century.[18] By the end of the century, 'alcoholism' had become the dominant term used in public discussions in Germany.[19] German encyclopaedias increasingly replaced the term 'drunkenness' (*Trunkenheit*) with 'addiction to drink' (*Trunksucht*) and 'alcoholism' (*Alkoholismus*).[20]

Many popular publications on alcoholism relied on the work of Abraham Adolf Baer (1834–1908), a prison doctor in Berlin, who also wrote on 'prison hygiene' and the 'anthropology of the criminal'.[21] In 1878 he published a book on alcoholism and its prevention, which was considered the 'beginning of a modern scientific discussion of the alcohol question'.[22] He called on the state to lead the 'fight against drunkenness ... through energetic and rational preventive and repressive measures'.[23] Above all, Baer identified irrationality and ignorance among the population as the cause of the problem. Knowledge and rationality would, according to him, become the antidote to alcoholism. 'The greatest enemy of this vice ... is a culture based on knowledge, cognition and morality; the more these spread among the people, the more surely the heavy curse of alcoholism will be wiped out and exterminated along with all the other bad habits.'[24] Baer's statement fitted squarely into the emerging discourse on what was referred to as the 'rationalisation' of society. In 1896 the sociologist and ethnographer Alfred Vierkandt wrote on the 'rationalisation of life' in modern society.[25] Werner Sombart used the same term in 1911 to describe modern society as shaped by capitalism.[26] Furthermore, rationalisation came to be seen as a defining characteristic in various areas: working life, birth control and modern culture in general.[27] It was thought that the spread of rationality was part of an unstoppable cultural development. However, as Eley et al. argue in *German Modernities* (2016), contemporaries considered the future as open, rather than being subject to the unfolding of traditional beliefs. It had to be actively shaped.[28] Some held the advance of civilisation itself responsible for the rise of alcoholism. In this view, the alcohol problem was understood as an inherent part of cultural progress.

In 1912, inspired by progressivist and new medical frameworks, the paediatrician Helene Breitung (later known as Helene Greeff, 1881–1951) developed teaching material to educate young people on abstinence. In her publication, which was published by the Guttempler Association, she claimed that 'drinking had never before been as much of an everyday habit as it is in today's civilised countries'.[29] She blamed breweries and distilleries for the increased consumption, as they produced ever-larger quantities of alcohol. Although she held that alcoholism had never been a social problem before the rise of the modern alcohol industry, she also claimed that society should heed the lessons from the histories of ancient cultures, which declined when they succumbed to drink 'at the peak of their power'.[30] The narrative of an impending decline of culture appeared in contemporary discourse once the euphoria of entering the new century had faded. Because progress had been anticipated, the fear of regression became typical of the rationalisation discourse. This fear seemed to justify increased intervention in the process of the perceived impending civilisationary decline. In his *The Human Motor: Energy, Fatigue, and the Origins of Modernity*, Anson Rabinbach outlines a similar narrative in regard to the working body in the widely used metaphor of the 'human motor'. This metaphor expressed confidence in science, but also led to a vague fear: the fear of 'fatigue' in the sense of losing energy and the strife for entropy, which Rabinbach sees as characteristic of the turn from the nineteenth century to the twentieth.[31]

The idea of cultural decay was not only influential to Breitung's thinking, but could also be found in other contemporary writing. The physiologist Gustav von Bunge (1844–1920) said that although drunkenness might be as old as history, alcoholism was not. Only modern production processes and 'perfectionised agriculture, progressing physics and chemistry combined with large capital' made large-scale production and distribution of alcohol possible.[32] The German psychiatrist Emil Kraepelin (1856–1926) agreed with Bunge that technical progress in regard to the efficiency of distilleries and breweries had increased to hitherto unknown heights.[33] Not only production, but also the alcohol content of beer had been optimised. Economic efficiency, scientific innovations and cultural change were increasingly suspected to cause the alcohol problem.

Indeed, the rate of beer consumption doubled between 1870 and 1890, while liquor consumption reached its peak between 1885 and 1887 but declined after taxes on spirits were raised in 1887.[34] Less liquor was drunk, and beer became more popular. Thus drinking became more moderate in the 1890s.[35] At the same time, contemporaries began to perceive alcoholism as a new phenomenon, for it contradicted their expectations of a progressive future. For many, progress meant not just technological but also moral progress in the sense that people would become more attuned to the power of reason. Conversely, drinking alcohol was considered irrational behaviour that would hinder society's progress.

Abraham Baer believed that alcoholism inflicted damage on the individual as well as on society. He used the metaphor of a 'social organism' (*socialer Organismus*) to express the intertwined relationship of society and its individuals.[36] Referring to Darwin, Baer highlighted that an individual's drunkenness posed a threat to all. This Neo-Lamarckian interpretation of Darwin led to the idea of the degeneration of society or even of mankind. Thus Baer provided an early impetus to the temperance movement that would soon re-utilise many of his arguments.[37] Experts, and in particular physicians and psychologists, led the German debate on alcohol, which was also raging in other countries. The Swiss psychiatrist Auguste Forel (1848–1931) had a major influence on German debates, as European writers' works were distributed by German publishers.[38] Others, such as the Austrian bacteriologist and hygienist Max von Gruber (1853–1927), taught in Germany and settled there.

Within the context of the debates on rationalisation, the influence of scientific expertise in all areas of life was expected, and the ensuing 'scientification' of the discourse on society and progress was welcomed. It was also held that mechanisation and technology, being the practical implementation of scientific knowledge, would improve society. Through bureaucratisation, a rational order of society was striven for. In the realm of economics, the principles of predictable and reasonable economic management were applied to social problems. Last but not least, the idea of a reasonable cultural development was firmly placed within the progressive history of Western rationalisation. These different facets of the rationalisation thesis were connected by the expectation of an imminent and revolutionary realisation of reason. At the same time, rationalisation was perceived as ambiguous. On the one hand, the process seemed to be inevitable, but on the other hand, it appeared to be pliable and manageable. These manifold ideas of rationalisation were finally incorporated by the German sociologist Max Weber (1864–1920) into a theoretical concept, which later formed the basis of modernisation theory.

Given the prominence of the discourse of rationalisation in Germany, it is not surprising that it also affected the way the 'alcohol question' was perceived. Alcoholism was understood as the result of a misguided rationalisation and as a force that brought the irrational back into the projected unfolding of social progress. The key elements of the debate on alcohol centred on, firstly, alcoholism as part of an ongoing, advancing process in society; secondly, 'mass society' and the 'irrationality of the crowd' as promulgators of drinking; thirdly, individual health as intertwined with public health; and, fourthly, the degeneration of the individual and of society as the result of alcohol consumption. Ideas about the rise of and competition between nation states and the creation of a 'New Man' arose alongside the abstinence movement. In the following section, these elements of the discourse will be investigated.

Alcoholism as an advancing process

Alcoholism came to be understood as the result of an evolving and ever-expanding process engendered by increased alcohol production and consumption in the wake of rationalisation. Technical improvements in alcohol production, such as Carl von Linde's cooling machine (1876), which facilitated beer production, and Lorenz Adalbert Enzinger's beer filter (1878), which enhanced the durability of beer, were seen to have facilitated higher alcohol consumption alongside industrialised working processes and a modern way of life. The increased rates, particularly before the 1880s, fuelled the rise of the abstinence movement, but medical perceptions of a spreading alcohol problem did not decrease with falling rates. The German-Baltic physiologist Bunge highlighted the wider, expanding impact of alcohol, which he saw as neither predictable nor manageable. In his 1886 inaugural lecture on the 'alcohol question' as the chair of physiological chemistry at the University of Basel, he pointed out: 'The abuse of alcoholic beverages leads to a whole host of diseases, and no organ of our body is preserved from its destructive effect.'[39] According to him, the unpredictability of these damaging processes made it impossible to control the effects of alcohol consumption on an individual's body. The consequences for society, understood as a 'collective body', were all the more unclear.

Emil Kraepelin used metaphors of progressive expansion to characterise the nature of alcoholism and its consequences for society.

> There can be no doubt that the alcoholic misery of our people is gigantic. We are dealing with an all-pervading alcohol poisoning, with a national epidemic. More and more, the most precious goods, intellectual and physical health, morality, happiness and prosperity fall apart.[40]

Using the metaphor of poisoning, Kraepelin expressed the fear that society was exposed to an irreversible process of decomposition that undermined its functionality. The metaphor of the epidemic evoked associations with the recent cholera epidemic in Hamburg in 1896, when bacteriological experts such as Robert Koch had been consulted.[41] However, while infectious diseases seemed to have become controllable through scientific knowledge, the alcohol problem remained diffuse and uncertain. To start with, it had to be identified and qualified as a problem. The metaphors of poisoning and epidemic helped to conceptualise the problem.

The Swiss psychiatrist Auguste Forel (1848–1931) described alcoholism as a slow and invisible process of intoxication. He stated that 'these effects develop so slowly when the doses are small and can proceed with such slightly visible disturbances that society gets accustomed to them and does not notice the degeneration which they generate'.[42] For him, the concern was that neither the individual nor society would notice the progressivity of alcoholism until it was too late. Forel symbolically transferred the physiologically describable poisoning of the individual to an alleged poisoning of society. Alcoholism became a metaphor for national disease and degeneration.[43] Forel regarded moderate and regular drinking in particular as a problem, as it poisoned incrementally, in small quantities, and led to a gradual increase in doses. This had two consequences, namely physical habituation to higher doses and the individual's adaption to the physical limitations and the symptoms of the poisoning. Applied to society, this meant that alcoholism would initially not be conspicuous, but society would gradually get used to widespread drinking and to an increasing number of alcoholics.

The slow but steady progressivity of alcoholism was described evocatively by the German physician Alfred Grotjahn (1869–1931), who taught social hygiene at the Charité University Clinic in Berlin. He focused on the consequences for the individual:

> The dangers to the heart, the blood vessels, the mucous membranes, the nervous organs and so on exposed to alcohol become particularly sinister through the fact that initially their extent is not noticed and pathological symptoms show up only after decades, but then [these symptoms] usually cannot be undone.[44]

Unlike many of his colleagues, Grotjahn argued for temperance and not for abstinence. He believed in the ability of medical progress and the rise of statistical methods to accurately determine the acceptable level of harmless alcohol consumption. Available statistics provided evidence of the alcohol problem. However, they were limited to the detection of the worst results of alcohol consumption, not of the many stages before. As Bunge put it: 'From the first glass to insanity, to crime, to despair and suicide there are a thousand stages of misery. Only the lowest ones are revealed in statistics.'[45] To people like Bunge, the full extent of alcohol-related problems was not yet fully understood. Therefore alcoholism was a process in society not to be underestimated.

Efficiency, rationalisation and the irrationality of the 'masses'

The question emerges as to why alcoholism had not been problematised as a societal issue before. Medical experts such as Bunge and Forel attributed the alcohol problem to the irrationality of the masses. *Masse* (the masses; the crowd) became a concept of political-social language in Germany in the nineteenth century, alongside *Klasse* (class), *Volk* (people) or *Nation* (nation). The term derived from the Greek word for dough and, unlike 'class', denoted the unformed crowd of the poor and uneducated.[46] The concept of the masses also expressed the fear in bourgeois circles of uncontrollable social problems. This perception changed significantly during the last few decades of the century, by which time everyone had become part of a mass society, regardless of social status, and particularly in regard to alcohol.[47] Alcoholism seemed to be an unavoidable result of modernity and cultural development, because efficient yet monotonous working conditions seemed to produce a need for regular drinking. These conditions affected a broad part of society – workers and office labourers alike. But unlike in the 1830s, indulgence in alcohol was not taken as an indicator of miserable working conditions, but as a threatening symbol of a way of life that had become prevalent throughout society.

The effects of technological progress were not the only issues discussed in relation to alcohol. In particular, the cognitive aspects of rationalisation were also addressed while the needs of a changing society challenged the individual. Bunge even suggested that the observed escape from modernity through alcohol might not simply originate from the irrationality of the masses, but instead from their discontent about and the dire consequences of rationalisation. In his view, people were wary of a technologically rationalised society that functions on the basis of calculated efficiency principles that led people to become 'cold, reasonable and calculating', and the world being ruled by 'cold calculation'.[48] For Bunge, alcoholism was not the result of bad living and working conditions as assumed by the socialists, but the result of imitation and cultural preferences: 'People drink because others drink.'[49]

Another social change observed alongside rationalisation was the increase in occupations that involved desk-based work, which came to be regarded as exhausting and as promoting regular drinking. Emil Kraepelin did research on human capability, measuring especially mental capability. He experimented with various substances (such as tea, coffee and morphine) to determine the ideal balance between exercise and fatigue in the work process, with a particular focus on mental fatigue.[50] Forel assumed that people believed they needed 'drugs because of modern culture and all the intellectual [*geistige*] work' they performed.[51] Paul Wurster (1860–1923), a German theologian, suggested that the accomplishments of science conflicted with the superstition of the people.[52] Irrational masses seemed to hamper scientific progress. Forel even suggested that 'Custom becomes indoctrination of the masses, and *a priori* an unquestioned belief in authority.'[53] He went on to say that people were accustomed to, or were looking for, well-established reasons and 'dumb excuses' to drink in order to 'bestow a semblance of logic, of rationality, of expediency on their illogical behaviour'.[54] Views like these expressed a suspicion that the masses thought and behaved in an irrational manner.

In his *Psychologie des foules* (Psychology of Crowds) of 1895, the psychologist and sociologist Gustave Le Bon (1841–1931) characterised 'the masses' or 'the crowd' as impulsive, irritable and incapable of reason, relying on sentiment rather than on clear judgement.[55] Le Bon's work was translated into German in 1908 by the philosopher Rudolf Eisler, by which time 'the masses' had already been conceptualised as 'irrational' and their relationship with alcohol was frowned upon.[56] The masses were seen as easily seduced by modern-style 'beer palaces' with 'electric lights and the sound of a full orchestra'.[57] The temptation of alcohol became affiliated with a system of technical innovation and economic profiteering. Irrational leisure pursuits and rationalised working time seemed to complement each other. The living conditions of the working classes had improved, and regular but moderate beer consumption had replaced the excessive consumption of spirits that usually happened on paydays. But as regular drinking came to be seen as a danger to individual health and society, the changes of modernity made it necessary for the state to educate people. As Bunge demanded: 'A good government should fight indefatigably and steadily against all stupidity and weaknesses of the masses.'[58] The idea of moderate but widespread alcohol consumption contradicted the principles of a rational modern society based on scientific knowledge.

Individual health and public health

The individual was understood to be directly connected to the collective. In this mutual relationship the individual became the key to improved public health. Drunkenness and moderate drinking were seen to endanger and degrade public health. Emil Kraepelin appealed to individuals' responsibility: 'The nation ... desperately needs the personal model of all those who are wise to free themselves from the terrible poison that undermines their health, morality and prosperity.'[59] Here, abstinence became a sign of solidarity, especially in the case of the *Trinkzwang* (obligation to drink socially) in German student associations for example. The moderate drinker was always seen to be in danger of becoming an alcoholic. And even if he or she did not, moderate drinking could still encourage others to drink and succumb to alcoholism. The predisposition to develop a 'pathological desire for repeated poisoning and larger doses' was seen to differ from person to person.[60] This led Bunge to conclude: 'The moderates are the seducers!'[61] For him, it was even worse to drink moderately than excessively, because moderate drinking perpetuated the drinking culture and insidiously damaged public health and thereby the *Volkskörper* or body politic. Abraham Baer had previously advanced this view when he investigated alcoholism with respect to its 'dispersion and impact on the individual and the social organism'.[62]

The perception of society as a 'social organism' drew to some extent on the cellular pathology of Rudolf Virchow (1821–1902). A famous physician and liberal politician, Virchow described the human organism as a *Zellenstaat* (state or nation of cells), in which the cells rely on each other and every cell contributes to the whole like a citizen contributing to the state. In popular scientific literature, Virchow's metaphor was also interpreted in the opposite way: the organism became a model for society. His metaphor resonated with the idea of the 'social organism', incorporating increasingly materialistic and biologistic interpretations. During the debate on the observed declining birth rate in Germany in 1912, the population began to be seen by the state as a biological resource to be preserved at all costs. The economist Rudolf Goldscheid (1870–1931) created the concept of *Menschenökonomie* (people or population economics), according to which the population was capital not to be wasted.[63] This idea was interwoven with Social Darwinian and eugenicist thinking and was prevalent well before the rise of National Socialism and its focus on the *Volkskörper*, culminating in totalitarianism and the needs of the individual being subordinated to the needs of the whole.

Before the rise of the Nazis, the relationship between the individual and the collective may have been less extreme, but drinking was not considered a private matter either.[64] The individual's responsibility for the wellbeing of society was also emphasised in the German *Lebensreformbewegung* (life reform movement) of the late nineteenth and early twentieth centuries, for example. This believed that the individual could change society by following a return to a lifestyle that was more at one with nature. In its vision 'life' was a spiritualistic concept in the Romantic tradition, and it appealed to intellectuals and bourgeois elite groups.[65]

From a more moral-pragmatic perspective, Kraepelin noted that in a society where alcohol was widely consumed, individuals were exposed to certain risks, such as becoming victims of accidents or violent crimes.[66] In a similar vein, Bunge therefore regarded his dedication to abstinence as a 'right to self-defence'.[67] In 1900 Heinrich Quensel, a civil servant in Cologne, also stressed the close link between the individual and society. He blamed alcohol for diminishing 'the entire capacity of the individual and of the whole of society'.[68] He was particularly concerned about economic disadvantages that affected not only the individual, but also the general public. These were manifest in the reduced productivity of the individual, increased costs of health insurance and a heightened risk of accidents. Quensel even regarded families as a type of collective that were prevented from making worthwhile investments if one member was an alcoholic. Alcohol thus also undermined future potential. In regard to the nation, Quensel postulated a general weakening of the *Volkskraft* (people's strength) because any cereals used for alcohol production were not available for *Volksnahrung* (people's food).[69] For him, alcoholism undermined the foundations of life. The money lost through alcohol would be better spent on the war fleet, Quensel suggested. Quensel's thinking and that of many of his contemporaries was guided by Social Darwinism, with the 'struggle for existence' and the 'survival of the fittest' becoming core principles. They saw alcoholism as a barrier to further social development. In the resulting eugenicist thinking, the individual was subordinated to the species and became the physical resource of a whole integrated societal entity.[70] From a demographic point of view, the population was the decisive factor on which the wealth of the nation was built, and, as Weipert has shown, efforts were made to improve this resource and increase its efficiency.[71]

Within this wider context, scientists, such as the Austrian bacteriologist and hygienist Max von Gruber (1853–1927), advocated a society of 'people voluntarily serving the whole'.[72] Gruber asked: 'Is our nation healthy in every respect?'[73] According to the metaphor of the *Volkskörper* or people's body, he understood any rise in the number of ill or weak individuals as a sign of a nation's disease. He referred to an increase in mental illnesses, disabilities and suicides, describing one-third of school-age children as sickly and weak, over 40 per cent of men as unfit for military service and a large number of young women as no longer able to breastfeed their children.[74] Morbidity statistics were part of the eugenicist reasoning Gruber pursued in his particularly severe form of racial hygiene. Gruber's main concern was the nation as a whole, not the individual. In 1909 he mused:

> Can the German people still be described as healthy despite all this? The *Volkskörper* will probably always have to bear a certain number of weaklings and cripples and sick people and parasites, and it can obviously bear them without suffering too much or even being fatally threatened. But they always constitute a heavy burden, which impairs its strength and ability to perform, and we must always pay attention to whether the evils grow or disappear.[75]

Degeneration: physical, mental and moral

The French psychiatrist Benedict Augustin Morel (1809–1873) had previously postulated the inheritability of bad characteristics, inborn or acquired (through poisoning, illness or adverse social environments). He predicted that they would develop progressively until the human race was extinguished.[76] On this basis, protagonists of abstinence postulated the heredity of mental illnesses acquired through alcoholic intoxication. This assumption chimed in well with the Neo-Lamarckian view that Abraham Baer had adopted during the 1870s:

> Everything that downgrades the individual's organism in its quality and degrades individuality has the consequence that the quality of the offspring also becomes qualitatively bad and inferior. What applies to an individual also applies to a majority of individuals, to the family, to the lineage, to the nation, to the race.[77]

Gustav Bunge shared the idea of transmitted deterioration:

> In spite of an originally immaculate hereditary material, the individual and the entire generation can fail because of subsequent germ defects, and they can fail so badly that not only this one individual or this one generation becomes worse or bad, but the whole lineage permanently and to its ultimate failure.[78]

Degeneration in this sense led to the extinction of the nation or, in eugenicist terms, the race. Stopping alcoholism became an urgent task for the nation.

The connection between the individual and society had become particularly significant because of the idea of degeneration that flourished alongside Neo-Darwinian and eugenicist thinking. Degeneration was regarded as the worst problem resulting from alcoholism. Kraepelin suggested that alcohol was 'one of the most important causes of degeneration we know'.[79] Statistics and physiological observations obtained from autopsies of alcoholics seemed to substantiate this suggestion. However, most descriptions of damages inheritable through alcoholism remained largely unclear about what exactly would be inherited. It was speculated that an irreparable deterioration would ensue in the individual's organism as well as in society. Bunge claimed that 'The fight against no other misery tolerates as little delay as the fight against drinking, because it is hereditable. The misery caused by alcohol cannot be reversed afterwards.'[80] A popular example of physical degeneration was the enlarged and adipose 'beer heart' (see Figure 6.1), which Quensel illustrated in his *Der Alkohol und seine Gefahren* (Alcohol and its

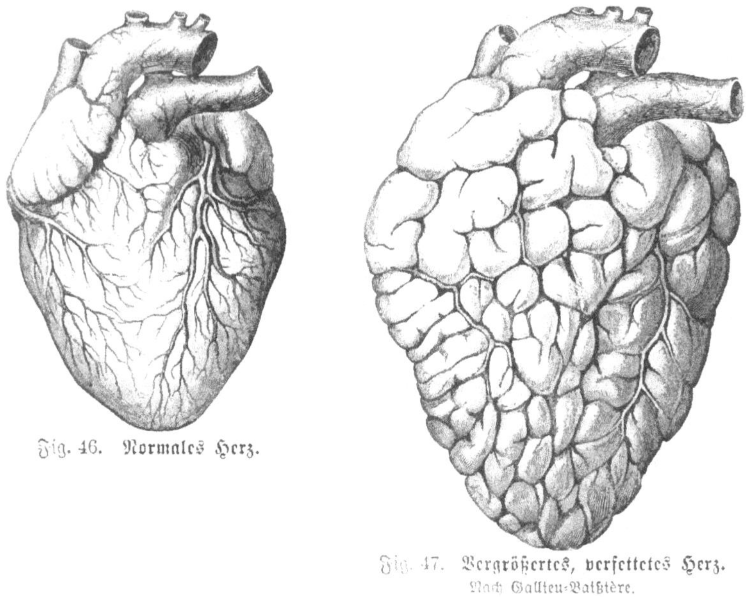

Figure 6.1 'The healthy heart and the "beer heart"'

Dangers).[81] Other popular medical self-help books used comparisons between diseased and healthy organs to raise awareness of the risks of regular drinking. In her famous publication *Die Frau als Hausärztin* (The Woman as Family Doctor) of 1911, the physician Anna Fischer-Dückelmann (1856–1917) exemplified with 'pictures from a drinker's life' (see Figure 6.2) the consequences of alcoholism for the general appearance of the drinker as well as the drinker's stomach and liver. Fischer-Dückelmann was one of the first female doctors practising in Germany. Her argument that moderate drinking would lead to alcoholism was based on statistical evidence.[82] She was not the only one to conclude that there was no such thing as harmless alcohol consumption.

In 1906 Auguste Forel coined the term 'blastophtory' to describe the 'poisoning of the germinating cells' by alcohol.[83] The Swiss physician Eduard Bertholet (1883–1965) pursued this thesis by physiologically investigating the effects of chronic alcoholism on the reproductive ability of men.[84] He identified four stages of

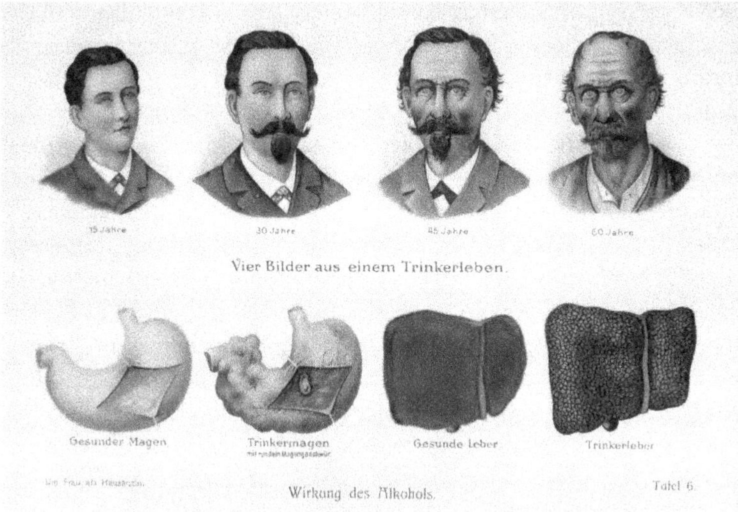

Figure 6.2 'Four pictures from a drinker's life'

alcohol-related fertility impairment. Those suffering from the two final stages he described as 'particularly dangerous for the future of the race, as they equip their offspring with many and varied infirmities'.[85] Bertholet described obesity and the loss of seminal filaments as typical damages to the reproductive organs caused by chronic alcoholism. The consequences for the offspring were vaguely summarised as weakened general constitution and reduced vitality. Bertholet conceded that other causes, such as tuberculosis, syphilis and a number of infectious diseases, could have a negative effect on reproductive ability. However, he stressed that their damaging effects 'could not be compared with the extremely severe degeneration caused by chronic alcoholism'.[86]

Not all alcoholics were equally affected by infertility, for only 17 per cent lacked the capacity to reproduce.[87] In Bertholet's view, the majority of alcoholics were therefore a problem for the health of society. Firstly, alcohol-induced damage to reproductive ability occurred gradually and was difficult to ascertain in the early phases. Secondly, according to him, alcoholics were particularly driven by their crude desires, frequently prone to *Eifersuchtswahn* (delusional jealousy) and hence all the more eager to reproduce.[88] For

Bertholet, not only contemporary society, but also the 'future of the race' was endangered by an accelerating process of genetic dissemination of the irrational.[89]

It is striking that the issue of alcoholism and pregnancy was not discussed widely. Bertholet focused predominantly on male reproductivity. The contemporary fear was that a man would damage the unborn child if it was conceived in drunkenness.[90] Overall, there was a gender bias in the alcohol debate, and it was mainly the effects of alcohol consumption on men that were investigated. Although it was less common for women to drink to excess, the overwhelming extent to which the alcohol debate concentrated on the male body, even within debates on reproduction, is striking. Max von Gruber took the extinction of the male line in Swedish noble families as an example of degeneration, pointing out that the sex ratio had gradually changed in favour of female descendants.[91] Male labour and soldiers and hence the economic and military capability of a nation seemed to weaken as well.[92] In regard to women, the ability to breastfeed and to give birth was considered to be affected by the alcohol problem, but it was assumed that morals still offered some protection against female alcoholism. As Gruber put it: 'In the abstinence or strict moderation of women we undoubtedly still have a valuable barrage at the moment against an even more rapid decay of the race.'[93] This supposition came to be challenged with the development of the women's emancipation movement and the expected participation of women in every part of social life. According to Kraepelin, degeneration had taken place at half of the expected rate on the basis that women consumed less alcohol than men. He considered that equality in drinking habits would be a deathblow for the people, so that 'the fate of our descendants would be sealed'.[94] This was especially so because alcoholism among women was regarded as having wider consequences in the shape of increased prostitution and sexually transmitted diseases. Moreover, female alcoholics were presented as particularly resistant to therapy, except hypnosis.[95] Kraepelin even perceived alcohol as an annihilator of masculine qualities such as 'clarity of thought, self-control, willpower and drive'.[96] At least since the Enlightenment, masculinity had been aligned with the rational. From the late nineteenth century, this connection was increasingly seen to have weakened, leading to a sense that society was disintegrating from the inside out.[97]

The technical and economic changes that rationalisation had brought about in society reminded Auguste Forel of 'an incurable internal infectious disease: emasculation, effeminacy and degeneration through sensual pleasures and destruction of ethics and of morals'.[98] According to Kraepelin, moral degeneration was visible in an individual's 'loss of joy in working', and in idleness, neglect of duty, divorce, economic distress, thievery and physical assault.[99] Degeneration was morally entwined with the decay of culture and tradition. The alcohol question became linked with the decline in birth rates, particularly from 1911 onwards, when a debate on birth rates coincided with the opening of the International Hygiene Exhibition in Dresden.[100] Both were interpreted as signifiers of moral decay. Von Gruber's work on alcohol and birth rates in particular represents the transition to racial hygiene. Together with Alfred Ploetz and Ernst Rüdin, he initiated the first exhibition of racial hygiene, which occurred at the same time as the International Hygiene Exhibition.[101] Gruber suggested: 'For me there is no doubt that the increasing tendencies to live unmarried and childless are only symptoms of this alcoholic depravation, and I consider this moral degeneration to be worse than any other causes of alcohol abuse!'[102]

During the late 1880s Bunge had already affirmed the contemporary idea that society was experiencing intellectual progress accompanied by moral decay. Although this process was perceived as a consequence of rationalisation, the ambition was to eliminate moral decay by rational means in order to effect intellectual and moral progress. But before this could be achieved, it was necessary to educate the public and press for total abstinence rather than mere moderation. As Bunge pointed out:

> Alcohol ... leads to the general crippling of the mind. ... The chronic, endemic anaesthesia and drowsiness does not allow the lack of morality to be recognised among the people. ... Where any desire for nobler pleasures emerges, it is washed away by the uninterrupted stream of beer.[103]

Only abstinence could ensure the moral progress of mankind.

Bunge was also at the forefront of debates on the link between moral and mental degeneration. The hereditary nature of mental illnesses was discussed particularly in regard to nervousness and delirium. Bunge noted: 'Almost all physicians agree that many of these diseases, especially the multiple nervous diseases acquired by alcohol – from the slightest nervousness to the most obvious insanity – are highly hereditary.'[104] As Radkau showed in *Das Zeitalter der Nervosität* (The Age of Nervousness) in 1998, alcohol was also seen to be involved in neurasthenia.[105]

Furthermore, a vaguely conceptualised tendency to drink, the addiction itself, was regarded as transferable to offspring. And even 'vice', in the form of moral degeneration, returned to the alcohol debate after an interlude when the idea of alcoholism as a disease had been predominant, concomitant to the medicalisation of the alcohol discourse following Magnus Huss's coining of the term 'chronic alcoholism' in 1849. The alcoholic once again became seen as immoral, albeit not within a purely religious framework. While lack of self-control had previously been considered as a sin, now hereditary alcoholism enshrined three forms of degeneration – physical, mental and moral.

Nearly three decades after Bunge, in 1912, Auguste Forel examined the effects of alcohol on mental illness in more detail. As a hypnosis expert and brain researcher, he considered 'brain degeneration' to be the most severe stage of alcohol abuse. Alcoholism was a slow and gradual process in which

> the drinker becomes more and more rough, sensually driven, brutal, ethically defect, untruthful, impudent until a small weakness ... leads to an outbreak of delirium. Chronic brain poisoning gets worse, deliria become continuous, and the patient dies of suicide or in a seizure or he becomes incurably insane and ends up in an asylum.[106]

As the inheritability of mental illness became a central aspect of his research, eugenicist thinking became increasingly important to his argumentation. As Bugmann has shown, Forel changed his 1891 designation of alcohol from 'brain poison' to 'racial poison' within just the few years in 1908.[107]

Nations in competition

Degeneration was seen to affect the physical and mental health of the nation, leading to a decay of morality in society. This stood in contrast to the idea of a progressive process of 'social evolution' in which the nations were in constant competition.[108] Kraepelin underlined this when he claimed: 'The demands on the nations in their hard struggle for existence are constantly growing.'[109] The German Emperor Wilhelm II emphasised the nation's need for 'strong nerves and a clear mind' in times of peace, but even more in times of war, because the next war was expected to be a 'modern war' and therefore completely different from previous wars.[110] The Emperor's words 'The nation that consumes the smallest amount of alcohol wins' became a popular slogan.[111] In this view inclining towards Social Darwinism, hereditary mental illnesses could possibly lead to extinction.

By the 1910s, attention to 'population' had become key to the survival of the nation in order to succeed in the competition with other nations. In Germany, the aspiration to become a global power was encapsulated in the terms *Weltgeltung* (world or global recognition) and *Weltpolitik* (world or global politics). A conflict between Western civilisation and German culture, in which the Germans had to succeed, was assumed.[112] With a world war looming on the horizon, a large and healthy population was therefore required to secure the nation's 'position as a great cultural power' and its autonomy in the future.[113] But even beyond a war, the 'struggle for existence' was considered to remain a vital issue. As Bunge put it in 1886,

> But it is not only the fight with cannons and bayonets that brings the foul to light. It also emerges in the no less murderous and merciless, so-called 'peaceful competition', which the nations fight against each other in economic matters. It is generally acknowledged that in the struggle of the Semitic race with the nations of Europe the sobriety and abstinence of the former is the main weapon.[114]

While ideas about racial competition and anti-Semitism were rife during the late German Empire, Jews such as the physician and

Zionist Max Nordau embraced similarly evolutionist and racist language by creating a positive stereotype: the *Muskeljude* (muscle or athletic Jew).[115] In 1911 the German sociologist Werner Sombart postulated a 'rationalisation of life' in Judaism.[116] Sombart claimed that the Jews had chosen a rational way of life through strict religious regulations, which had a beneficial effect on their efficiency and the preservation of the population. His ideas were highly controversial and problematic. Even contemporaries were not sure whether his work, which was full of racist statements and attributions, could be interpreted philo-Semitically or anti-Semitically. Importantly, the debates reveal the complexity of contemporary assumptions about an all-pervasive rationalisation process and prevalent concerns about population growth. Alcohol discourse could not but be affected by these varied ideas. For example, Bunge suggested that anti-Semites should 'refrain from disgusting beer drinking' in order to enter into the 'peaceful competition' to increase labour and population.[117] As in the debates about birth rates, competition in reproduction, in which the survival of a nation was built on an increase in population, was alluded to here.

The competition between nations also had ramifications in the sphere of colonialism. Here abstinence seemed to provide advantages. Bunge noted:

> It is known that the German in America, despite all Germanic virtues, disappears among the other nations mainly because he is so inseparably attached to his beer mug. In the 'peaceful competitions' of the nations, this race, which does not want to let go of alcohol, will be mercilessly trampled underfoot.[118]

According to Bunge, alcohol had posed an obstacle to successful colonisation long before the German Empire announced its colonial ambitions in 1897. Moderate alcohol consumption impeded the influence of German immigrants in the emerging USA and hence the progress of the entire American nation. German immigrants were held responsible for making regular beer consumption in North America socially acceptable and for unsettling the exemplary progress of the temperance movement.[119] Nevertheless, America and England were regarded as Germany's major competitors and as exemplary when it came to temperance. The Christian abstinence campaigner Paul Wurster suggested in 1911 that Germany had to catch up in order to compete on the global market and improve the *Volkskraft und Volksgesundheit* (the people's and the nation's power and health).[120] Even the creation of a 'New Man' was mooted to prevent degeneration and extinction.

The ideal of a 'New Man' became particularly prevalent in totalitarian systems during the twentieth century. Radical as well as conservative ideologies pursued this kind of human self-optimisation. This kind of thinking, which reached its peak in twentieth-century totalitarian Germany, had originated in the 1890s, when high hopes were pinned on the role of the younger generation.[121] In 1910 Kraepelin appealed to young people to remain abstinent:

> In the struggle against alcohol, we need the help of a new generation. … They will be responsible for curbing the terrible misery that alcohol produces in our nation, for draining the sources of poison that flood our veins. A new generation must grow up whose brain is not stifled by a hangover, which with a clear glance recognises the misery of our people, and with a firm hand eradicates the insolent parasite that every year cheats innumerable thousands among us out of health and good fortune![122]

Constant vigilance could be achieved only through educational work. The young were supposed to generate 'goal-oriented fighters' who would not only fight against the temptations of alcohol, but also participate in the competition of cultures.[123] Gruber mirrored these ideas in 1909 when he demanded the 'production of a physically, mentally and morally capable humanity' as well as 'enthusiasm for human perfection'.[124] His desire for perfecting humankind through outside intervention matched his idea of racial hygiene and eugenics nearly two decades before the rise of National Socialism.

Abstinence was clearly not regarded as a value in itself by people like Kraepelin, and Forel had warned that abstinence should not become idolised. Like progress in cultural development, it served to 'achieve higher purposes'.[125] Forel clarified what he was aiming at: 'We don't want to become contemplative ascetics, but lively, active people who can love, sing, exercise, ride, fight, and then certainly win the struggle for existence.'[126] His aspirations to improve humanity and cultural development formed the theoretical basis for radical measures such as forced sterilisation of patients in the Burghölzli psychiatric institution, which Forel managed.[127]

Science was expected to correct undesirable cultural developments. In Forel's words, 'It is a difficult and important task of the future social sciences to adapt family life more and more to the higher social interests of all people. This is unavoidable in the further development of our social body.'[128] Forel's trust in the power of science was demonstrated not least by the fact that he motivated his students to test the positive effects of abstinence for themselves. In fact, in the 1890s, Forel implemented the kind of mass educational work that Bunge had demanded a decade earlier.[129] He addressed his student listeners in Uppsala as 'human material' that should carefully choose suitable women as the 'breeding choice of the future'.[130] Teaching staff were urged to convey the message of abstinence to pupils.[131] Such appeals to youth embodied the hope that the alcohol problem could be solved through science and education. They were located firmly within eugenicist thinking.

The idea of alcohol as a 'nerve poison' that infiltrates the life forces led the protagonists of abstinence to the conclusion that a fundamental renewal of life was necessary. Just as evolution seemed to demand constant adaptation, cultural progress could be achieved through the education of young people. In 1910 the judge and member of the Guttempler temperance movement Hermann Popert (1871–1932) wrote a novel featuring a teetotal hero named Helmut Harringa who became a popular model for this way of living. Harringa, a North Frisian, represents the 'Deutschtum der Werdenden' (Germanness of the new generation to be).[132] He repeatedly encounters the negative effects of alcohol abuse throughout the plot. The novel was part of the emerging *völkische Bewegung* (people's national movement) and was well received in the *Jugendbewegung* (Youth Movement).[133] The teacher Robert Theuermeister followed a similar path in his novels directed at young people. Under the pseudonym Karl Albert Schöllenbach, in 1915 he published the novel *Wilm Heinrich Berthold*, which was partly autobiographical and was focused on an abstinent protagonist.[134] Although his work has fallen into oblivion, Theuermeister is considered an important author of the Youth Movement.[135] Abstinence had been a theme in literature earlier. In 1889 the famous novelist and dramatist Gerhart Hauptmann (1862–1946) wrote a drama in which the protagonist Loth leaves the love of his life because he fears the alcoholic degeneration of her family.[136] Hauptmann's socially critical drama constitutes an important contribution to literary naturalism, and he received international recognition when he was awarded the Nobel Prize for Literature in 1912. He was close to the life reform movement at Monte Verità, where alternative ways of life were explored.[137]

Conclusion

The alcohol debates among medical experts during the period from the 1870s to the 1910s followed from the ideas promulgated by Abraham Baer. Baer's successors anticipated that the detrimental effects of alcohol would accelerate more quickly than he had assumed. Alcoholism was seen as shackled to modern life and a misguided process of rationalisation. It was also feared that alcoholism would develop its own momentum and thwart the prospect of a progressive and rational future. Alcoholism was described as an insidious process. Mass culture was held responsible for the promotion of widespread alcohol consumption. Because the damage caused by alcohol consumption had been scientifically proven, drinking was considered an irrational behaviour of the masses based on bad habits and customs. Modern lifestyles led to alcoholism because alcohol offered an escape from increased technological rationalisation.

For many experts the solution to the alcohol problem lay in the mutual relationship of the individual and public health. Some promoted abstinence for the sake of solidarity, while others refused to regard drinking as merely a private matter. Within the wider context of emerging ideas of a 'social organism' and a *Volkskörper*, the way alcoholism was perceived changed considerably. Eugenicist thinking entered the discourse on alcohol, and the needs and actions of the individual became subordinated to the wellbeing of the whole. While during the alcohol debates of the 1830s and 1840s drunkenness was identified as the root of social problems, from the 1870s to the 1910s it was seen as a cause of degeneration.

Degeneration took many shapes and forms. Physical decay, the 'beer heart', long-term addiction and bad sperm cells were seen as signs of physical degeneration. The decline of culture and of the modern lifestyle – especially among women – was attributed to moral degeneration. Mental degeneration, caused by inheritance of mental diseases and addiction itself, was considered particularly serious. These ideas also had an effect on and fostered certain politics. Within the context of the 'competition of nations', a rational lifestyle became essential. Abstinence would facilitate colonisation and ensure the survival of the nation and 'the race' in the future. In order to achieve this goal, it was necessary to educate the young generation to remain abstinent. Finally, as Social Darwinian and eugenicist thinking became central to debates on alcohol, the ideal of a 'New Man' emerged, and abstemious heroes appeared even in contemporary popular literature.

The debates that raged over a period of about four decades can arguably be seen to have culminated in the idea of the rationalisation of the irrational. The aim was to turn the irrational 'masses' into a controlled and controllable population. The discourse on the 'rationalisation of birth control' was closely enmeshed with the discussions on alcohol. Mental illnesses and many other diseases were considered avoidable through abstinence rather than mere moderation. The iconic International Hygiene Exhibition in Dresden in 1911 aimed to create further insights into disease causation and, not least, into the link between mental illness and alcohol. The individual became responsible for the health of the nation. Alcoholism could be thwarted, and thus the nation's mind could be saved.

Notes

1 In a broader context, I examine the significance of the discourse on rationalisation around 1900 in my PhD project, which is part of the research project 'Semantische Transformationen im 20. Jahrhundert' headed by Christian Geulen and sponsored by the DFG (German Research Foundation).

2 Heinrich Tappe, *Auf dem Weg zur modernen Alkoholkultur. Alkoholproduktion, Trinkverhalten und Temperenzbewegung in*

Deutschland vom frühen 19. Jahrhundert bis zum Ersten Weltkrieg (Stuttgart: Franz Steiner Verlag, 1994); Hasso Spode, *Die Macht der Trunkenheit: Kultur- und Sozialgeschichte des Alkohols in Deutschland* (Opladen: Leske & Budrich, 1993); Wolfgang Schivelbusch, *Das Paradies, der Geschmack und die Vernunft. Eine Geschichte der Genußmittel* (Frankfurt am Main: Fischer, 1992). For a biopolitical perspective on abstinence see Mirjam Bugmann, *Hypnosepolitik. Der Psychiater August Forel, das Gehirn und die Gesellschaft (1870–1920)* (Cologne, Weimar, and Vienna: Böhlau, 2015), 8. Bugmann interprets abstinence as an instrument for biopolitical intervention.

3 For conceptual history approaches see Reinhart Koselleck, 'Einleitung', in Reinhart Koselleck, Werner Conze and Otto Brunner (eds), *Geschichtliche Grundbegriffe. Historisches Lexikon zur politisch-sozialen Sprache in Deutschland*, vol. 1 (Stuttgart: Klett-Cotta, 1972), xiii–xxvii. With regard to the twentieth century see Stefan-Ludwig Hoffmann, Kathrin Kollmeier, Willibald Steinmetz, Philipp Sarasin, Alf Lüdtke and Christian Geulen, 'Geschichtliche Grundbegriffe reloaded?', *Contributions to the History of Concepts*, 7, no. 2 (2012), 78–128. Alcohol has rarely been a separate topic in the history of concepts. Recently, alcohol has been discussed from a conceptual history perspective in the context of public health: Johannes Kananen, Sophy Bergenheim and Merle Wessel (eds), *Conceptualising Public Health: Historical and Contemporary Struggles over Key Concepts* (Abingdon and New York, 2018).

4 Tappe, *Auf dem Weg zur modernen Alkoholkultur*, 306, 331, 338.

5 Ibid., 310.

6 Hasso Spode, *Die Macht der Trunkenheit*, 204–5.

7 Tappe, *Auf dem Weg zur modernen Alkoholkultur*, 354–5.

8 Spode, *Die Macht der Trunkenheit*, 255.

9 Tappe, *Auf dem Weg zur modernen Alkoholkultur*, 300–5.

10 Ibid.

11 Ibid., 354–5, 280.

12 Spode, *Die Macht der Trunkenheit*, 217–34.

13 Ibid., 13–14, 199–202.

14 Judith Große, Francesco Spöring and Jana Tschurenev, 'Einleitung: Sittlichkeitsreform, Biopolitik und Globalisierung', in Judith Große, Francesco Spöring and Jana Tschurenev (eds), *Biopolitik und Sittlichkeitsreform: Kampagnen gegen Alkohol, Drogen und Prostitution 1880–1950* (Frankfurt and New York: Campus, 2014), 7–46, at 20–1; Harry G. Levine, ,The discovery of addiction: changing

conceptions of habitual drunkenness in America', *Journal of Studies on Alcohol*, 39, no. 1 (1978), 143–74.

15 Christoph Wilhelm Hufeland, *Ueber die Vergiftung durch Branntwein* (Berlin, 1802), 6, 8. Translations are by the author except where otherwise stated.

16 Constantin von Brühl-Cramer, *Ueber die Trunksucht und eine rationelle Heilmethode derselben. Geschrieben zur Beherzigung für Jedermann. Mit einem Vorwort von Dr. C.W. Hufeland* (Berlin: In der Nicolaischen Buchhandlung, 1819), iv, viii.

17 Ibid.

18 Magnus Huss, *Chronische Alkoholskrankheit oder Alcoholismus Chronicus. Ein Beitrag zur Kenntnis der Vergiftungs-Krankheiten, nach eigener und anderer Erfahrung*, trans. Gerhard van dem Busch (Stockholm and Leipzig: C.E. Fritze, 1852), ii, 3.

19 Spode, *Die Macht der Trunkenheit*, 124–33.

20 'Trunkenheit', in *Pierer's Universal-Lexikon der Vergangenheit und Gegenwart*, 4th edn, vol. 17 (Altenburg: Verlagsbuchhandlung H.A. Pierer, 1863), 877; 'Trunksucht', in *Meyers Großes Konversations-Lexikon. Ein Nachschlagewerk des allgemeinen Wissens*, 6th edn, vol. 19 (Leipzig and Vienna: Bibliographisches Institut, 1908), 758–9; 'Alkoholismus', in *Brockhaus' Kleines Konversations-Lexikon*, 5th edn, vol. 1 (Leipzig: F.A. Brockhaus, 1911), 44. Furthermore, the noun 'alcoholic' (*Alkoholiker*) emerged at the end of the century to describe a 'person addicted to alcoholic drinks'. 'Alcoholic, adj. and n.', in *Oxford English Dictionary Online*, 3rd edn (Oxford: Oxford University Press, 2012), www.oed.com/viewdictionaryentry/Entry/4706 (accessed 24 March 2020).

21 Abraham Adolf Baer, *Der Verbrecher in anthropologischer Beziehung* (Leipzig: Verlag von Georg Thieme, 1893); Abraham Adolf Baer, *Die Gefängnisse, Strafanstalten und Strafsysteme. Ihre Einrichtung und Wirkung in hygienischer Beziehung* (Berlin: T.C.F. Enslin, 1871).

22 'Mäßigkeits- und Abstinenzbestrebungen', in *Meyers Großes Konversations-Lexikon. Ein Nachschlagewerk des allgemeinen Wissens*, 6th edn, vol. 13 (Leipzig and Vienna: Bibliographisches Institut, 1906), 409–12.

23 Abraham Adolf Baer, *Der Alcoholismus, seine Verbreitung und Wirkung auf den individuellen und socialen Organismus, sowie die Mittel, ihn zu bekämpfen* (Berlin: Verlag von August Hirschwald, 1878), 546.

24 Ibid.

25 Alfred Vierkandt, *Naturvölker und Kulturvölker. Ein Beitrag zur Socialpsychologie* (Leipzig: Duncker & Humblot, 1896), 406.

26 Werner Sombart, *Die Juden und das Wirtschaftsleben* (Leipzig: Duncker & Humblot, 1911), 261.

27 Julius Wolf, *Der Geburtenrückgang. Die Rationalisierung des Sexuallebens in unserer Zeit* (Jena: Gustav Fischer, 1912), 3.

28 Geoff Eley, Jennifer L. Jenkins and Tracie Matysik, 'Introduction: German modernities and the contest of futures', in Geoff Eley, Jennifer L. Jenkins and Tracie Matysik (eds), *German Modernities from Wilhelm to Weimar: A Contest of Futures* (London and New York: Bloomsbury, 2016), 1–29, at 3.

29 Helene Breitung, *Unterrichtsstunden für abstinente Jugendvereine* (Heidelberg: Neutraler Guttempler-Verlag, 1912), 25.

30 Ibid.

31 Anson Rabinbach, *The Human Motor: Energy, Fatigue, and the Origins of Modernity* (Berkeley and Los Angeles: University of California Press, 1990), 1–19.

32 Gustav von Bunge, *Die Alkoholfrage: Ein Vortrag. Nebst einem Anhang: Ein Wort an die Arbeiter* (Basel: Neuland-Verlag, 1921 [1886]), 21.

33 Emil Kraepelin, *Alkohol und Jugend. Nach einem Vortrag vor den Oberklassen der Heidelberger Mittelschulen* (Basel: Verlag der Schriftstelle des Alkoholgegnerbundes, 1913), 11.

34 Alfred Heggen, *Alkohol und bürgerliche Gesellschaft im 19. Jahrhundert. Eine Studie zur deutschen Sozialgeschichte* (Berlin: Colloquium-Verlag, 1988), 118; Judith Baumgartner, 'Antialkoholbewegung', in Diethart Kerbs and Jürgen Reulecke (eds), *Handbuch der deutschen Reformbewegungen. 1880–1933* (Wuppertal: Hammer, 1998), 141–54, at 142–3; Hasso Spode, 'Germany', in Jack S. Blocker, Jr, David M. Fahey and Ian R. Tyrrell (eds), *Alcohol and Temperance in Modern History: An International Encyclopedia* (Santa Barbara, Denver and Oxford: ABC-CLIO, 2003), vol. 1, 257–63.

35 Tappe, *Auf dem Weg zur modernen Alkoholkultur*, 228–31.

36 Baer, *Der Alcoholismus*, 141–377.

37 As early as 1882, Baer is quoted as a reference in the article on alcoholism in the prominent *Brockhaus* encyclopaedia. 'Alkoholismus', in *Brockhaus' Conversations-Lexikon. Allgemeine deutsche Real-Encyklopädie in sechzehn Bänden*, 13th edn, vol. 1 (Leipzig: F.A. Brockhaus, 1882), 427–9.

38 Many of Forel's books were first published in Germany, e.g. *Der Hypnotismus. Seine Bedeutung und seine Handhabung. In kurzgefasster Darstellung* (Stuttgart: Ferdinand Enke, 1889); *Hygiene der*

Nerven und des Geistes im gesunden und kranken Zustande (Stuttgart: Ernst Heinrich Moritz, 1905); *Die sexuelle Frage. Eine naturwissenschaftliche, psychologische, hygienische und soziologische Studie für Gebildete* (Munich: Ernst Reinhardt, 1907).

39 Bunge, *Die Alkoholfrage*, 21.

40 Emil Kraepelin, *Alkohol und Jugend. Nach einem Vortrag vor den Oberklassen der Heidelberger Mittelschulen* (Basel: Verlag der Schriftstelle des Alkoholgegnerbundes, 1913), 9.

41 Richard J. Evans, *Death in Hamburg: Society and Politics in the Cholera Years, 1830–1910* (Oxford: Clarendon Press, 1987).

42 Auguste Forel, *Hygiene of Nerves and Mind in Health and Disease*, trans. Herbert Austin Aitkins (New York and London: The Knickerbocker Press, 1907), 194.

43 More recently, Susan Sontag has used the term 'illness as metaphor'. However, Forel's usage of the metaphor of national disease involved a more straightforward relocation of focus, from the individual's illness on to society, involving social decay. Although Forel associated alcoholism also with moral decline, his primary concern was not with the effects on the individual.

44 Alfred Grotjahn, *Alkohol-Genuß, Alkohol-Mißbrauch: Ein hygienisches Merkbüchlein für das werktätige Volk* (Berlin and Paris: Verlag Joh. Sassenbach, 1900), 4.

45 Bunge, *Die Alkoholfrage*, 14.

46 Reinhart Koselleck, Fritz Gschnitzer, Karl Ferdinand Werner and Bernd Schönemann, 'Volk, Nation, Nationalismus, Masse', in Koselleck, Conze and Brunner (eds), *Geschichtliche Grundbegriffe*, vol. 7 (Stuttgart: Klett-Cotta, 1992), 141–431, at 246, 366–8.

47 Stefanie Middendorf, 'Masse', version 1.0, *Docupedia-Zeitgeschichte*, 5 November 2013, http://docupedia.de/zg/middendorf_masse_v1_de_2013 (accessed 19 October 2020).

48 Bunge, *Die Alkoholfrage*, 22.

49 Ibid., 27.

50 Rabinbach, *The Human Motor*, 150–2. Emil Kraepelin published several studies on measuring physical and mental work (e.g. he had students do simple addition tasks): Emil Kraepelin, *Ueber geistige Arbeit* (Jena: Gustav Fischer, 1894); Emil Kraepelin, *Ueber die Beeinflussung einfacher psychischer Vorgänge durch einige Arzneimittel. Experimentelle Untersuchungen* (Jena: Gustav Fischer, 1892); Emil Kraepelin and August Hoch, *Über die Wirkung der Theebestandtheile auf körperliche und geistige Arbeit* (Leipzig: Wilhelm Engelmann, 1895).

51 Auguste Forel, *Die Trinksitten. Ihre hygienische und sociale Bedeutung, ihre Beziehungen zur akademischen Jugend* (Stuttgart: Verlag von Ferdinand Enke, 1891), 10.
52 Paul Wurster, *Kurzgefasste Geschichte der Antialkoholbewegung im 19. Jahrhundert* (Reutlingen: Mimir, 1911), 22.
53 Forel, *Die Trinksitten*, 22–3.
54 Ibid.
55 Gustave Le Bon, *Psychologie des foules* (Paris: Félix Alcan, 1895), 24. An English translation was published as *The Crowd: A Study of the Popular Mind* (London: T. Fisher Unwin, 1896).
56 Gustave Le Bon, *Psychologie der Massen*, trans. Rudolf Eisler (Leipzig: Verlag Werner Klinkhardt, 1908).
57 Bunge, *Die Alkoholfrage*, 21.
58 Ibid.
59 Kraepelin, *Alkohol und Jugend*, 7.
60 Forel, *Hygiene of Nerves and Mind*, 194.
61 As cited in Baumgartner, 'Antialkoholbewegung', 147. Forel agreed with his statement on moderate drinking: 'In short, temperance as a common habit leads with mathematical exactness to immoderation and to a slow, unnoticed physical and moral degeneration of the nation.' Forel, *Die Trinksitten*, 10.
62 Baer, *Der Alcoholismus*.
63 Thorsten Halling, Julia Schäfer and Jörg Vögele, 'Volk, Volkskörper, Volkswirtschaft – Bevölkerungsfragen in Forschung und Lehre von Nationalökonomie und Medizin', in Rainer Mackensen and Jürgen Reulecke (eds), *Das Konstrukt 'Bevölkerung' vor, im und nach dem 'Dritten Reich'* (Wiesbaden: VS Verlag für Sozialwissenschaften), 388–428; Matthias Weipert, *'Mehrung der Volkskraft': Die Debatte über Bevölkerung, Modernisierung und Nation 1890–1933* (Paderborn, Munich and Vienna and Zürich: Schöningh, 2006), 143–4.
64 Weipert, *'Mehrung der Volkskraft'*, 141.
65 In England, a similar movement did not have this holistic commitment. See Thomas Rohkrämer, 'Gab es eine Lebensreformbewegung in England?', in Marc Cluet and Catherine Repussard (eds), *'Lebensreform'. Die soziale Dynamik der politischen Ohnmacht. La dynamique sociale de l'impuissance politique* (Tübingen: Francke, 2013), 319–35.
66 Kraepelin, *Alkohol und Jugend*, 10–11.
67 Bunge, *Die Alkoholfrage*, 20.
68 Heinrich Quensel, *Der Alkohol und seine Gefahren. Zugleich ein Beitrag zur Bekämpfung der Alkoholsucht als Volkskrankheit* (Cologne: Greven & Bechthold, 1900), 7.

69 Ibid., 23–4.
70 Peter Weingart, Jürgen Kroll and Kurt Bayertz, *Rasse, Blut und Gene. Geschichte der Eugenik und Rassenhygiene in Deutschland* (Frankfurt am Main: Suhrkamp, 1992), 18.
71 Weipert, *'Mehrung der Volkskraft'*, 233–5.
72 Max von Gruber, *Volkswohlfahrt und Alkoholismus* (Berlin: Deutscher Verlag für Volkswohlfahrt, 1909), 3.
73 Ibid.
74 Ibid., 5.
75 Ibid.
76 Weingart, Kroll and Bayertz, *Rasse, Blut und Gene*, 47–50.
77 Baer, *Der Alcoholismus*, 268.
78 Bunge, *Die Alkoholfrage*, 19.
79 Kraepelin, *Alkohol und Jugend*, 7.
80 Bunge, *Die Alkoholfrage*, 28.
81 Quensel, *Der Alkohol*, 15.
82 Anna Fischer-Dückelmann, *Die Frau als Hausärztin* (Stuttgart: Süddeutsches Verlags-Institut, 1911).
83 Auguste Forel, 'Vorwort', in Eduard Bertholet, *Die Wirkung des chronischen Alkoholismus auf die Organe des Menschen, insbesondere auf die Geschlechtsdrüsen. Autorisierte Übersetzung mit Ergänzungen von Dr. med. Alfred Pfleiderer. Mit einem Vorwort von Prof. Dr. August Forel* (Stuttgart: Mimir, 1913), 7; Natalia Gerodetti, *Modernizing Sexualities: Towards a Socio-Historical Understanding of Sexualities in the Swiss Nation* (Bern: Peter Lang, 2005), 175–9; Jakob Tanner, '"Keimgifte" und "Rassendegeneration". Zum Drogendiskurs und den gesellschaftlichen Ordnungsvorstellungen der Eugenik', *Itinera*, 21 (1999), 249–58.
84 Bertholet, *Die Wirkung*, 35. The reason for this was the idea of being part of a process in which it was now necessary to secure the 'future of the race' by making it possible to pass on the positive traits that had been produced so far, and to maintain the potential of a further development of the race: 'In their wonderfully fine structure, these gametes enclose the whole future and power of our race and they are, in short, the seat of the "hereditary engrams", i.e., the seat of everything that has developed and is to continue to develop by way of inheritance of the characteristic features of our race.' Ibid., 66. Like Gruber, Bertholet ascribed the basis of all possible cultural development to the germ cells. If these foundations were damaged or even destroyed, cultural development would not take place.
85 Ibid., 52.

86 Ibid., 59–60.
87 Ibid., 67.
88 Ibid., 68.
89 Ibid., 52.
90 Joachim Radkau, *Das Zeitalter der Nervosität. Deutschland zwischen Bismarck und Hitler* (Munich and Vienna: Carl Hanser Verlag, 1998), 168.
91 Gruber, *Volkswohlfahrt und Alkoholismus*, 11–16.
92 Ibid., 5; Quensel, *Der Alkohol*, 23–4.
93 Gruber, *Volkswohlfahrt und Alkoholismus*, 27.
94 Kraepelin, *Alkohol und Jugend*, 7–8.
95 Bertholet, *Die Wirkung*, 72–4. On the rare treatment of female alcoholics in the Burghölzli asylum directed by Forel see Bugmann, *Hypnosepolitik*, 156–7.
96 Kraepelin, *Alkohol und Jugend*, 3–4.
97 Cornelia Klinger, 'Von der Gottesebenbildlichkeit zur Affentragödie. Über Veränderungen im Männlichkeitskonzept an der Wende zum 20. Jahrhundert', in Ulrike Brunotte and Rainer Herrn (eds), *Männlichkeiten und Moderne. Geschlecht in den Wissenskulturen um 1900* (Bielefeld: transcript, 2008), 25–36, at 25–7.
98 Forel, *Die Trinksitten*, 28.
99 Kraepelin, *Alkohol und Jugend*, 8.
100 Karl Oldenberg, 'Ueber den Rückgang der Geburten- und Sterbeziffer', *Archiv für Sozialwissenschaft und Sozialpolitik*, 32 (1911), 319–77; Julius Wolf, *Der Geburtenrückgang. Die Rationalisierung des Sexuallebens in unserer Zeit* (Jena: Gustav Fischer, 1912); Max Hirsch, 'Der Geburtenrückgang. Etwas über seine Ursachen und die gesetzgeberischen Maßnahmen zu seiner Bekämpfung', *Archiv für Rassen- und Gesellschaftsbiologie einschließlich Rassen- und Gesellschaftshygiene*, 5, no. 8 (1911), 628–54; Alfred Grotjahn, *Soziale Pathologie. Versuch einer Lehre von den sozialen Beziehungen der menschlichen Krankheiten als Grundlage der sozialen Medizin und der sozialen Hygiene* (Berlin and Heidelberg: Hirschwald, 1911).
101 Weingart, Kroll and Bayertz, *Rasse, Blut und Gene*, 206–7.
102 Gruber, *Volkswohlfahrt und Alkoholismus*, 30.
103 Bunge, *Die Alkoholfrage*, 21.
104 Ibid., 12.
105 Radkau, *Das Zeitalter der Nervosität,* 167.
106 Forel, *Die Trinksitten*, 18.
107 Bugmann, *Hypnosepolitik*, 52.
108 With special regard to economics, Rudolf Goldscheid discussed

the connection between cultural development and national competition. See Rudolf Goldscheid, *Entwicklungswerttheorie, Entwicklungsökonomie, Menschenökonomie. Eine Programmschrift* (Leipzig: Verlag Werner Klinkhardt, 1908); with regard to demography see Grotjahn, *Soziale Pathologie*, 487, 499.

109 Kraepelin, *Alkohol und Jugend*, 16.

110 As cited in Alexander Lion and Maximilian Bayer, *Jungdeutschlands Pfadfinderbuch*, 5th edn (Berlin and Heidelberg: Springer-Verlag, 1914), 156.

111 Ibid.

112 Jörg Fisch, 'Zivilisation, Kultur', in Brunner, Conze and Koselleck (eds), *Geschichtliche Grundbegriffe*, vol. 7, 679–774.

113 Gruber, *Volkswohlfahrt und Alkoholismus*, 8.

114 Bunge, *Die Alkoholfrage*, 18.

115 Christoph Schulte, *Psychopathologie des Fin de Siècle. Der Kulturkritiker, Arzt und Zionist Max Nordau* (Frankfurt: Fischer, 1997), 274.

116 Werner Sombart, *Die Juden und das Wirtschaftsleben* (Leipzig: Duncker & Humblot, 1911), 261–81; Jerry Z. Muller, 'Kapitalismus, Rationalisierung und die Juden – Zu Simmel, Weber und Sombart', in Nicolas Berg (ed.), *Kapitalismusdebatten um 1900 – Über antisemitisierende Semantiken des Jüdischen* (Leipzig: Leipziger Universitätsverlag, 2011), 23–48, at 43–6; Friedrich Lenger, 'Werner Sombarts "Die Juden und das Wirtschaftsleben" (1911) – Inhalt, Kontext und zeitgenössische Rezeption', in Berg (ed.), *Kapitalismusdebatten um 1900*, 239–53.

117 Bunge, *Die Alkoholfrage*, 18–19.

118 Ibid., 19.

119 See Wurster, *Kurzgefasste Geschichte*, 22.

120 Ibid., 23.

121 Arnd Bauerkämper, 'Der Neue Mensch', version 1.0, *Docupedia-Zeitgeschichte*, 4 July 2017, http://docupedia.de/zg/bauerkaemper_neue_mensch_v1_de_2017 (accessed 1 May 2019); Gottfried Küenzlen, *Der Neue Mensch. Eine Untersuchung zur säkularen Religionsgeschichte der Moderne*, 2nd edn (Munich: Wilhelm Fink Verlag, 1994), 153–60.

122 Kraepelin, *Alkohol und Jugend*, 16.

123 Ibid.

124 Gruber, *Volkswohlfahrt und Alkoholismus*, 31–2.

125 Forel, *Die Trinksitten*, 25.

126 Ibid.

127 Francesco Spöring, '"Du musst ein Apostel der Wahrheit werden": Auguste Forel und der sozialhygienische Antialkoholdiskurs, 1886–1931', in Große, Spöring and Tschurenev (eds), *Biopolitik und Sittlichkeitsreform*, 111–44, at 142; Jakob Tanner, *Geschichte der Schweiz im 20. Jahrhundert* (Munich: C.H. Beck, 2015), 86–7.

128 Forel, *Die Trinksitten*, 26.

129 Bunge, *Die Alkoholfrage*, 21.

130 Forel, *Die Trinksitten*, 29.

131 Breitung, *Unterrichtsstunden*; Gerhard Burk, *Die Erziehung unserer Jugend zu alkoholfreier Kultur und Lebensanschauung. Ihre Notwendigkeit und praktische Durchführung dargelegt auf Grund von Wissenschaft und Erfahrung* (Reutlingen: Mimir, 1911); Richard Ponickau, *Alkoholfreie Schulausflüge. Gesammelte Aufsätze* (Leipzig and Gohlis: Verein Abstinenter Philologen, 1911). On the connection between teachers and the abstinence movement see Spöring, '"Du musst ein Apostel der Wahrheit werden"', 130–1.

132 Ferdinand Avenarius, 'Vorwort', in Hermann Popert, *Helmut Harringa. Eine Geschichte unserer Zeit*, 14th edn (Dresden: Köhler, 1911).

133 Kai Detlev Sievers, 'Antialkoholismus und Völkische Bewegung. Hermann Poperts Roman "Helmut Harringa"', *Internationales Archiv für Sozialgeschichte der deutschen Literatur*, 29, no. 1 (2004), 29–54.

134 Karl Albert Schöllenbach [Robert Theuermeister], *Wilm Heinrich Berthold. Allerlei von der siebenjährigen Wanderfahrt eines jungen Lehrers in das neue Heimatland deutscher Jugend* (Leipzig: Strauch, 1915).

135 Malte Lorenzen, *Zwischen Wandern und Lesen. Eine rezeptionshistorische Untersuchung des Literaturkonzepts der bürgerlich deutschen Jugendbewegung 1896–1923* (Göttingen: Vandenhoeck & Ruprecht, 2016), 266–70.

136 Gerhart Hauptmann, *Vor Sonnenaufgang. Soziales Drama* (Berlin: C.F. Conrad's Buchhandlung, 1889).

137 Gunter Reiss, 'Vor Sonnenaufgang', *Kindlers Literatur Lexikon Online*, 3rd edn (Stuttgart and Weimar: Verlag J.B. Metzler, 2009), www.kll-online.de (accessed 1 May 2019).

7

'Disciples of Asclepius' or 'advocates of Hermes'? Psychiatrists and alcohol in early twentieth-century Greece

Kostis Gkotsinas

In 1903 the Second Pan-Hellenic Medical Conference, held in Athens, included a session on 'alcohol-induced diseases in Greece', with papers by two members of the then small community of Greek psychiatrists. While the speakers denounced the health damage caused by alcohol use, in the ensuing discussion a neurologist stated instead that alcohol 'is not a poison, but a nutritional element useful to the normal functioning of the human organism'.[1] His intervention provoked an indignant reaction of a colleague: 'We did not gather here as merchants, but as doctors with the one and only holy and great duty: to enlighten society as the disciples of Asclepius and not as the advocates of Hermes, the God of profit'. The debate evinces a dissonance within the psychiatric corps, divided between proponents of total abstinence and advocates of moderate use who made a distinction between fermented and distilled beverages.

What arguments were employed by each side, the 'disciples of Asclepius' and the 'advocates of Hermes'? What were the reasons for the divergent attitudes of Greek psychiatrists towards alcohol? And were these attitudes a Greek particularity or did they correspond to a broader network of ideas on alcohol circulating across Europe at the beginning of the twentieth century? In order to answer these questions, one must analyse the discourses on, and the attitudes of Greek psychiatrists towards, alcohol and alcoholism within their broader political, economic, social, cultural and intellectual context. Thus far, the secondary bibliography on alcohol production and consumption in the Hellenic world or, in more recent times, within the Greek state has delved into a wide array of issues: the history of the vine plant, winemaking techniques or wine culture, from Antiquity, through the Byzantine period and the years of Venetian and Ottoman rule, to the twentieth century;[2] the perspective of the agrarian economy with special emphasis on the cultivation and exportation of currants in the nineteenth century;[3] the development of the alcohol industry and the trade in alcoholic products in the eastern Mediterranean in the second half of the nineteenth century and the beginning of the twentieth;[4] and, finally, the social and cultural implications of alcohol production and consumption, with the constructive contribution of anthropological studies to fruitful research fields, such as practices of commensality, gendered attitudes towards alcohol or representations and symbolic charges of a given alcoholic beverage, for example, whisky in contemporary Greece.[5]

Intriguingly, there has been not much interest in discourses against alcohol in the Greek case, although such discourses did exist. This omission was perhaps due to the fact that the denunciation of alcohol and its effects was not as vociferous as in other countries and, ultimately, did not gain momentum. Nonetheless, efforts to curb drinking were not doomed in advance, and their contextualised analysis illustrates the history of both alcohol in Greece and the groups that adopted an anti-alcohol rhetoric, such as the psychiatric body. The development of the latter has interested historians and psychiatrists alike in recent decades and inspired studies of institutions, actors and scientific trends. But, once more, the question of alcohol, albeit central to the works of some early psychiatrists and neurologists, remains to be investigated.

Before doing so, it would be useful to briefly address two issues: first, the patterns of alcohol production and consumption during the nineteenth century in Greece and, second, the development of the psychiatric discipline at the turn of the twentieth century. After setting the background, we can explore how the members of the nascent scientific discipline of psychiatry, who sought to put their expertise into practice and to assert their authority, increasingly perceived 'immoderate' alcohol consumption as a pathology. To this end, this chapter examines the introduction and ascendance of the term 'alcoholism' in Greek scientific and non-scientific vocabulary, the symptoms attributed by neurologists and psychiatrists to the 'chronic intoxication from alcohol', the therapies and the measures proposed to cure or prevent this 'social malady' and, finally, the crystallisation of two major positions towards alcohol within the ranks of anti-alcohol crusaders (total abstinence versus moderate use).

Alcohol in Greek society

For millennia, wine has constituted an essential calorie supplement and an important component of the everyday diet in the Mediterranean: according to an 1840 source, a wealthy merchant in Athens bought 3.2 kg of bread, 2.2 l of wine and 1.2 kg of meat for his family every day.[6] But wine was also a central component of social life and religious ceremonies in the eastern Mediterranean, from the worship of Dionysus and Bacchus to the Eucharist. In the Greek case, this meant that alcohol consumption was sanctioned both by the heritage of ancient Greece, where modern Greeks sought cultural references and legitimisation of their present, and by the second pillar of modern Greek identity, so to speak, Christianity, whose holy texts contain many references to the grape product.[7] Apart from wine, the production of distilled drinks (such as raki) is attested in the region from the late Byzantine period onwards, so that by the nineteenth century spirits had also joined daily practices and social rituals.

In other words, when the modern Greek state was created in 1830, it inherited a tradition of alcohol production, commerce and consumption. The Bavarian administration, appointed by the three Great Powers (France, Britain, Russia) that guaranteed the new state's independence, did not fail to notice the economic prospects of alcohol. For this reason, a series of measures was adopted to encourage production (importation of vines, grants for scholars to study winemaking abroad, invitations to foreign oenologists and the creation of a model winery in Athens).[8] In the same vein, private initiative resulted in the foundation of the first wineries, breweries and ouzo or tsipouro (the equivalents of arak) distilleries in the 1850s and 1860s. Some of these efforts ultimately failed, but others bore fruit, and in the following decades, Greek wineries and distilleries multiplied in symbiosis with the currant economy.

In fact, whereas Greek currants were exported mainly to Britain until the 1860s, their production increased rapidly after the 1870s *phylloxera* blight that destroyed French vineyards, in order to cover the needs of the French wine industry. However, when a few years later French vineyards recovered, excessive quantities of Greek currants remained unsold and rotted in warehouses. Wineries and distilleries constituted a means of channelling this surplus and of mitigating the consequences of an acute social issue, while the Greek state intervened with measures like the creation of the Wine & Spirits Company in 1906, in an attempt to absorb the surplus currant production. These trends determined the character of wine production (wine made from currants was preferred to that from grapes) and contributed to the creation of the Greek cognac industry.[9]

In this manner, by the end of the century, the three branches of the alcohol industry (winemaking, beer brewing and cognac distillation) were growing, and Greek industries supplied the coasts of the eastern Mediterranean. Those who believed that industrial development was a necessary condition for the financial recovery of the Greek state, especially after the bankruptcy of 1893, placed their hopes on the distilling and winemaking sector. In 1894 for instance, Othon Rousopoulos (1856–1922), the founder of the Industrial and Commercial Academy, imagined the country's future in the following decade thus: 'I see in every corner colossal wine depots, containing rows of wine bottles filled with exquisite wines and constituting *a kind of bulwark against economic decay*.'[10]

Beyond the dreams of a thriving Greek industry and economy, one must not forget that commodities like alcohol constitute a substantial source of state revenue. As early as 1834, the Greek state imposed a land tax on wine, and at the end of the century, successive governments imposed consumption taxes on alcohol; interestingly enough, a part of the revenues generated from these taxes was allocated to the National Defence Fund, created after the defeat against the Ottoman Empire in 1897 to finance the modernisation of the Greek army.[11] In this general context, it is not surprising that the authorities prioritised accommodating the viticulturists and the electorate of grape-producing constituencies, or the demands of brewers, distillers, winemakers or grocers, who, on more than one occasion, addressed petitions to the authorities to promote their interests and to seek favourable conditions for pursuing and expanding their activities.[12]

On the consumption end, according to the neurologist and psychiatrist Simonidis Vlavianos (1873–1946), 'until 1870, even until 1880, the Greek, most of the Greeks, ignored what alcohol is, making almost exclusively pharmaceutical use of raki, which only a minority knew how to produce, and of cognac; what is more, our parents partook in wine moderately and scarcely sacrificed to Bacchus'.[13] However, in the last quarter of the nineteenth century, per capita consumption of alcoholic beverages apparently rose, partly as a result of the growth of local production.[14] Another factor that contributed to the spread of alcohol consumption was its medical uses in a society that hesitantly became more medicalised. Indeed, during the nineteenth century and later, alcohol was used as a raw material in tonic preparations, and various 'medical' wines (vins médicinaux) were prescribed for a vast array of illnesses and pathological conditions, ranging from fever to anorexia and weakness. A 1884 pharmacopoeia based on a French publication contained more than thirty preparations containing wine, while the cognac industry developed rapidly, purportedly after the drink was generously administered as medicine during the typhus epidemic of 1881–82 in the capital; an advertisement in a 1891 newspaper claimed that 'many hospitals use [Metaxa cognac] as a medicine for the suffering and the recovering'.[15] More generally, broader socio-cultural shifts concerning the management of leisure time, the emergence of new entertainment forms and the growing popularity of places of both consumption and socialisation, such as tavernas and coffee shops, contributed to the diffusion of alcohol; this was reflected in various cultural products, from popular songs to operetta and from literature to theatre, where the character of the 'drunkard' entered the scene. For instance, in a short story by Alexandros Papadiamantis (1851–1911), published on 1 January 1895, a carpenter and father of five spends his Sundays and half of his wage drinking, despite his family's misery – a recurrent theme in anti-alcohol literature.[16] At the same time, we encounter positive depictions of alcohol consumption, for example, in a revue staged from August 1894 to October 1895 involving a group of fashionable youngsters singing: 'Golden, golden youth / drink, drink wine / and thus the early years merrily go by.'[17]

The development of psychiatry in Greece

These developments coincided with the first timid steps of psychiatry in Greece.[18] When the Greek state became independent from the Ottoman Empire in 1830, it lacked not only resources and industrial infrastructure, but also health and educational institutions. It is no coincidence that the first psychiatric hospital in Greece was founded beyond the borders of the small state: in 1838 the British administration of the Ionian Islands created, in a suburb of Corfu's capital, a psychiatric institution, which was inherited by the Greek state when the Ionian Islands were transferred to it in 1864.[19] For two decades, it was Greece's only psychiatric hospital, essentially a mental asylum, until in the mid-1880s a private donation led to the creation of the Dromokaition psychiatric hospital in Athens, built according to French plans and hosting initially eighty-five patients.[20] In other words, until the turn of the twentieth century the therapeutic options were extremely limited. This began to change at the beginning of the century with the creation in 1904 of the Aiginiteion, the psychiatric clinic of the University of Athens (again thanks to a private donation for want of public funds), the functioning of a few municipal and communal asylums in smaller cities and on islands (Thessaloniki, Syros, Kefalonia, Chios, Chania, Lesbos) and the founding of a dozen private clinics, as well as the establishment of Athens Public Psychiatric Hospital in the 1920s.[21] Thus, without taking into account private clinics, the total bed capacity reached 4,000 on the eve of World War II.[22]

Destined to train personnel for the state mechanism and institutions, the University of Athens was inaugurated in 1837 (it remained the country's only university for a century), and one of its four initial faculties was a faculty of medicine. However, a chair of 'Neurology and Phrenic [Mental] Maladies' was created only at the end of the nineteenth century, in 1897, and entrusted to Professor Michail Katsaras (1860–1939), who held it until 1930. Even so, Greek students who were attracted by this emerging discipline had to pursue their studies abroad, which many of them did, by visiting mainly France and Germany, the two leading schools of thought in psychiatry at the time as well as the two major cultural references for Greek society. Beyond the Greek neurologists' and psychiatrists' curricula vitae, the impact of these foreign influences can be traced in the translations of foreign manuals (Heinrich Schüle's *Handbuch der Geisteskrankheiten* (Handbook on Mental Disorders, 1878), Benjamin Ball's *Leçons sur les maladies mentales* (Lessons on Mental Maladies, 1880–83) or Emmanuel Régis's *Manuel pratique de médecine mentale* (Practical Manual of Mental Medicine, 1885),[23] in the names given to clinics, like Dr Simonidis Vlavianos's Maison de Santé, or the references cited by Greek experts in their writings and lectures, which covered an extended bibliography and, as a rule, kept up with developments in the psychiatric field abroad, following the changing trends and shifting paradigms. To be sure, more often than not foreign models were grafted rather than assimilated, as Dimitris Ploumpidis points out, and the use of psychopathological and nosographic criteria lacked uniformity.[24] Thus terms and notions coined in Western and Central Europe were translated and used according to the particular foreign academic ties of the individual authors and without input from patient observation, since the latter was rare before the development of psychiatric institutions.

Be that as it may, neurologists and psychiatrists gradually took charge of mental health, which in the previous centuries had been entrusted to religious institutions, such as monasteries. Among other issues, like their counterparts in Europe, they took interest in the question of alcohol and its effects on the human body. The aforementioned Vlavianos (one of the prominent figures of Greek psychiatry, who had studied in Paris, had founded the first psychiatric and neurological journal in 1902 and was the director of a private clinic) gave a speech on alcoholism and its disastrous consequences in December 1907, in which he claimed, 'we neurologists and psychiatrists of Greece, then all the other physicians, will be morally responsible if we do not halt the progressing and growing tide of evil with everything within our powers.'[25] The growing evil in question was precisely 'alcoholism', the subject of Vlavianos's doctoral dissertation[26] and a concept that had found its way into

Greek scientific writings and public discourse at the end of the nineteenth century.

The introduction and use of the 'alcoholism' concept

In 1819, the German-Russian physician Constantin von Brühl-Cramer (d. 1821) published a treatise on what he termed *Trunksucht*, which was translated as 'dipsomania', and suggested an approach to addiction as a disease rather as the result of immorality.[27] At the end of the nineteenth century, Tilemachos Mitaftsis, associate professor of nervous and mental maladies at the University of Athens, ranked 'dipsomania' among the impulses of 'degenerates' and went on to describe a difference between the 'dipsomaniac' and the 'habitual wine drinker and alcoholic' ('καθ' έξιν οινοπότην και αλκοολικόν'): the latter consumed alcohol on an everyday basis and preferred a specific alcoholic beverage, while the former had paroxysms and consumed enormous quantities of any liquid.[28] In fact, the difference between 'dipsomania' and 'alcoholism' was more profound, as Hasso Spode argues: Brühl-Cramer's approach constituted a shift in scientific paradigms and an emancipation from moral considerations.[29]

This does not necessarily apply to 'alcoholism', since according to Katsaras's manual, which for decades served as a reference work, 'In the case of wine drinking it is a question of a moral flaw, whereas in the case of dipsomania of a morbid conscious and unrestrained urge to drink.'[30] The term 'alcoholism' was coined in the mid-nineteenth century, by the Swedish doctor Magnus Huss (1807–1890), who, elaborating on previous theories, united the negative effects of alcohol on the human body in one nosographic category. The term proved successful and spread rapidly across Europe, being used also in Greece by the end of the nineteenth century. Although a 1892 Greek-English dictionary featured only entries like 'drunkenness', 'inebriation', 'intoxication' (μέθη) and 'given to drinking, drunken' (οινόφλυξ), two years later Mitaftsis's Greek translation of Schüle's manual included a chapter entitled 'Alcoholism and alcoholic insanity'.[31] And in a less scholarly context, a series of articles published in December 1897 by the daily newspaper *Akropolis* reported on 'The great social plagues in Europe', namely 'Alcoholism, madness, suicides', which the reporter significantly located away from Greece.[32]

It is true that at the turn of the twentieth century, these formative years for Greek psychiatry, other terms and variants were also in use to describe this new pathology, for example, 'oenopneumatism' (*οινοπνευματισμός*), 'oenopneumatosis' (*οινοπνευμάτωσις*), 'oenopneumatiasis' (*οινοπνευματίασις*) or 'absinthism' {*αψινθισμός*) for the particular cases of absinthe or liqueur consumption.[33] Nonetheless, these fumbling terminological attempts, like 'dipsomania', did not prevail and by the 1910s the terms 'alcoholism' and 'alcoholic' were well established and used by specialists and non-specialists alike. As a professor of linguistics in the University of Athens wrote to Vlavianos asking him to endorse the use of 'alcoholism' and its derivatives, the term 'has already become a possession not only of science, but of our common language as well'.[34] In other words, the vocabulary and conceptual framework were set for the study and description of 'chronic intoxication from alcohol'.

Symptomatology of 'chronic intoxication from alcohol'

The interest of neurologists and psychiatrists in the issue of alcohol was certainly stimulated by their training abroad, their participation in international conferences,[35] the study of foreign bibliography and later that of texts published in Greek; the first psychiatric periodical publication, the *Ψυχιατρική και Νευρολογική Επιθεώρησις* (Psychiatric and Neurological Review), hosted articles on alcoholism from its first issue in September 1902.[36] But their attention was aroused equally by the first hospitalisations for 'alcoholic insanity' in psychiatric institutions (thirty-four cases were recorded in the Dromokaition hospital from 1887 to 1892) and eventually by the publication of statistics concerning deaths attributed to chronic or acute alcohol intoxication.[37]

Drawing on their experience from psychiatric hospitals, clinics and private practice, Greek psychiatrists started conducting their own observations.[38] But more often than not, they drew their examples and arguments from the rich foreign literature, as is proved by their quotes, references and citations of sources and statistics from France, Switzerland, Prussia (and later Germany), Scandinavia, Britain and the USA. Such references served both as a display of erudition and scientific competence and as an indisputable confirmation of the writers' claims. In any case, in their texts and lectures they addressed the question of 'alcoholism' and described the various health issues associated with alcohol. These accounts regularly distinguished between, on the one hand, 'drunkards', who experienced 'acute alcoholism', and, on the other, 'alcoholics', who were subject to 'chronic alcoholism'. This distinction is illustrated, for instance, by the questionnaire that the editor of the *Psychiatric and Neurological Review*, Vlavianos, addressed to its readers in the second issue of October 1902, in order to collect data concerning alcohol consumption and alcoholism in Greece.[39] The first two of the forty-seven questions enquired which alcoholic beverages were consumed and whether there were 'drunkards' (acute alcoholics) and chronic alcoholics in the readers' respective localities.

The latter were of more interest to scholars, who enumerated the various physical and psychic alterations and lesions provoked by alcohol consumption.[40] According to their accounts, at the initial stages alcoholics experienced a decrease in memory and an increase in headaches, vertigo, insomnia, nightmares, delusions, hallucinations, irritability and mood swings. The escalation of consumption was presented as an unavoidable path that led to further trouble, including both organic disorders (for example, stomach ulcers, cirrhosis, heart hypertrophy, arteriosclerosis, vision problems, erectile dysfunction, etc.) and neurological or psychological disorders. More precisely, in the context of a predominantly neurological approach, emphasis was placed on alterations of the nervous centres and brain functions, affecting perception, mobility and the intellect (tremors, atony, anaesthesia, bouts of epilepsy, general progressive palsy, neuropathy). Another set of symptoms was closely linked to a psychiatric interpretation of alcoholism and included what specialists termed acute or chronic alcoholic phrenitis or insanity, *delirium tremens*, dementia, moral insanity, mental alienation, bouts of hysteria, etc. According to a more elaborate schema, chronic alcoholism would lead to acute psychosis (divided into subacute alcoholic phrenitis or oniric delirium, acute alcoholic phrenitis or acute alcoholic hallucinatory delirium, and ultra-acute alcoholic phrenitis or *delirium tremens*) or to chronic psychosis (in the form of Korsakoff syndrome or alcoholic dementia).[41] Ultimately, alcoholics would meet their demise as a result of apoplexy or a weakened constitution that led to tuberculosis, pneumonia and other common pathologies.

But psychiatrists and neurologists did not limit themselves to recording the organic and psychic disorders caused by alcoholism. Ascribing to themselves the role of defenders of Greek society, they almost invariably detailed the broader consequences of alcohol on society, for they estimated that it was above all a 'social poison'.[42] In the first place, they stressed the economic repercussions of alcohol misuse, which were twofold: on the one hand, the cost of alcohol was blamed for diverting workers' incomes and draining family budgets, leading to pauperisation (see Figure 7.1); on the other hand, and on a larger scale, they calculated the financial consequences of alcoholism for the state, in terms of lost labour days, of aid to paupers, of maintenance costs for prisons, reformatories, hospitals, clinics and asylums, or of higher mortality rates.[43]

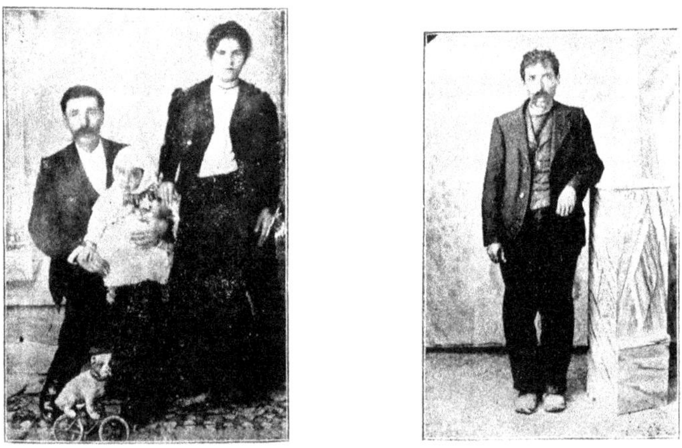

Εἰκ. 3.—Κ. Γ. . . οἰκογενειάρχης, πρὶν ἢ γίνῃ ἀλκοολικός. (Συλλογὴ ἡμετέρα   Εἰκ. 4.—Ὁ ἴδιος Κ. Γ. . . . γενόμενος ἀλκοολικός. (Συλλογὴ ἡμετέρα

Figure 7.1 'Image 3. K.G.... Family man, before he became an alcoholic. Image 4. The same K.G.... having become an alcoholic.'

Another danger linked with pauperisation and stemming from the ill-effects attributed to alcohol was the rise of criminality, a menace for the lives and properties of Greek citizens. To back up this opinion, authors invoked penitential statistics that were principally foreign, given the lack of official Greek statistics. And, as if the impact of alcoholism on contemporaries was not enough, there lay a danger for future generations, since psychiatrists were, among other things, convinced of the catastrophic hereditary effects of alcohol consumption. This belief was associated with the widespread and popular theory of degeneration, which was based on the Lamarckian principle of the heredity of acquired characteristics. In fact, the terms 'degenerate' (*εκπεφυλισμένος*) and 'degeneration' (*εκφυλισμός*) are encountered in the decade following the publication of Morel's *Traité des dégénérescences physiques, intellectuelles et morales* in 1857.[44] By the end of the nineteenth century the adjective 'degenerative' (*εκφυλιστικός*) was employed to qualify a delirium, a tendency or a frenzy, and the Greek neurologist Mitaftsis, as already mentioned, wrote his PhD on 'the degenerates'. In this work, which was prefaced by Jean-Baptiste Charcot, son of the famous Salpêtrière neurologist, Mitaftsis listed 'dipsomania' among the psychic stigmas that were believed to constitute pathological psychic manifestations. In other words, Mitaftsis adopted the point of view of Morel, who began the list of the principal causes of degeneration with intoxicating agents like alcohol, hashish and opium.[45] Thus the link between alcohol and degeneration had been established since the second half of the nineteenth century and remained popular well into the following century.

Moreover, this association was developed within a broader intellectual climate of eugenic aspirations and racial ideas that were widespread in Europe at the time.[46] In this context, the threat of alcoholism cast its shadow over the 'Greek nation', which 'at the first steps of its rebirth and national rehabilitation ... ought to maintain its vital forces in good condition, in order to use them in due time to fulfil its truly great mission'.[47] Therefore alcoholism was perceived as a national danger, jeopardising national or even 'racial' survival and destiny, and all the more so because Greeks were believed to be particularly exposed to the psychic and psychological effects of alcohol, owing to the 'nervous nature of the Greek race'.[48]

Therapeutic responses

As therapists, psychiatrists and neurologists set forth a variety of therapeutic responses to address the physical and psychological effects of habitual drinking. These responses combined traditional approaches that can be traced back to Hippocratic practices (such as a diet devised to purify and fortify the patient's organism, and hydrotherapy)[49] with the latest methods recommended by European colleagues, namely the administration of various substances expected to counter the action of alcohol (for example, strychnine injections, 'anti-ethylene', or antiserum therapy).[50] Certain therapists advocated also the recourse to hypnosis and hypnotic suggestion – during this transitional period many articles in the *Psychiatric and Neurological Review* were dedicated to the study of hypnotism, while psychoanalysis remained largely unknown to Greek scholars and the public.[51]

However, because alcoholism was considered an issue that extended beyond strictly medical grounds, the authorities on the matter wished to equally address its social consequences. As a part of a broader hygienist programme, they called for a series of measures. One set involved state intervention and legislation. Prohibition was considered as an option, and Greek authors referred to similar measures adopted in various US states even before the passage of the Volstead Act in 1919 – but even the more uncompromising among them conceded that strict prohibition was contrary to Greek habits, tastes and traditions.[52] Other potential legislative measures included modifying the closing time of public houses, increasing the price of or limiting the permits to run such establishments and raising taxes on alcoholic beverages in general or distilled products in particular. In fact, in 1899 a bill was submitted to parliament proposing the re-enactment of taxation on alcohol, which had been suspended after the country's bankruptcy in 1893.[53] One of the main arguments invoked to support the taxation of consumption rather than that of production was that such legislation would help combat alcoholism. However, as the parliamentary record shows, MPs' main concern was how to generate state income and how not to incommode the alcohol industry and the viticulture sector.[54] For that reason, other suggestions like the creation of a state monopoly on alcohol never materialised, contrary to the treatment of other products like salt, matches or rolling paper. Similarly, while many recommended the creation of asylums for immoderate consumers who were diagnosed as alcoholics, the finances of the Greek state, as mentioned above, were meagre and hardly allowed the creation of a public psychiatric hospital even as late as the 1920s.

Finally, apart from measures destined to crack down on producers, sellers and consumers, another set of measures was prophylactic, that is, they aimed to prevent alcoholism through lectures, publications, special courses in schools on the dangers of alcohol, sports, the formation of temperance leagues, the creation of popular clubs and meeting places where no alcohol would be served, and overall the amelioration of living and eating conditions for the working classes, as poverty was considered not only a consequence of alcoholism, but also one of the principal causes for its spread.[55] Indeed, some actions were taken in the direction of prevention and propaganda. For example, the Athena-Health Fraternity, founded in 1907, included in its statute the 'combating of meat eating, smoking, alcoholic drinks'.[56] And a decade later, in 1917, the Supreme Directorate of Public Education issued a circular encouraging the circulation among elementary and high schools across the country of the brochure *The Disastrous Effects of Alcoholic Beverages and Tobacco* in order to combat and eradicate 'habits destined assuredly to sap the soul and body of youngsters and lead to imperil the existence of our race'.[57] Nevertheless, it is evident that these propositions required substantial means and a large consensus in order to produce concrete, durable results and, ultimately, have an impact.

Total abstinence versus moderate use

However, the anti-alcohol front that was formed in the early twentieth century was not uniform. According to the gynaecologist Moysis Moyseidis, writing in 1935, there were three camps in the battlefield over alcohol: the anti-alcohol extremists, who condemned alcohol in every form; the friends of wine and beer, who propagandised for their consumption; and, between them, the anti-alcohol moderates, who accepted the reasonable use of fermented, but not of distilled, drinks: one such example was the professor of food chemistry of the University of Athens, who believed that 'drinking a glass of wine or beer in a pleasant meeting is not harmful; on the contrary, it offers a pleasant relief from life's everyday struggles'.[58] For his part, Moyseidis considered that the moderates were closer to 'scientific truth' and that, at the same time, they respected the economic, social and psychological aspects of the matter – hinting thus at the importance of the specific socio-cultural context in Greece on scholarly discourses.[59]

Overall, one would expect that among the detractors of alcohol, neurologists and psychiatrists would have been particularly eager to adopt a more intransigent point of view on the matter of drinking. Contrary to physicians, who could have recourse to alcoholic preparations in their medical practice, psychiatrists treated alcohol as the root of many mental and neurological conditions. Moreover, the crusade against alcohol offered neurologists and psychiatrists the grounds to assert their expertise and their scientific and professional autonomy to physicians as psychiatry made its first steps in Greece at the turn of the twentieth century.

However, things were more complex. Leaving aside eventual turf wars between members of the medical profession, opinions on the nature and the extent of the anti-alcohol fight diverged even within the limited circle of Greek psychiatrists. Opposed to the proponents of total abstinence, the advocates of moderate use often put forward a distinction between fermented and distilled beverages, arguing that the consumption of the former had either a recreational and social function or a nutritional value. Eventually wine or beer consumption could be presented as a bulwark against alcoholism in the strict sense of the term, which they believed was provoked by distilled beverages containing starch (based, for instance, on cereals, potatoes or beets). On the other hand, the proponents of total abstinence considered that the amount of ethanol contained in beverages was irrelevant, as the substance remained a poison. Therefore the drunkard and the chronic alcoholic simply represented different degrees of the same condition, and their harmful habit should be eradicated at all costs and by all means.

An episode that highlights the opposition between the advocates of the two approaches is the one cited in the beginning of this chapter and recorded in the proceedings of the Second Pan-Hellenic Medical Conference held in 1903.[60] The rising concern about alcoholism was reflected in the inclusion of a session on 'alcohol-induced diseases in Greece', with two papers presented by the assistant directors of the Dromokaition psychiatric hospital: Michail Katsaras and Michail Yianniris (1865–1956), a psychiatrist who had studied in Greece and France and who would later become director of the hospital. They both denounced the damage to health caused by alcohol use, although Katsaras was more pessimistic in his account, while Yianniris presented statistics that allowed him to consider that the numbers were not yet alarming in Greece, thanks mainly to the nature and quality of drinks consumed and of the living conditions in the country. However, in the discussion that followed, Georgios Karyofyllis, a neurologist who later founded his own private clinic, argued that alcohol 'is not a poison, but a nutritional element' which helps its consumers breath and digest better, and is indicated for the treatment of tuberculosis, typhus, post-partum septicaemia or cases of acute psychosis and post-partum mania. To back up his views, he also referred to foreign scientific expertise, quoting, among others, the sixth memoir of the American National Academy of Sciences, 'An experimental inquiry regarding the nutritive value of alcohol', published the previous year in Washington – a good illustration of the fact that Greek psychiatrists kept abreast with contemporary scientific publications, even from across the Atlantic.[61]

His intervention provoked an indignant reaction from Vlavianos, who was a fervent opponent of alcohol consumption, ranking himself among the 'disciples of Asclepius' who were on a mission to enlighten society. He admonished his colleague Karyofyllis for defending commercial interests linked with alcohol, stating that in many cases of neurasthenia, epilepsy or general palsy due to alcohol, practitioners tended to record the result instead of the cause. Finally, he proposed the creation of a pan-Hellenic anti-alcohol association. Other physicians objected equally to Karyofyllis's medical argumentation.[62]

Nonetheless, the matter was far from settled. A similar debate was repeated three decades later, this time by means of published texts. Spyridon Dontas (1878–1958), professor of physiology at the University of Athens, had already contributed in 1934 an article on 'Le vin comme aliment' (Wine as a nutrient) to the French journal *Bulletin international du vin*, the organ of the Office International du Vin.[63] On the occasion of his acceptance to the Academy of Athens in 1935, he gave a speech entitled 'Wine against alcoholism' (which was also published as a brochure by the Ministry of Agriculture with a foreword by its general secretary). In his speech, after enumerating the harmful effects of spirits, he praised the properties of wine, claiming that 'the appropriate way to control, insofar as possible, alcoholism is the broader diffusion of the use of natural wine, to replace the harmful alcoholic drinks. The moderate use of natural wine, which is plentiful in Greece, and in particular of the healthy resinated wine, is beneficial to the organism, causing no harm. Especially for those who work and are insufficiently fed, wine is a necessary nutritional supplement.'[64]

Such points of view were not specific to Greece. In other wine-producing countries, like France, temperance advocates promoted wine over distilled beverages as well.[65] But, as was the case elsewhere, such views triggered the ire of the inflexible part of the psychiatric profession. Thus Dontas's publication led to a response from Konstantinos Katsaras (1886–1958), a neurologist who had studied in Germany, was the director of a private clinic situated near Piraeus, the Greek capital's port, and was the son of Michail Katsaras. His own text, published in 1936, was eloquently entitled *Wine and Alcoholism*. In it, he refuted the nutritional benefits of wine and alcohol in general and asked his colleagues to cease 'the extremely dangerous scientific propaganda' in favour of wine consumption, proposing instead the consumption of grape juice (see Figure 7.2).[66] Contrary to the opinion expressed by Dontas in another article, where he compared wine to quinine and alcoholism to malaria, Katsaras argued that wanting to combat alcoholism with wine was similar 'to wanting to put out the blaze with fire, or to throwing gunpowder or oil on an open fire!'[67]

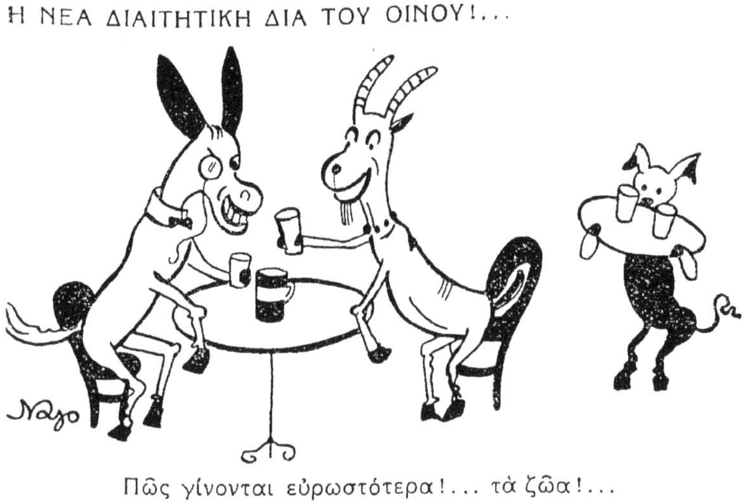
Η ΝΕΑ ΔΙΑΙΤΗΤΙΚΗ ΔΙΑ ΤΟΥ ΟΙΝΟΥ!...
Πῶς γίνονται εὐρωστότερα!... τὰ ζῶα!...

Figure 7.2 'THE NEW NUTRITION WITH WINE! ... How brutes become stronger! ...'

However, these turf wars and scientific debates were not irreconcilable. In 1938 the Supreme Hygienic Council constituted a committee to study how to encourage currant and wine consumption. Its conclusions were that there should be a campaign to promote the use of currants in industry and a systematic fight against alcoholism, based on the principles that the consumption of a small quantity of wine with every meal is useful for every healthy person, since wine excites the appetite, facilitates digestion, fortifies the organism and encourages a pleasant psychic disposition. What was more interesting than the committee's conclusions was its composition. Apart from Spyridon Dontas, it consisted of the General Technical Advisor of Hygiene in the relevant ministry and the professors of therapeutics, of hygiene, and of neurology and psychiatry in the University of Athens, as well as a psychiatrist who for nearly forty years had denounced the dangers of alcohol and promoted the role of the 'disciples of Asclepius' in the fight against alcoholism: Dr Simonidis Vlavianos, by that time President of the Athens Medical Association.[68]

Conclusion

How should we interpret the participation of Vlavianos in the committee and his endorsement of an indulgent approach towards wine drinking? Was it a sign of pragmatism, opportunism, or simple resignation? Already in 1910, he was professing: 'Let our symbol be total abstinence [*abstinence totale*] and then moderate use [*modération*]. The latter succeeds, the former triumphs.'[69] In other terms, he did not rule out a less intransigent tactic in his fight against alcoholism. On the whole, the attitude of Vlavianos and of his colleagues in denouncing the consequences of alcoholic beverages was shaped by their studies and scientific training, by their professors and readings, by their personal observations as they practised and, as alcohol-related hospitalisations occurred, by their professional interests, as well as by their social and cultural ties. Therefore, their opinions expressed their desire to assert their scientific expertise and their anxiety about what they perceived as a menace to society at the same time.

However, they lived and worked in a society with the characteristics of what some anthropologists term a 'wet culture', that is, a society where production and consumption of alcohol was fully integrated in social and cultural practices. What is more, alcohol represented significant financial and fiscal benefits, which were even associated with national interests for the Greek state. As a result, and as in other European countries, the campaigners against alcohol, divided on the question of total abstinence or moderate use, failed to form a common front and influence public policies. And as psychiatrists and neurologists gradually attained recognition in the eyes of the medical profession and of public and state institutions (as demonstrated by the inclusion of two psychiatrists in the 1938 committee), they proved more willing to 'water down their wine' and to retreat from their more uncompromising stance.

Notes

The research project 'A last drink? Alcohol and anti-alcoholism in Greece (1870–1940)' was funded by the Research Centre for the Humanities (RCH) for the year 2018, with the support of the Stavros Niarchos Foundation.

RESEARCH CENTRE for the HUMANITIES

ΙΣΝ/SNF

ΙΔΡΥΜΑ ΣΤΑΥΡΟΣ ΝΙΑΡΧΟΣ
STAVROS NIARCHOS FOUNDATION

1 K. Papagiannis (ed.), *Πρακτικά του Β' Πανελληνίου Ιατρικού Συνεδρίου* [Proceedings of the Second Pan-Hellenic Medical Conference] (Athens: M. Saliveros, 1903), 246–7: 'δεν είνε δηλητήριον, αλλά θρεπτικόν στοιχείον χρήσιμον εις την κανονικήν λειτουργίαν του ανθρωπίνου οργανισμού ... ημείς ενταύθα δεν συνήλθομεν ως έμποροι αλλ' ως ιατροί καθήκον έχοντες εν και μόνον ιερόν και υψηλόν, να διαφωτίσομεν την κοινωνίαν ως μύσται του Ασκληπιού και ουχί ως οπαδοί του κερδώου Ερμού.' The original quotes in the footnotes are in Katharevousa, the purist Greek used in official documents, religious circulars, academic writing and teaching until the 1970s. All translations are by the author.

2 A. Matthaiou, 'Το κρασί ως βασικό είδος διατροφής στην Τουρκοκρατία' [Wine as a basic nutrient under Ottoman rule], in *Ιστορία του ελληνικού κρασιού* [History of Greek Wine] (Athens: ETBA, 1992), 183–90; M. Sivignon, 'Les vignes et les vins de la Grèce contemporaine', in J.-L. Mayaud (ed.), *Clio dans les vignes. Mélanges offerts à Gilbert Garrier* (Lyon: Presses universitaires de Lyon, 1998), 231–50; J. Jouanna, L. Villard and D. Béguin (eds), *Vin et santé en Grèce ancienne* (Athens: École française d'Athènes, 2002); E. Grammatikopoulou (ed.), *Οίνος: Πολιτισμός και κοινωνία* [Wine: Civilisation and Society] (Athens: National Hellenic Research Foundation, 2006).

3 S. Petmezas, 'L'économie agricole grecque face à la longue crise de la première globalisation', *Historical Review/La revue historique*, 10 (2003), 85–106; G. Meloni and J. Swinnen, 'Standards, tariffs and trade: the rise and fall of the raisin trade between Greece and France in the late nineteenth century and the definition of wine', LICOS Discussion Paper no. 386, Katholieke Universiteit Leuven, 2017, https://www.econstor.eu/bitstream/10419/172038/1/875994148.pdf (accessed 26 April 2019).

4 C. Agriantoni, 'Η Ελληνική Οινοβιομηχανία το 19ο αιώνα: από την Αναζήτηση της Ποιότητας στο σταφιδίτη' [The Greek wine industry in the nineteenth century: from the quest for quality to wine from currants], in *Ιστορία του ελληνικού κρασιού*, 133–44; N. Bakounakis, *Το κρασί του Γουσταύου, Αφήγημα οινικών περιπετειών* [Gustav's Wine: Narrative of Wine Adventures] (Athens: Kastaniotis, 1997).

5 P. Allen, 'Apollo and Dionysus: alcohol use in modern Greece', *East European Quarterly*, 18, no. 4 (1985), 461–80; E. Papataxiarchis, 'Friends of the heart: male commensal solidarity, gender, and kinship in Aegean Greece', in P. Loizos and E. Papataxiarchis (eds), *Contested Identities: Gender and Kinship in Modern Greece* (Princeton: Princeton University Press, 1991), 156–79; D. Gefou-Madianou, 'Exclusion and unity, retsina and sweet wine: commensality and gender in a Greek agrotown', in D. Gefou-Madianou (ed.), *Alcohol, Gender and Culture* (London and New York: Routledge, 2002), 108–36; T. Bampilis, *Greek Whisky: The Localization of a Global Commodity* (New York: Berghahn Books, 2013).

6 F. Braudel, *Civilization and Capitalism, 15th–18th Century*, vol. 1: *The Structures of Everyday Life, the Limits of the Possible* (London: William Collins, 1981), 232–7; E. Liata, *Τιμές και αγαθά στην Αθήνα (1839–1846)* [Prices and Commodities in Athens (1839–1846)] (Athens: MIET, 1984), 66, cited in Matthaiou, 'Το κρασί ως βασικό είδος διατροφής στην Τουρκοκρατία', 189, n. 35.

7 M. Iossifides, 'Wine: life's blood and spiritual essence in a Greek Orthodox convent', in Gefou-Madianou (ed.), *Alcohol, Gender, and Culture*, 80.

8 Bakounakis, *Το κρασί του Γουσταύου*, 45–8.

9 Agriantoni, 'Η Ελληνική Οινοβιομηχανία το 19ο αιώνα', 140.

10 Industrial and Commercial Academy, *Τα Εγκαίνια του Οινοποιείου* [The Inauguration of the Winery] (Athens: Nomikis, 1900), 5: 'Βλέπω εις πάσαν αυτής γωνίαν οιναποθήκας κολοσσιαίας, ενεχούσας συστοιχίας οινοδοχείων πλήρων θεσπεσίων οίνων και αποτελούσας *είδος προπυργίου κατά της οικονομικής καχεξίας*.' Underlining in the original.

11 *Gazette of the Government of the Greek Kingdom*, Law 3027, art. 2C, 21 June 1904, p. 363.

12 *Αναφορά των Αμπελοκτημόνων του Νομού Αττικής περί Ενδεικνυομένων Μέτρων προς Προστασίαν της Οινοπαραγωγής προς την σεβ. Βουλήν των Ελλήνων* [Attica Viticulturists' Petition on the Appropriate Measures for the Protection of Wine Production to the Honourable Greek Parliament] (Athens: P. Leonis, 1908), 11.

13 S. Vlavianos, *Ο αλκοολισμός* [Alcoholism] (Athens: Kratous, 1907), 33:

'μέχρι του 1870, ακόμη και μέχρι του 1880 ο Έλλην, το πολύ μέρος των Ελλήνων, ηγνόει τι εστί οινόπνευμα, χρήσιν δε μόνον σχεδόν φαρμακευτικήν εποιείτο της ρακής, ης την παρασκευήν κατ' οίκον μικρά τις μερίς εξέμαθε και του κονιάκ· ου μην αλλά και του οίνου μετρίως μετελάμβανον οι γονείς ημών και τας θυσίας τω Βάκχω σπανιωτάτας προσήνεγκον.'

14 M. Yianniris, 'Η παραφροσύνη εν Ελλάδι' [Insanity in Greece], *Ψυχιατρική και Νευρολογική Επιθεώρησις* [Psychiatric and Neurological Review], 1, no. 5 (1903), 155.

15 M. Mangakis (ed.), *Πρακτικά του Πανελληνίου Ιατρικού Συνεδρίου* [Proceedings of the Pan-Hellenic Medical Conference], vol. 2 (Athens: P.D. Sakellarios, 1902), 35; V. Pintos, *Φαρμακοποιία* [Pharmacopoeia] (Athens: A. Koromilas, 1884), 1285–6; 'Ζήτημα Υγείας' [Questions of health], *Εφημερίς* [Journal], 6 November 1891, p. 3: 'ποιούσιν χρήσιν και πλείστα νοσοκομεία ως φαρμάκου διά τους πάσχοντας και αναρρωννύοντας'.

16 A. Papadiamantis, 'Πατέρα στο σπίτι' [A father at home], *Ακρόπολις* [Acropolis], 1 January 1895, reprinted in *Άπαντα* [Collected Works], ed. N. Triantafyllopoulos, vol. 3 (Athens: Domos, 2007), 89–94. Papadiamantis is one of the most prominent figures of Greek literature and a representative of the late nineteenth-century literary trend termed 'ethography', which focused on social mores and everyday life situations, echoing the contemporary realist and naturalist movements.

17 Th. Hadjipantazis and L. Maraka (eds), *Η Αθηναϊκή Επιθεώρηση* [The Athenian Revue], A2 (Athens: Hestia, n.d.), 74–5: 'Νιότη χρυσή, χρυσή / πίνε κρασί, κρασί, / και με χαρά περνούν τα νιάτα.' The 'Athenian revue' was an assortment of sketches satirising current affairs and combining songs with prose. The revue 'A bit of everything' cited here was the first of this genre.

18 The following draws mainly on the seminal work of D. Ploumpidis, *Ιστορία της Ψυχιατρικής στην Ελλάδα: Θεσμοί, Ιδρύματα και Κοινωνικό Πλαίσιο, 1850–1920* [History of Psychiatry in Greece: Institutions, Hospitals, and Social Context, 1850–1920] (Athens: Exantas, 1995). For non-Greek-speaking readers, see C. Synodinou, 'La Grèce', in J. Postel and C. Quétel (eds), *Nouvelle histoire de la psychiatrie* (Paris: Dunod, 2004), 541–9; D. Ploumpidis, A. Karavatos and G. Christodoulou, 'The development of psychiatry in Greece from the late 18th century to the mid-twentieth century', in G. Christodoulou, D. Ploumpidis and A. Karavatos (eds), *Anthology of Greek Psychiatric Texts* (Athens: Beta Medical Arts, 2011), xxix–xl.

19 Ministry of the Interior, *Στατιστική του εν Κερκύρα Φρενοκομείου του Έτους 1877* [Statistics of Corfu Mental Hospital for the Year 1877] (Athens:

Ethnikon Typographeion, 1878), 3–4; I. Triantafylloudis, 'Δημογραφική Αποτύπωση των Νοσηλευθέντων στο Ψυχιατρικό Νοσοκομείο Κέρκυρας (1838–2000)' [Demographic footprint of patients in Corfu Psychiatric Hospital (1838–2000)] (PhD dissertation, Ionian University, 2017), 79–88.

20 F.B. Sanborn, 'Insanity in Greece: the hospital of Athens', *Journal of Mental Science*, 39, no. 166 (1893), 338–43; V. Karamanolakis, 'Το Δρομοκαΐτειο Φρενοκομείο, 1887–1903: Όψεις της Εγκατάστασης ενός Ιδρυματικού Θεσμού' [Dromokaition Mental Hospital, 1887–1903: aspects of the creation of an asylum institution], *Μνήμων* [Mnemon], 20 (1998), 45–66; D. Kritsotaki and V. Lekka, 'Lay narratives of mental illness at the Dromokaition Hospital, 1900–1920', in Marius Turda (ed.), 'Private and public medical traditions in Greece and the Balkans', *Deltos: Journal of the History of Hellenic Medicine*, special issue (2012), 51–5; M. Fiste et al., 'Dromokaition Psychiatric Hospital of Athens: from its establishment in 1887 to the era of deinstitutionalization', *Annals of General Psychiatry*, 14, no. 7 (2015), https://annals-general-psychiatry.biomedcentral.com/track/pdf/10.1186/s12991-015-0047-1 (accessed 26 April 2019).

21 A.P. K[ouzis], 'Αιγινήτειον Νοσοκομείον' [Aiginiteion Hospital], in *Μεγάλη Ελληνική Εγκυκλοπαίδεια* [Great Hellenic Encyclopaedia], vol. 2 (Athens: Pyrsos, 1927), 485; K. Filandrianos, *Δημόσιο Ψυχιατρείο Αθηνών: Το Δαφνί ... μία Φανταστική Πολιτεία* [Athens Public Psychiatric Hospital: Dafni ... an Imaginary Republic] (Athens: n.pub., 1977); E. Missouridou, 'Το Ψυχιατρικό Νοσοκομείο Αττικής και η Ιστορία της Ψυχιατρικής Νοσηλευτικής στην Ελλάδα' [Attica Psychiatric Hospital and the history of psychiatric nursing in Greece], *Nosileftiki*, 47, no. 3 (2008), 294–303.

22 Statistique Générale de la Grèce, *Annuaire statistique de la Grèce, 1939* (Athens: Ethnikon Typographeion, 1940), 388.

23 H. Schüle, *Κλινική πραγματεία περί φρενικών νόσων* [Clinical Treatise of Phrenic Maladies], trans. T. Mitaftsis (Athens: Paliggenesia, 1894) was translated from the French edition with extensive additions from the manuals of Ball and Régis (see Christodoulou, Ploumpidis and Karavatos, *Anthology of Greek Psychiatric Texts*, 506).

24 D. Ploumpidis, 'An outline of the development of psychiatry in Greece', *History of Psychiatry*, 4, no. 14 (1993), 243.

25 S. Vlavianos, 'Ο αλκοολισμός και αι ολέθριαι αυτού συνέπειαι' [Alcoholism and its disastrous consequences], *Ψυχιατρική και Νευρολογική Επιθεώρησις* [Psychiatric and Neurological Review], 6, no. 4 (1907), 128: 'εσμέν ηθικώς υπεύθυνοι οι νευρολόγοι και ψυχίατροι της Ελλάδος, είτα δε και

πάντες οι άλλοι ιατροί, αν μη ανακόψωμεν το προϊόν και αύξον ρεύμα του κακού διά πάσης προσπαθείας.'

26 Vlavianos, *Ο αλκοολισμός*.

27 C. von Brühl-Cramer, *Über die Trunksucht und eine rationelle Heilmethode derselben* [On Dipsomania and a Rational Therapy of It] (Berlin: Nicolai, 1819); F.-W. Kielhorn, 'The history of alcoholism: Brühl-Cramer's concepts and observations', *Addiction*, 91, no. 2 (1996), 121–8.

28 T.A. Mitaftsis, *Οι έκφυλοι* [The Degenerates] (Athens: Sp. Kousoulinou, 1899), 92.

29 H. Spode, *Die Macht der Trunkenheit: Kultur- und Sozialgeschichte des Alkohols in Deutschland* [The Force of Drunkenness: Cultural and Social History of Alcohol in Germany] (Opladen: Leske und Budrich, 1993), 127–33.

30 M. Katsaras, *Παθολογία των νεύρων και ψυχιατρική* [Nerve Pathology and Psychiatry], vol. 2 (Athens: Alexandros Papageorgiou, 1898), 547: 'Εν μεν τη οινοποσία πρόκειται περί ελαττώματος ηθικού, εν δε τη διψομανία περί νοσηράς ενσυνειδήτου και ακατασχέτου προς πόσιν ορμής.'

31 A. Kyriakides, *A Greek–English Dictionary* (Nicosia: The Owl, 1892), 293, 332; Schüle, *Κλινική πραγματεία περί φρενικών νόσων*, 460–89 (chapter title: 'Αλκοολισμός και αλκοολικαί φρενοβλάβειαι').

32 'Αι μεγάλαι κοινωνικαί πληγαί εν Ευρώπη. Ο αλκοολισμός, η τρέλλα, αι αυτοκτονίαι' [The great social plagues in Europe: alcoholism, madness, suicides], *Ακρόπολις* [Akropolis], 10, 11 and 12 December 1897.

33 S. Koumanoudis, *Συναγωγή Νέων Λέξεων υπό των Λογίων Πλασθεισών από της Αλώσεως μέχρι των καθ' ημάς Χρόνων* [Collection of New Words Formed by Scholars from 1453 to this Date], vol. 1 (Athens: P.D. Sakellarios, 1900), 41, 718.

34 S. Vlavianos, 'Ο αλκοολισμός' [Alcoholism], *Ψυχιατρική και Νευρολογική Επιθεώρησις* [Psychiatric and Neurological Review], 8, nos 5–6 (1910), 4.

35 S. Vlavianos, 'Le traitement de l'alcoolisme par l'hypnotisme', in Dr Legrain and Dr Boissier (eds), *Compte rendu du VIIe Congrès international contre l'abus des boissons alcooliques*, vol. 2 (Paris: Union française antialcoolique, 1900), 169–74; S. Vlavianos, 'L'alcoolisme en Grèce', in Legrain and Boissier (eds), *Compte rendu du VIIe Congrès*, 305–7.

36 G. Anton, 'Αλκοολισμός και Κληρονομικότης' [Alcoholism and heredity], *Ψυχιατρική και Νευρολογική Επιθεώρησις* [Psychiatric and Neurological Review], 1, no. 1 (1902), 10–15.

37 Yianniris, 'Η παραφροσύνη εν Ελλάδι', 153; *Μηνιαίον Δελτίον Θανάτων εν 12 πόλεσι της Ελλάδος εχούσαις Πληθυσμόν ανώτερον των 10000 Κατοίκων* [Monthly Bulletin of Deaths in 12 Greek Cities with a Population above 10,000 Inhabitants] (Athens: Ethnikon Typographeion, 1899–1908).

38 For example, S. Vlavianos, 'Περίπτωσις Υποξέος Αλκοολικού Παραληρήματος Ιαθέντος' [A case of cured sub-acute alcoholic delirium], *Ψυχιατρική και Νευρολογική Επιθεώρησις* [Psychiatric and Neurological Review], 4, nos 9–10 (1906), 268–70.

39 S. Vlavianos, 'Αντιαλκοολική εκστρατεία' [Anti-alcohol campaign], *Ψυχιατρική και Νευρολογική Επιθεώρησις* [Psychiatric and Neurological Review], 1, no. 2 (1902), 29–32.

40 Katsaras, *Παθολογία των νεύρων και ψυχιατρική*, vol. 2, 650–6; A. Armodios, 'Ο Αλκοολισμός υπό Υγιεινήν και Κοινωνιολογικήν Έποψιν' [Alcoholism from a health and sociological viewpoint], *Ψυχιατρική και Νευρολογική Επιθεώρησις* [Psychiatric and Neurological Review], 2, no. 2 (1903), 40–4; I. Tastsoglou, 'Ο Αλκοολισμός και αι εξ αυτού Ψυχοπάθειαι παρ' ημίν' [Alcoholism and consecutive psychopathies in Greece], *Ο Πρακτικός Ιατρός* [The Practical Physician], 9, no. 1 (1931), 3–4.

41 K.A. Mitaftsis, *Ψυχιατρική* [Psychiatry] (Athens: P. Leoni, 1932), 225–37. Konstantinos Mitaftsis, a neurologist and psychiatrist, was the younger brother of Tilemachos Mitaftsis.

42 Armodios, 'Ο Αλκοολισμός υπό Υγιεινήν και Κοινωνιολογικήν Έποψιν', 40.

43 S. Vlavianos, 'Ο Αλκοολισμός υπό Οικονομολογικήν Έποψιν' [Alcoholism from an economic viewpoint], *Ψυχιατρική και Νευρολογική Επιθεώρησις* [Psychiatric and Neurological Review], 1, no. 4 (1902), 116–18.

44 Koumanoudis, *Συναγωγή Νέων Λέξεων*, 347.

45 Mitaftsis, *Οι έκφυλοι*, 92; B.-A. Morel, *Traité des dégénérescences physiques, intellectuelles et morales de l'espèce humaine et des causes qui produisent ces variétés maladives* (Paris: J.B. Baillère, 1857), 79–170.

46 D. Pick, *Faces of Degeneration: A European Disorder, c. 1848–c. 1918* (Cambridge: Cambridge University Press, 1989); S. Trubeta, *Anthropology, Race and Eugenics in Greece (1880s–1970s)* (Leiden and Boston: Brill, 2013), 203–39.

47 A. Armodios, 'Ο Αλκοολισμός υπό Υγιεινήν και Κοινωνιολογικήν Έποψιν' [Alcoholism from a health and sociological viewpoint], *Ψυχιατρική και Νευρολογική Επιθεώρησις* [Psychiatric and Neurological Review], 2, no. 3 (1903), 80: 'Το Ελληνικόν έθνος, μόλις ευρισκόμενον εις τα πρώτα βήματα της αναγεννήσεως και εν τη εθνική αυτού αποκαταστάσει … οφείλει να διατηρήση ακμαίας τας ζωτικάς δυνάμεις, ίνα χρησιμοποιήση

αυτάς εν καιρώ τω δέοντι προς εκπλήρωσιν της όντως υψηλής αυτού αποστολής.'

48 M. Katsaras, 'Περί των εξ οινοπνεύματος παθήσεων εν Ελλάδι' [On the maladies caused by alcohol in Greece], in Papagiannis (ed.), *Πρακτικά του Β' Πανελληνίου Ιατρικού Συνεδρίου*, 209: 'νευρική φύσις της ελληνικής φυλής'.

49 Hydrotherapy or hydropathy is the therapeutic use of water, mainly cold, in full or local baths, showers, ablutions, compresses, massages etc. See N. Tsampoulas and S. Pezopoulos, *Κλινική υδροθεραπεία και λουτροθεραπεία* [Clinical Hydropathy and Balneotherapy] (Athens: D. Petsalis, 1931), v–vii; R. Price, 'Hydropathy in England 1840–70', *Medical History*, 25 (1981), 269–80 (for drugs and alcohol see 276); J. Bradley, 'Medicine on the margins? Hydropathy and orthodoxy in Britain, 1840–60', in Waltraud Ernst (ed.), *Plural Medicine, Tradition and Modernity, 1800–2000* (London: Routledge, 2002), 19–39.

50 Vlavianos, 'Ο αλκοολισμός' (1910), 169–76.

51 For example, S. Damoglou, 'Ο Υπνωτισμός ως Θεραπετικόν Μέσον' [Hypnotism as a therapeutic means], *Ψυχιατρική και Νευρολογική Επιθεώρησις* [Psychiatric and Neurological Review], 3, no. 4 (1904), 115–20. On the introduction of psychoanalysis in Greece, see D. Karydaki, 'Freud under the Acropolis: the challenging journey of psychoanalysis in twentieth-century Greece (1915–1995)', *History of the Human Sciences*, 31, no. 4 (2018), 13–37.

52 Katsaras, 'Περί των εξ οινοπνεύματος παθήσεων εν Ελλάδι', 225.

53 *Εφημερίς των Συζητήσεων της Βουλής* [Journal of Parliamentary Debates], 5 July 1899, p. 1317; Ministry of Finance, *Φορολογία, Παραγωγή και Κατανάλωσις των Οινοπνευμάτων και του Ζύθου μετά Στατιστικών Πινάκων* [Taxation, Production, and Consumption of Spirits and Beer with Statistical Tables] (Athens: Ethnikon Typographeion, 1905), xii–xiv.

54 'Η Φορολογία των Οινοπνευμάτων' [The Taxation of Alcohols], *Άστυ* [Asty], 6 July 1899, p. 3.

55 G. Metaxas, 'Ο Αλκοολισμός εν Κοζάνη της Μακεδονίας' [Alcoholism in Kozani, Macedonia], *Ψυχιατρική και Νευρολογική Επιθεώρησις* [Psychiatric and Neurological Review], 1, no. 6 (1903), 173–4; Vlavianos, 'Ο αλκοολισμός' (1910), 177–82.

56 'Αδελφότης 'Αθηνά-Υγεία' [Athena-Health fraternity], *Ψυχιατρική και Νευρολογική Επιθεώρησις* [Psychiatric and Neurological Review], 5, no. 5 (1907), 151.

57 Supreme Directorate of Public Education, *Circular to the Inspectors General and Inspectors of Elementary Schools*, no. 1458/1977, 25

February 1917, concerning Prof. N. Panas, *Τα Ολέθρια Αποτελέσματα των Οινοπνευματωδών Ποτών και του Καπνού* [The Disastrous Effects of Alcoholic Beverages and Tobacco] (Athens: n.pub., 1914): 'έξεων προωρισμένων ασφαλώς να υποσκάπτωσι την ψυχήν και το σώμα των νέων και περιαγάγωσιν εις κίνδυνον την ύπαρξιν της φυλής ημών'.

58 S. Galanos, *Τα Αλκοολούχα Ποτά: Ιστορία, Παρασκευή, Σύστασις και Ενέργεια αυτών επί του Οργανισμού του Ανθρώπου* [Alcoholic Beverages: History, Fabrication, Composition and Action on the Human Organism] (Athens: Ekdotiki, 1926), 80: 'ποτήριον οίνου ή ζύθου πινόμενον εις ευχάριστον συγκέντρωσιν δεν είνε επιβλαβές, αλλ' απεναντίας συντελεί εις την επίτευξιν ευχαρίστων ωρών αναπαύσεως από των καθημερινών αγώνων της ζωής'.

59 M. Moyseidis, 'Το Οινόπνευμα και τα Οινοπνευματώδη Ποτά από Απόψεως Υγιεινής' [Alcohol and alcoholic drinks from a health viewpoint], *Υγεία* [Health], 12, no. 2 (1935), 21–2.

60 Papagiannis (ed.), *Πρακτικά του Β' Πανελληνίου Ιατρικού Συνεδρίου*, 208–51.

61 W.O. Atwater and F.G. Benedict, 'An experimental inquiry regarding the nutritive value of alcohol', *Memoirs of the National Academy of Sciences*, 8, no. 6 (1902), 231–397.

62 Papagiannis (ed.), *Πρακτικά του Β' Πανελληνίου Ιατρικού Συνεδρίου*, 246–7.

63 S. Dontas, 'Le vin comme aliment', *Bulletin international du vin*, 7, no. 76 (1934) 50–4. On the *Bulletin*, see K. Munholland, '"Mon docteur le vin": wine and health in France, 1900–1950', in M. Holt (ed.), *Alcohol: A Cultural and Social History* (Oxford and New York: Berg, 2006), 82.

64 S. Dontas, 'Ο οίνος κατά του αλκοολισμού' [Wine against alcoholism], *Πρακτικά της Ακαδημίας Αθηνών* [Proceedings of the Academy of Athens], session of 14 March 1935, pp. 129–30: 'ο κατάλληλος τρόπος προς μετριασμόν, κατά το δυνατόν, του αλκοολισμού είναι η ευρυτέρα διάδοσις της χρήσεως του φυσικού οίνου, προς αντικατάστασιν των βλαβερών οινοπνευματωδών ποτών. Η μετρία χρήσις του αφθονούντος εν Ελλάδι φυσικού οίνου και ιδίως του υγιεινού ρητινίτου είναι ωφέλιμος εις τον οργανισμόν, χωρίς να φέρη βλάβην. Εις τους εργαζομένους μάλιστα και ανεπαρκώς τρεφομένους ο οίνος είναι αναγκαίον συμπλήρωμα της τροφής.'

65 See, for example, R. Brunet, *La valeur alimentaire et hygiénique du vin* (Paris: Librairie agricole de la Maison rustique, 1914).

66 K. Katsaras, *Οίνος και αλκοολισμός* [Wine and Alcoholism] (n.p.: Pyrsos, 1936), 22, 26–7: 'σταματήσατε την επικινδυνωτάτην επιστημονική σας

προπαγάνδα διά του συστήματος της κρασοθεραπείας, του 'μετρίως' και 'λελογισμένως' υπέρ της καταναλώσεων του οίνου'.

67 S. Dontas, 'La doctrine du vin', *Bulletin international du vin*, 9, no. 97 (1936), 100; Katsaras, *Οίνος και αλκοολισμός*, 16: 'σαν να θέλωμε να σβήσωμε την πυρκαϊά με τη φωτειά, ή ν' αποφασίσωμε να ρίξωμε μπαρούτι ή λάδι σ' αναμμένη φωτειά!'

68 S. Dontas, 'Le referendum médical en Grèce sur la valeur alimentaire hygiénique et thérapeutique du vin', *Bulletin international du vin*, 11, no. 116 (1938), 23–4.

69 S. Vlavianos, 'Ο Ανταλκοολικός Αγών εν Ελλάδι' [The fight against alcohol in Greece], *Ψυχιατρική και Νευρολογική Επιθεώρησις* [Psychiatric and Neurological Review], 8, nos 5–6 (1910), 1–2: 'Το σύμβολον ημών έστω η απόλυτος εγκράτεια [*abstinence totale*] και είτα η εν μέτρω χρήσις [*modération*]. Το δεύτερον επιτυγχάνει, το πρώτο θριαμβεύει.'

8

The fear of the immoderate Muslim: alcohol, civilisation and the theories of the *École d'Alger*, 1933–1962

Nina S. Studer

From the beginning of the military conquest of the region, the majority of French observers noted that Algerian Muslims had strictly adhered to the Qur'anic prohibition of alcohol before the advent of the French.[1] This assumption was demonstrably untrue. Alcohol was consumed by Jewish, Christian and Muslim groups in Algeria before the French conquest, as it was in other Muslim regions, such as, for example, the Mughal Empire.[2] The prohibition of alcohol in the Qur'an is clear, yet, as argued by Shahab Ahmed in his recent book *What is Islam?*, historically, Muslims did not always translate the consumption of alcohol into a loss of religious identity.[3]

French colonial psychiatrists writing in the nineteenth and twentieth centuries, however, were mostly unaware that parts of the Muslim population had been drinking alcohol in Algeria for centuries. Many French authors found the idea of abstinence deeply perplexing and 'non-French' on account of the complex interconnections between France's national identity and certain forms of alcohol, as demonstrated by the historian Kolleen Guy and the anthropologist Marion Demossier.[4] Yet not all of the Muslims they encountered in Algeria adhered to this total abstinence, which French observers interpreted as a new development. Consequently, they understood themselves as living through a period of rapid change in this respect, with more and more formerly abstinent Muslims ostensibly starting to drink increasing amounts of alcohol. Understandably, they documented their observations of this 'new' phenomenon of alcohol-drinking Muslims in their publications and theorised about its origins and possible consequences. The French doctor Louis Lataillade, for example, blamed contact with France for this process of gradual alcoholisation among Muslims in his 1936 dissertation:

> For if, during one century [i.e. the century after the conquest of Algiers in 1830], French civilisation has been able to begin to halt old scourges in North Africa – syphilis, malaria – it has, on the other hand, imported new, previously unknown ones – alcoholism, tuberculosis. Consequently the contract which binds the colonising people to the colonised now only becomes more rigorous and demanding.[5]

The narrative of alcohol having been unknown in the region until it was imported by the French came to the fore soon after the conquest of Algiers in 1830. Consequently, in the mid-twentieth century, psychiatric experts such as those affiliated with the influential psychiatric school of thought commonly called the *École d'Alger*, established by the French psychiatrist Antoine Porot in Algeria from the 1920s onwards,[6] were able to anchor reports of their personal experiences with Muslim alcoholic patients in a large body of nineteenth-century and early twentieth-century literature that recorded an assumed steady rise of alcohol consumption among Muslims during colonisation.[7] Despite the fact that the *École d'Alger* based their texts on the findings of earlier experts, the narrative that the colonised Muslim had recently discovered alcohol – and thus that excessive drinking presented a pressing new problem – remained dominant throughout the last thirty years of the colonisation of Algeria; an anachronism that seems to have been unapparent to colonial authors.[8]

World War I, during which Algerian Muslim soldiers fought and drank alongside the French, had, according to many colonial authors, further accelerated Muslim alcohol consumption in Algeria.[9] Nevertheless, it was the establishment of psychiatric institutions on North African soil in the 1930s, which will be discussed below, that brought a sea change in the eyes of French authors writing about the alcohol consumption of the colonised Muslim. They found themselves suddenly confronted with a sharp increase in Muslim patients. A range of mental illnesses, including alcoholism, which had formerly been regarded as rare among colonised Algerians,[10] were now increasingly framed as ubiquitous.[11]

This chapter examines how French colonial psychiatrists wrote about social and economic alcohol-related problems among colonised people between the first establishment of a psychiatric institution in Algeria in 1933 and Algerian independence in 1962. How did they explain the reported increase in alcohol consumption, and how were sentiments of guilt – related to their own involvement in the introduction of alcoholism into what was, allegedly, a formerly sober region – expressed in their publications? Did the French colonial psychiatrists of the twentieth century truly believe that France was to blame for alcoholism and alcohol-related criminality among Muslims? Had France's celebrated *mission civilisatrice* been, in the specific context of alcohol consumption, a corrupting influence on Algerian Muslims? Finally, this chapter asks whether the framing of 'immoderation' as a medically and psychiatrically defined character trait – presumed to be shared by all Muslims – had an impact on colonial descriptions of Algerians' alcohol consumption.

The source material analysed for this chapter was written by French colonial doctors interested in alcohol and by French colonial psychiatrists who either belonged to, or were contemporaries of, the *École d'Alger*. The source material consists of monographs, articles, dissertations and conference papers from the 1930s to 1962. Publications by Algerian Muslims, either in French or in Arabic, will not be covered in this chapter, as presenting the centuries-spanning discourse of Muslim religious, legal and medical scholars on this issue is far beyond the scope of a single chapter. This chapter focuses solely on Orientalist psychiatric viewpoints pertaining to alcohol-drinking Algerian Muslims in the French colony.[12] It should be added that, while publications of French colonial psychiatry in general, and the *École d'Alger* in particular, have been a site of research for a number of historians, psychiatric theories about the alcohol consumption of colonised Algerians have been mostly neglected.[13]

This chapter is divided into four parts. The first part provides the historical background of psychiatric developments during the 1930s. It maps the impact of the theories proposed by the *École d'Alger* on the study of alcoholism in the region. The second part examines the idea that Algerian Muslims, who allegedly had not consumed any alcohol before French colonisation, took to drinking alcohol only in an attempt to imitate their colonisers. This imitation was, in the time period studied in this chapter, often contextualised by the theory of 'assimilation', whose ideals had by that time already been largely discarded. The third part of this chapter focuses on the notion that alcoholism was a particularly serious problem in the Algerian context, because, as was proposed by members of the *École d'Alger*, Muslims inherently lacked any moderation. Finally, the last section discusses the idea, prevalent among French colonists, that alcohol-drinking Muslims were more prone to criminality and violence than any other group in colonial Algeria, and consequently presented a greater social problem to the settler society of Algeria.

The *École d'Alger* and alcoholism

The period between the founding of the first psychiatric institution in 1933 and Algeria's independence from France in 1962 was the time when the *École d'Alger* flourished and influenced the methods, treatments and theories of French metropolitan psychiatry. The historian Richard Keller argued in his 2007 book *Colonial Madness* that the publications of the *École d'Alger* in this specific time period 'reflected the hardening of racial lines that characterized Algeria in the interwar years as a distinct mentality emerged among the so-called *pieds-noirs*, or French Algerian settlers'.[14] The French discussion on alcoholism among Muslims in Algeria was consequently dominated by psychiatrists of a particularly racialised mindset, which had a long-lasting impact on the framing of the issue.[15]

While French hospitals had been established in Algeria since 1830,[16] the first colonial psychiatric institution, the hospital of Blida-Joinville, was founded (by Antoine Porot) only in 1933.[17] Before the establishment of Blida-Joinville, a small number of psychiatric patients – both colonisers and colonised – were shipped from Algeria to asylums in France for treatment.[18] Most of the alcoholic patients shipped to France from Algeria were Europeans.[19] French experts in the metropolitan institutions wrote only occasionally about what they perceived to be an increase in alcoholism among their Muslim patients.[20] The opening of Blida-Joinville also meant that psychiatric experts writing about mental illnesses among colonised Muslims now lived and worked on Algerian soil,[21] and, as Charlotte Chopin has shown, colonial doctors and psychiatrists of the *École d'Alger* both embodied and justified settler values.[22]

Blida-Joinville was an institution that welcomed men and women, and settler and colonised patients, with colonised Algerians making up the largest proportion of the patient population. Between 1933 and 1940, Muslims made up the largest group of the hospital population (49.29 per cent), while 43.66 per cent of patients were 'European' and 7.1 per cent 'Jewish'.[23] In many of the colonial texts, immense pride was expressed in the achievement of having founded a psychiatric institution in Algeria. The psychiatrists Maurice Desruelles and Henri Bersot, for example, stated in a 1939 article that 'This psychiatric hospital is one of the most beautiful achievements of the schemes of assistance in Algeria and does great honour to the colony and its government.'[24] Yet despite praise like this, not all was as had been hoped. When it was officially opened in 1938, Blida-Joinville had a capacity of 1,200 beds, divided into four departments, for both French and Algerian patients.[25] This proved quickly inadequate for the needs of the colony. Many Muslims, who previously would never have brought their family members into a colonial institution because of the risk of them being transported across the sea, now admitted their loved ones to the care of the French psychiatrists in Blida-Joinville. Consequently Blida-Joinville quickly became overcrowded.[26]

The psychiatrists of the *École d'Alger* who worked in the departments of Blida-Joinville published a series of articles on the diagnoses assigned to these 'new' patients, which included 'alcoholism'. These studies were based on the theory of 'North African primitivism', namely the theory that colonised people acted and reacted in ways that were markedly different from French behaviour.[27] Antoine Porot and the psychiatrists of the *École d'Alger* were notably criticised for this by the psychoanalyst and political philosopher Frantz Fanon, who worked in psychiatric institutions in both Algeria and Tunisia in the 1950s.[28]

Antoine Porot's son and student, Maurice Porot, and his colleague Jean Gentile, conducted a study in 1941 into "Alcoholism and Mental Problems in the Algerian Muslim Native".[29] They noted that 54 per cent of Muslim patients with mental illnesses in Blida-Joinville had consumed alcohol at some point in their lives, and that these patients ranged from one-time consumers to people who drank every day.[30] Antoine Porot used this study to underline the idea that there had been a shocking increase in alcoholism among Algerian Muslim patients in the twentieth century and suggested in 1943 that '60 per cent of the natives interned in Blida are alcoholics'.[31] A rough estimation combining Antoine Porot's statement with the numbers provided by Charles Bardenat, mentioned above, and the 1,200-bed capacity of Blida-Joinville during this time period leads to startling numbers: Antoine Porot seems to have been suggesting that in 1943 around 360 Muslim alcoholics were interned in Blida-Joinville.

Antoine Porot's reference for the figure of 60 per cent was the article written by Maurice Porot and Jean Gentile, and specifically their statement that 54 per cent of Muslim patients had had some contact with alcohol before hospital admission.[32] Yet by rounding up and presenting all alcohol drinkers as outright alcoholics, he severely misconstrued the numbers provided by his two students. The numbers are also seen to be flawed if compared with data provided in other publications. In 1954 three French psychiatrists of the *École d'Alger*, G.-A. Manceaux, Jean Sutter and Yves Pélicier, stated that 6 per cent of all Muslim patients in French psychiatric institutions in Algeria were alcoholics.[33] This amounted to just 10 per cent of the total suggested by Porot a decade earlier.

The figures provided by French colonial psychiatrists on the increase in alcoholism usually related to Muslim men. The alcohol consumption of Muslim women was routinely neglected by colonial authors, who believed that only marginalised Muslim women, detached from their families, would turn to alcohol. Consequently, the women whose alcohol consumption and alcoholism were recorded in the sources were mostly those described as 'prostitutes' and 'dancers' – with little or no proof provided for these claims – or as domestic workers.[34] Maurice Porot and Jean Gentile, for example, excluded female alcohol consumption completely from their 1941 study, arguing that 'The extreme rarity of alcoholism among Muslim women (apart from prostitutes) made us confine this survey to men only.'[35] Because of such preconceptions, the non-gendered descriptions of drinking habits in the source material have to be read as male unless it is stated otherwise.

Because of a lack of reliable statistical evidence about alcohol consumption and alcoholism rates in the published psychiatric sources, it is difficult to substantiate whether the ostensibly well-documented increase was just a postulated increase (linked to miscalculation, the spread of psychiatric institutions in the region and an intensifying interest in the diagnosis of alcoholism) or was due to an actual increase in numbers (linked to a greater availability of alcohol under French rule).[36] Yet it is clear that most of the French psychiatric experts writing between the 1930s and Algeria's independence in 1962 were convinced that they were observing and recording a gradual loss of inhibition towards alcohol in the Muslims around them. The leaders of the *École d'Alger* in particular believed there to be an actual increase in both consumption and over-consumption of alcohol among Muslims, and wrote about it accordingly.

Mission corruptrice?

The idea that alcohol was introduced not only into Algeria but into the whole Maghreb by the French was the cornerstone of psychiatric theories about the alcohol consumption of colonised Muslims. Consequently, their alcohol consumption was always understood as something imported and copied. French colonial doctors and psychiatrists often blamed the French for the advent not only of alcohol but also alcoholism in the Maghreb, and expressed a certain feeling of guilt about the existence of alcoholic Muslims. Many suspected that the bad example of European settlers – especially of the non-French, namely the Italians, Spaniards and Maltese in Algeria – was responsible for the rising levels of alcohol consumption among the colonised Muslim population.[37] This interpretation of the situation was troublesome to the French in general and to French doctors and psychiatrists in particular. The psychiatrist Raoul Vadon, for example, stated somewhat dejectedly in his 1935 dissertation on 'Medical assistance for psychopaths in Tunisia', that, while he was working in Algeria, alcohol was easily accessible to Tunisian Muslims, 'thanks to the contribution of our so-called civilisation'.[38]

France's colonial empire was based on the ideals of the *mission civilisatrice*, the assumption that the colonisation of a region by France would markedly improve the lives of the colonised, and, as Nancy Gallagher demonstrated in her 1983 book *Medicine and Power in Tunisia*, European medicine was an 'integral part of the French *mission civilisatrice*'.[39] Many colonial doctors and psychiatrists wholeheartedly adopted the *mission civilisatrice* and believed that their role was as much to improve the health of the colonisers and the colonised as to educate and elevate the colonised on both an intellectual and a moral level. Colonising Algeria meant, in the eyes of many of the French psychiatrists studied for this chapter, civilising Algeria. By the 1930s, France had been 'civilising' Algeria for a century. In this narrative of success, the question of France's influence on the rising alcohol consumption among Muslims and the consequences of overconsumption presented a moral challenge. Was alcoholism among the colonised a necessary evil born of their contact with French civilisation? Dr H. Foley of the *Pasteur Institute of Algeria*, for example, described in 1938 a clear link between civilisation and alcoholism in an article on medical issues in the rural south of Algeria:

> As in all countries of the world, alcoholism spread among the Algerian Natives with civilisation. If it is still unknown among the nomadic Arabs, and, in general, among most of the inhabitants of the Sahara, its progress can be observed in the localities populated by Europeans, in the garrison towns, and, particularly, among the Natives who have lived in France or in the Tell [the Tell Atlas range in Algeria], among the former military, the prostitutes.[40]

The 'civilisation' spreading among Algerians mentioned by Foley was, in his eyes, clearly the hoped-for result of the efforts of the *mission civilisatrice*; it was *French* civilisation spreading in the colony. Yet the projected positive effect of French influence was apparently also the 'cause' of alcoholism among those they tried to 'civilise'.

French psychiatrists were convinced that proximity to French culture caused the colonised Muslim to drink. They held the view that Muslim city dwellers on the Mediterranean coast had begun to indulge in alcohol because of their exposure to French people and institutions, while those in the countryside were, so to speak, outside the reach of this apparently 'corrupting' proximity to France. In particular, it was believed that Algerian Muslims whose work brought them into direct contact with French drinkers, such as soldiers, porters, servants and 'prostitutes',[41] witnessed and then copied the bad example of the French settlers, who, according to many disapproving psychiatric experts, drank too much. In 1959, for example, the psychiatrists Jean Sutter, Maurice Porot and Yves Pélicier were convinced that only those Algerians who had been in contact with France had started to drink: 'The religious interdiction of drinking alcohol is still respected by the vast majority of rural Muslims. Those of the towns, on the other hand, indulge more and more in alcohol and often with a considerable immoderation.'[42]

There is evidence that alcohol consumption was indeed more prevalent among Algerian Muslims in the colonial cities. French psychiatrists were, however, seemingly unaware of the fact that the upheaval of colonisation itself had, in the words of the psychologist Ihsan al-Issa of 2000, brought about 'the destruction of traditional village life' in Algeria.[43] Al-Issa argued that this process had brought many poor Algerians into the cities, where they could no longer rely on the social networks of their villages, which, in turn, caused many to develop mental illnesses. Alcoholism was one.

From the beginning of the colonisation of Algeria, French authors had debated whether the spread of civilisation necessarily went hand in hand with a rise in alcoholism. One group of French observers believed that alcoholisation – which they often directly or indirectly connected to either Christianity or secularism – was necessary to achieve civilisation. A 1913 newspaper article on 'Alcoholism in Morocco', for example, exclaimed that alcoholism was 'The barometer of civilisation!'[44]

The questions of whether it was possible to 'civilise' Algerian Muslims without alcoholising them, and whether 'civilisation' was even achievable without the involvement of alcohol, were closely linked to one of the main debates in regard to French colonialism since the beginning of the conquest of Algeria: the contest between the contrasting theories of 'assimilation' and 'association'.[45] Although they were very different in outlook, both of these concepts were based on the ideals of the *mission civilisatrice*. As the historian Patricia Lorcin explained in 1995 in Imperial Identities, both theories had 'civilisation' as their alleged end goal.[46]

In the nineteenth century, French colonial psychiatrists had actively engaged in the discussion of whether assimilation could work on Muslim Algerians, namely if they could ever 'progress' enough to turn into Frenchmen, or whether France should push 'association', or the parallel and asynchronous development of the different races in the Algerian context. The debate about assimilation versus association was often bound up with drinking habits. In the nineteenth century, there were claims that the adoption of alcohol as a drink of choice was a sign of Algerians being at least 'capable' of assimilation.[47] In the twentieth century, however, evolutionary theories led a majority of psychiatric authors to the conviction that had long been propagated by many of the anti-assimilationist settlers in Algeria:[48] Algerian Muslims could never be turned into Frenchmen, as they were just too different.[49] Pierre Pinaud, for example, declared in his 1933 medical dissertation on 'Alcoholism among Arabs in Algeria' that, despite both belonging to the 'white race', Algerian Muslims and French people were inherently different and that this difference could, apparently, not be bridged.[50]

The psychiatrists of the *École d'Alger* were clearly in favour of a strong theory of association. While they interpreted alcohol consumption among colonised Muslims as essentially France's fault, they did not consider drinking an indicator of assimilability. Colonised Muslims could never hope to become French in any way, and still less so through alcohol, as they drank it 'wrongly' – both too much of it and the wrong drinks – as will be discussed in the next part of this chapter. The perceived increase in the number of alcohol-drinking Muslims was construed as a sign of North African 'primitivity'. It should be added here that this argumentation and vocabulary were also adopted by some Muslim writers of this period. The prolific Algerian author Mohammed Soualah, for example, lamented in 1937 that alcohol and alcoholism were spreading 'rapidly' in the Maghreb, before stating that, because of alcohol, 'this beautiful North African race, strong, sober and prolific, is undergoing a veritable physical and moral downfall'.[51]

'Immoderation specific to the primitives'

From the 1930s onwards, when writing about alcohol, French colonial psychiatrists focused on over-consumption to such a degree that they used the term 'alcoholism' even when they referred to moderate drinking, as in the case of the article by Antoine Porot quoted above. The fact that a Muslim 'drank alcohol' was very often interpreted as evidence of 'alcoholism'. The notion that Muslims were incapable of moderate consumption was explained either by the assumption that those who, knowing that they broke religious precepts, felt the need to profit to the utmost from their transgression, or by postulation of an inherent trait among Muslims for immoderation.[52] The latter was far more prevalent, especially among the theories of the *École d'Alger*. Maurice Porot and Jean Gentile even went as far as stating in their 1941 article that '*The Muslim who drinks, does not drink moderately* … .'[53] The authors based this assertion on their experience at Blida-Joinville. They confirmed Antoine Porot's earlier suggestions of 1918 and those of an article co-authored with Don Côme Arrii in 1932 that the drinking habits of Algerian Muslims were driven by an 'immoderation specific to the primitives', which supposedly made alcohol consumption among Muslims all the more dangerous.[54] In 1943 Antoine Porot wrote: 'Periodically, alarms are raised [about the problem of alcoholism in Algeria], especially regarding the danger that is posed to the natives who rush towards alcohol with an immoderation specific to all primitives.'[55]

Porot's view was that it was 'immoderation' that made alcohol consumption dangerous. He never suggested that people should be abstinent and believed that moderate drinking was a sign of civilised Frenchness. Porot did not subscribe to the views promulgated by the French abstinence movement, which had formed during World War I.[56] Instead, he conformed to a long-established consensus in

France, where people had always regarded abstinence as somewhat suspicious and as essentially non-French. As the historian Patricia Prestwich put it in 2003: 'In the late nineteenth century, those who voluntarily abstained from all alcohol were considered eccentric and prone to other non-French preoccupations, such as vegetarianism, animal rights and Protestantism.'[57]

Many colonial psychiatrists during the time period covered by this chapter agreed with Porot, suggesting that it was this inherent immoderation, rather than the increased availability of alcohol connected with the French conquest, that caused the medical, economic and social alcohol-related complications that apparently plagued Algeria. Immoderation was described in the psychiatric sources as a shared, inherited character trait of a 'race' – which variously included all 'Arabs', all Muslims, all colonised people and all 'primitives'. Psychiatrists of the *École d'Alger* even propagated the theory of a North African 'primitive mentality' that included both immoderation and proneness to addiction as two of its main criteria.[58] Immoderation was seen to be exacerbated by the abstinence of generations of Algerian Muslims before European influence. As Antoine Porot and Don Côme Arrii perceived: 'The native is hypersensitive to alcohol because of his individual or ancestral unaccustomedness [to drinking] … .'[59]

Was the drinking behaviour of Algerian Muslims persistently immoderate or was this observation just a racist prejudice shared by French authors? On the basis of the psychiatric source material from the colonial period, it is impossible to answer this question. Nessim Znaien has suggested in a 2020 chapter on 'Drinking and production patterns of wine in North Africa during French colonisation, *c.* 1830–1956' that there was indeed a clear increase in the consumption of wine among all groups in Algeria after 1900, including among Muslims.[60] An increase in wine consumption might indicate an increase in over-consumption. Similarly, the problems caused by overcrowding at the psychiatric hospital of Blida-Joinville, and Maurice Porot's and Jean Gentile's research in 1941 that seemed to show that over half of male Muslim inpatients had consumed alcohol at least once in their lives, may have caused colonial psychiatric experts to assume an increase in immoderate drinking.

The information in the source material, however, is merely anecdotal and cannot be extrapolated to broader patient and non-patient populations. The most thorough investigation into the forms of alcohol consumed by individual Algerians can be found in Pierre Pinaud's 1933 dissertation, in which he described Muslim patients confined in mental institutions and certified as 'alcoholics', as well as Muslim alcohol consumers among the general public, as drinking litres of wine every day,[61] consuming excessive amounts of aperitifs and anisettes at 'all hours of the day'[62] and absorbing 'excessive amounts' of beer.[63] One of the cases he mentioned in his dissertation was a Muslim man whom he had personally looked after and who, at the end of Ramadan, had consumed enormous amounts of alcohol. Allegedly, this man had drunk 'in an hour, six bottles of red wine'.[64] Although Pinaud was not part of the *École d'Alger*, his personal experiences led him to subscribe to the idea that alcohol consumption among Muslims was immoderate almost by definition.

Lack of moderation was not described in any detail in the source material; the *École d'Alger* interpreted it as an inborn character trait that did not seem to warrant explanation and definition.[65] Pinaud, on the other hand, explained 'immoderation' in relation to the pressure felt by Algerians during the process of colonisation, when new models of social and religious behaviour emerged. He noted in 1933:

> An essential point, which strikes one from the beginning of this study, is the immoderation with which the native indulges in alcohol. With him, there are no half measures: either he respects the wise precepts of the Qur'an and will abstain all his life from bringing any fermented beverage to his lips; or, if he starts drinking, he will soon exceed fair and reasonable measures. There are only very few Arabs who maintain a rational and moderate consumption of alcohol similar to that of many Europeans.[66]

This 'immoderation specific to the primitives', to use Porot's favourite formulation again, was, allegedly, shown not only in the amounts consumed by the Algerian Muslims, but also in their choice of drink. French authors often lamented that Algerian Muslims usually did not choose to drink wine, which was essentially seen as harmless by most French authors, including doctors and psychiatrists.[67] Instead they chose stronger liquors, such as anisettes, and absinthe before its prohibition in 1915. It should be added, however, that this interpretation of Muslim drinking habits was extremely one-sided. Many Algerian Muslims did drink wine, as shown, for example, in Pinaud's dissertation, where he described cases of Muslim patients drinking four to five litres of wine a day.[68] Despite such evidence, most of the colonial psychiatrists believed that Algerian Muslims had chosen to consume mainly 'bad alcohol', i.e. everything stronger than wine and beer. This taste for 'bad alcohol' led, allegedly, to situations that were dangerous both to the drinkers and to the rest of society, as will be discussed in detail in the fourth part of this chapter. Even Pinaud, perhaps the least prejudiced voice on this issue among the authors studied in this chapter, conceded that the consumption of anisettes posed a particularly serious problem for Algerian Muslims. For him, anisettes were an extreme drink due to the 'essential oils' used in their production, which had historically been blamed for the strong effects of absinthe.[69] Their consumption added a further level of danger to the quantitative immoderation of Algerian Muslims and to the 'fact' that their bodies were not yet generationally adapted to the consumption of alcohol:

> But the natives seem more particularly affected [by the overconsumption of anisettes]. This is, we believe, the result of an idiosyncrasy [of the drink, i.e. the 'essential oils'], unique no doubt, and a less robust resistance to this poison combined with an exaggerated consumption. The cases of acute intoxication assume particularly grave forms among the Arabs …[70]

The idea of immoderation among Muslims in regard to both choice of drink and quantity consumed was, however, nothing new. The historian Rudi Matthee showed in 2014 that since the sixteenth century Muslim alcohol consumption had been described as excessive.[71] The harking back to earlier ideas was not unusual. While being enormously influential, most of the ideas that the *École d'Alger* propagated in the twentieth century had, indeed, existed for some time, as is noted by Richard Keller.[72]

The tragedy of alcoholised criminality

According to Richard Keller, the idea that North Africans were excessively violent was another theme that the *École d'Alger* had adopted from the publications of nineteenth-century French colonial psychiatrists.[73] The *École d'Alger* suggested that the observed increase in immoderate alcohol consumption among Muslims heightened the threat posed by Muslims even further. In this they agreed with the French settlers, who were deeply fearful of Muslims in general and Muslim drunkenness in particular. As Peter Dunwoodie, a professor of French literature, suggests, after 1912 'newspaper campaigns exploited widespread fears that France faced a major social crisis' in Algeria.[74] These fears were focused on the figure of the 'dangerous Algerian', the suspected rapist and murderer.[75] Pinaud alluded to these same sensational newspaper reports in his 1933 dissertation when he claimed that 'it is enough to consult any newspaper in order to observe the considerable number of criminal acts, attacks and murders committed by natives in a state of drunkenness'.[76]

The characterisation of North African men as dangerous *per se* has recently been critiqued by a group of Tunisian psychiatrists, who have claimed that French colonial psychiatry framed North Africa as 'a space of wild violence and of sexual perversity, as well as of madness'.[77] In the eyes of the psychiatrists of the *École d'Alger*, the perceived danger was intensified if North Africans were drunk. Antoine Porot and his student Jean Sutter even connected alcohol and criminality to the 'primitive mentality' of all Muslims. They claimed that nothing was more likely than alcohol 'to reveal the criminal impulsivity which we have already reported as one of the dominant traits of the native soul'.[78] In their eyes, alcohol intensified a predisposition towards criminality and violence inherent in North Africans. The idea of alcohol as a catalyst for crime in North Africans was also taken up by some North Africans themselves. The aforementioned Algerian writer Mohammed Soualah, for example, stated in 1937 that the consumption of anisettes destroyed Maghrebi families, as it drove North African 'men, degraded, [to] commit crimes'.[79]

In his 1937 dissertation, Jean Sutter epitomised this sense of fear, shared by his fellow settlers and, as shown by Soualah's example, also some Algerians, painting a vivid picture of 'everyday' drunken violence among Algerian Muslims:

> It is conceivable that their primitive temperament, the mental debility so frequent in them, creates conditions particularly favourable to brutal, impulsive reactions, often imprinted with veritable savagery. Every day, in the cities, at the doors of the cafés or the bars, disputes start, which, very quickly, degenerate into brawls; they play with the knife or with the baton, or even the gun, and this lasts until the arrival of the police, until the desperate flight to another tavern, a new fight.[80]

In Sutter's worldview, alcohol ignited a violent savagery in North Africans, which might otherwise have remained hidden. Consequently, alcohol posed a distinct threat to Algerian society. As the French psychiatric experts believed that a large percentage of all criminal acts were committed by Muslim men under the influence, the reported rising alcohol levels among Muslims must have appeared alarming. Antoine Porot warned readers in a section of the 1952 version of the *Handbook for Clinical and Therapeutic Psychiatrists* titled 'Chronic Alcoholism': 'Our findings as medical experts in North Africa have allowed us to establish a parallelism between the extension of alcoholism and the increase in criminality stemming from it: from 24 per cent in 1929 to 50 per cent in 1940.'[81] These numbers, which included alcoholism and criminality among both Muslim and French patients, were undeniably alarming. Yet given how carelessly Antoine Porot used the statistics on alcohol consumption in Blida-Joinville composed by Maurice Porot and Jean Gentile, these figures must be taken with a large pinch of salt, especially as he did not provide source references for them. In any case, Porot's claim of a doubling of alcohol-fuelled criminality in just a little over ten years confirmed existing views that the safety of French settlers in Algeria was threatened. Even though violence was most often directed towards those in close proximity to the drinkers – namely families, friends and neighbours – French settlers, frightened by sensationalist newspaper articles on Muslim violence, pictured themselves as the potential victims of thefts, assaults and even murders by drunk Algerian Muslims.

Alcohol was not only seen to pose a danger to the drinker on account of its detrimental medical and psychiatric effects, and to society because of associated alcohol-fuelled violence and crime, but was also seen to jeopardise the wellbeing of future generations – Muslim and European alike.[82] In the context of Algeria, this was also understood as a problem among the French.[83] French settlers in particular were often framed as failing France's *mission civilisatrice* by not producing capable, strong and healthy children. As the historian Daniel Pick suggested in his *Faces of Degeneration*, in the nineteenth century alcoholism was framed as one of the main factors causing or at least furthering 'racial degeneration', lowering birth rates and thus 'endangering the European races'.[84] While theories of hereditary degeneracy were strongly criticised and largely discredited in French psychiatry in the early twentieth century, as discussed, for example, by Ian Dowbiggin in *Inheriting Madness*,[85] French colonial doctors and psychiatrists were, nevertheless, still influenced by them. In colonial Algeria, degeneration was seen as a pressing issue, as European settlers felt threatened by the colonised population surrounding them.

The idea of racial degeneration through alcoholism was also at the core of the postulated decline of the Algerian Muslim, a 'race' that was seen to have once possessed a wide range of noble qualities. Pierre Pinaud mused:

> We have improved the conditions of existence of this population [the Algerian Muslims], but we have imposed on them many of our vices. It is up to us to save them. … A tighter regulation of the consumption of alcohol must be imposed, or we risk soon seeing this race, which was so great and strong, mother of our civilisation, accelerate its march into the abyss under the yoke of this redoubtable poison [alcohol].[86]

Pinaud conformed here to the Orientalist narrative of Muslim regions as civilisations in decline.[87] In the context of the Maghreb, these narratives usually insisted that the perceived decline had started at an unspecified period, long in the past, while Pinaud believed its cause to lie in the introduction of alcohol to the region.

Conclusions: when others drink

French colonial psychiatrists, whose publications were used as the source material for this chapter, wrote as experts for an expert audience, even though the ideas expressed in their texts often reflected and justified settler notions about colonised Algerians – especially when it came to the allegedly inherent Muslim immoderation and tendency to violence.[88] It can be argued that the opinions expressed in the publications of the *École d'Alger* were a distillation of a distinct *pieds-noirs* mentality and that they should be read as a clear defence of settler interests.

By the 1930s, the discussion about whether alcohol consumption among Muslims could ever be an acceptable sign of assimilation was over. The consensus was that the 100 years of French presence in the colony had proven that assimilation was not possible for the simple reason that it had, allegedly, not occurred. The way colonised Muslims misused alcohol was taken by the psychiatrists of the *École d'Alger* as the ultimate proof of their un-assimilability. Even authors such as Pinaud, who concluded in their publications that the alcohol consumption of Algerian Muslims showed a certain degree of assimilation on their part, stated that they had assimilated 'wrongly'. Reports on Algerian alcohol drinkers have to be understood as case studies, composed by the settler-psychiatrists of the *École d'Alger* to prove the un-assimilability of colonised Muslims.

Between 1930 and 1962 there was surprisingly little variety in the views of French colonial psychiatrists on the subject of Muslim alcohol consumption. Psychiatrists of the *École d'Alger* tended to dominate wider views on alcohol and alcoholism. There were only a few dissenting French voices on issues surrounding alcohol-drinking Muslims. The best example of an exception is Pierre Pinaud, whose nuanced 1933 medical dissertation on 'Alcoholism among Arabs in Algeria' was based on his personal experiences in Algeria before the establishment of Blida-Joinville, and unlike the main authors writing on the psychiatric diagnosis of alcoholism among Algerian Muslims in the 1930s, he seems not to have had any personal or professional connection to Antoine Porot.

As shown in this chapter, Pinaud's views diverged from the principal theories of the *École d'Alger* in many respects, especially in regard to the explanation for excessive consumption and in regard to the question of guilt. He described the immoderation in consumption that he observed among Algerian drinkers not as a racial characteristic, as the *École d'Alger*'s theories of a primitive mentality suggested, but as a result of breaking Islam's religious norms.[89] As he did not understand 'immoderation' to be a racial characteristic, he did not blame it for the rise in alcoholism, but instead put responsibility for this rise on the force that introduced alcohol into the region: France's colonial empire itself. In Pinaud's eyes, France was directly accountable for the 'degeneration' of Algerian Muslims, which he clearly deplored.[90]

Publications of the *École d'Alger* and, to a certain extent, Pinaud's own works expressed the view that there was an increase in alcohol consumption among colonised Algerians, which necessarily led to alcoholism on account of Muslims' alleged innate immoderation and taste for particularly harmful drinks. The increase was seen to have caused overcrowding in the psychiatric institution of Blida-Joinville as well as a fear of Muslim violence and criminality among the European settlers. The perceived threat was fuelled both by financial worries about the expansion and upkeep of overcrowded psychiatric institutions in Algeria and by sensationalist reports in settler newspapers on crimes committed by drunk Muslims.

The psychiatrists of the *École d'Alger* recorded their findings in a world where decolonisation was occurring all around them. Their tendency to adhere to a settler mentality, combined with a certain defensiveness due to the fact that most of them wrote texts that could be read as pro-colonial in an increasingly anti-colonial world, found its way into their theories on alcohol consumption. Their focus on the violence committed by drunk Algerian Muslims, for example, must be understood as a justification of continued French presence and control in Algeria, on both an ideological and a practical level.

Finally, most of the colonial psychiatrists of the *École d'Alger* expressed the paradoxical view that France had introduced alcohol and alcoholism into the region, yet still blamed Algerian Muslims for both their alcoholism and the criminality allegedly caused by it. This paradox was due to the fact that, in the eyes of these authors, it was an innate immoderation that caused both alcoholism and drunken assaults, not alcohol itself. Therefore France's *mission civilisatrice* was not truly to blame for the problems caused by the introduction of alcohol, as France had no influence on the character traits of the 'un-assimilable' colonised Muslim. In their view, by introducing alcohol, France had given the Algerian Muslims a tool of progress, a means of attaining civilisation, but the Algerian Muslims were incapable of grasping it, and their allegedly innate immoderation turned alcohol, a symbol of Frenchness and civilisation, into a catalyst for violence and degeneration.

Notes

1 The clearest prohibition of alcohol in the Qur'an can be found in Sura 5:90–1. Pierre Pinaud, for example, explicitly referred to this passage in the introduction to his 1933 medical dissertation on 'Alcoholism among Arabs in Algeria'. He admittedly quoted the wrong verse number (5:92), but he still showed an understanding of the Muslim sources that most other colonial authors did not seem to possess. P. Pinaud, 'L'alcoolisme chez les Arabes en Algérie' (medical thesis, University of Bordeaux, 1933), 9. Most colonial authors just vaguely stated that alcohol was forbidden in the Qur'an. For both Algeria and the rest of the Maghreb during this time period, see, for example: A. Porot and D. Arrii, 'L'impulsivité criminelle chez l'indigène algérien: ses facteurs', *Annales médico-psychologiques*, 2 (1932), 588–611, at 599f, https://archive.org/details/BIUSante_90152x1932x02/mode/2up (accessed 20 August 2021); G. Hardy, 'L'alimentation des indigènes au Maroc', *La géographie*, 58, nos 3–4 (1932), 143–58, at p. 145; M. Desruelles and H. Bersot, 'L'assistance aux aliénés en Algérie depuis le XIXe siècle', *Annales médico-psychologiques*, 2 (1939), 578–96, at 594, https://archive.org/details/BIUSante_90152x1939x02/mode/2up (accessed 20 August 2021).

2 The Jewish population of Algeria produced several alcoholic drinks. Others were imported from Europe, or fermented or distilled by Muslims. Local forms of alcohol that predated the French conquest of Algeria and were consumed throughout the whole colonial period were usually neglected in French publications, which chose to interpret alcohol in Algeria as a purely imported good. In fact, only a handful

of mentions of traditional, locally produced alcoholic liquors, such as palm wine and fig and date liquors, can be found in the publications of French colonial doctors and psychiatrists during the time period studied for this chapter. See Pinaud, 'Alcoolisme', 36f.; H. Foley, 'Aperçu de la pathologie indigène dans les territoires du Sud algérien', in L. Aufrère et al. (eds), *La vie dans la région désertique Nord-tropicale de l'ancien monde* (Paris: P. Lechevalier, 1938), 275–305, at 301f. On the consumption of alcohol in the Mughal Empire, see S. Honchell, 'The story of a drunken Mughal: Islam, alcohol and imperial ambition', *Social History of Alcohol and Drugs: An Interdisciplinary Journal*, 25 (2015), 4–28, at 5–7.

3 S. Ahmed, *What is Islam? The Importance of Being Islamic* (Princeton and Oxford: Princeton University Press, 2016), 57–73.

4 The additional layers of this alcohol-based identity in a colonial context, however, have until now been mostly neglected. See, for example, K.M. Guy, *When Champagne Became French: Wine and the Making of a National Identity* (Baltimore: Johns Hopkins University Press, 2003); K.M. Guy, 'Rituals of pleasure in the land of treasures: wine consumption and the making of French identity in the late nineteenth century', in W. Belasco and P. Scranton (eds), *Food Nations: Selling Taste in Consumer Societies* (New York: Routledge, 2002), 34–47; M. Demossier, *Wine Drinking Culture in France: A National Myth or a Modern Passion* (Cardiff: University of Wales Press, 2010).

5 L. Lataillade, 'Coutumes et superstitions obstétricales en Afrique du Nord' (medical thesis, University of Algiers, 1936), 161. This and all subsequent translations are by the author. Very similar quotes can also be found in Pinaud's 1933 and Sutter's 1937 dissertations on Algeria: Pinaud, 'Alcoolisme', 15f.; J. Sutter, 'L'épilepsie mentale chez l'indigène nord-africain (étude clinique)' (medical thesis, University of Algiers, 1937), 75f.

6 While the founding text of the *École d'Alger* is commonly taken to be Antoine Porot's 1918 article 'Notes de psychiatrie musulmane' (Notes on Muslim psychiatry), the *École d'Alger* was truly established only after psychiatric institutions had been built on North African soil in the 1930s. See A. Porot, 'Notes de psychiatrie musulmane', *Annales médico-psychologiques*, 9 (1918), 377–84, https://archive.org/details/BIUSante_90152x1918x09/mode/2up (accessed 20 August 2021).

7 French twentieth-century authors and in particular those of the 1930s were deeply influenced by earlier publications. See S. Graebner, '"Unknown and unloved": the politics of French ignorance in Algeria, 1860–1930', in P. Lorcin (ed.), *Algeria and France 1800–2000: Identity,*

Memory, Nostalgia (Syracuse: Syracuse University Press, 2006), 49–62, at 54.

8 All of the 'classics' of early colonial psychiatry in the region mentioned the religious prohibition of alcohol and the increase in alcohol consumption and alcoholism among Muslims after French colonisation. See A. Kocher, 'De la criminalité chez les Arabes au point de vue de la pratique médico-judiciaires en Algérie' (medical thesis, University of Lyon, 1883), 72; A.J. Meilhon, 'L'aliénation mentale chez les Arabes: études de nosologie comparée', *Annales médico-Psychologiques*, 4 (1896), 27–40, 204–20, at 210, https://archive.org/details/BIUSante_90152x1896x04/mode/2up (accessed 20 August 2021); A. Voisin, 'Souvenirs d'un voyage en Tunisie (1896)', *Annales médico-psychologiques*, 4 (1896), 89f., at 90, https://archive.org/details/BIUSante_90152x1896x04/mode/2up (accessed 20 August 2021).

9 See Pinaud, 'Alcoolisme', 15f.; P. Maréschal and Chaurand, 'La paralysie générale en Tunisie', in P. Combemale (ed.), *Congrès des médecins aliénistes et neurologistesde France et des pays de langue française* (Paris: G. Masson, 1937), 247–54, at 250, https://archive.org/details/BIUSante_110817x1937/mode/2up (accessed 20 August 2021); Sutter, 'Épilepsie mentale', 83f.

10 See Desruelles and Bersot, 'Assistance', 590; Pinaud, 'Alcoolisme', 39. Some of the colonial experts even went so far as to explicitly claim that alcohol-related medical and psychiatric problems had been unknown among North African Muslims until relatively recently. Foley, 'Aperçu', 302.

11 It should be added, however, that in the time period studied for this chapter, a minority of authors still adhered to the idea that Algerian Muslims did not drink any alcohol and consequently never, or only rarely, developed alcoholism. See Maréschal and Chaurand, 'Paralysie générale', 248.

12 The voices of the colonised do, however, form part of my broader project of analysing descriptions of drinking habits in the colonial Maghreb.

13 See J.-M. Bégué, 'French psychiatry in Algeria (1830–1962): from colonial to transcultural', *History of Psychiatry*, 7 (1996), 533–48; R. Berthelier, *L'homme maghrébin dans la littérature psychiatrique* (Paris: L'Harmattan, 1994); A. Bullard, 'The truth in madness', *South Atlantic Review*, 66, no. 2 (2001), 114–32; A. Bullard, 'The critical impact of Frantz Fanon and Henri Collomb: race, gender, and personality testing of North and West Africans', *Journal of the History of*

the Behavioral Sciences, 41, no. 3 (2005), 225–48; R. Collignon, 'La psychiatrie coloniale française en Algérie et au Sénégal', *Revue Tiers Monde*, 47, no. 187 (2006), 527–46; R. Keller, 'Madness and colonization: psychiatry in the British and French empires, 1800–1962', *Journal of Social History*, 35, no. 2 (2001), 295–326; R. Keller, 'Pinel in the Maghreb: liberation, confinement, and psychiatric reform in French North Africa', *Bulletin of the History of Medicine*, 79, no. 3 (2005), 459–99; R. Keller, *Colonial Madness: Psychiatry in French North Africa* (Chicago and London: University of Chicago Press, 2007); A. Möbius, 'Zur Entwicklung der Psychiatrie in Tunesien (1956–1997) unter besonderer Berücksichtigung des Lebenswerkes von Sleïm Ammar' (medical thesis, University of Cologne, 2001).

14 Keller, *Colonial Madness*, 138.

15 The psychiatric methods and theories propagated by psychiatrists either belonging to the *École d'Alger* or influenced by it had a far-reaching impact on both psychiatry and broader society: it is arguable that after-effects of their theories on what they saw as a typically North African form of primitivism can still be felt today. On the durability and influence of the *École d'Alger*, see R. Berthelier, 'À la recherche de l'homme musulman', *Sud/Nord*, 1, no. 22 (2007), 127–46, at 137; M. Vaughan, 'Introduction', in S. Mahone and M. Vaughan (eds), *Psychiatry and Empire* (Basingstoke: Palgrave Macmillan, 2007), 1–16, at 7; F. Gouriou, 'Psychopathologie et migration: repérage historique et épistémiologique dans le contexte français' (PhD dissertation, University of Rennes, 2008), 50.

16 The first French hospitals built in Algerian cities under French command after the conquest were military hospitals, led by military doctors and staffed by military personnel. The first duty of French military doctors was care for French troops. The first medical concern towards the colonised was the 'transmission and eradication of disease'. P. Lorcin, 'Imperialism, colonial identity, and race in Algeria, 1830–1870: the role of the French Medical Corps', *Isis*, 90, no. 4 (1999), 653–79, at 654f. See also Keller, *Colonial Madness*, 11f.

17 On the delayed establishment of colonial psychiatric institutions in Algeria, see also Keller, 'Madness and colonization', 304f. Although patients had been treated at the psychiatric hospital of Blida-Joinville in northern Algeria since July 1933, it was officially opened at the 1938 meeting of the Congrès des Médecins Aliénistes et Neurologistes de France et des Pays de Langue Française in Algiers. A. Porot, 'L'œuvre psychiatrique de la France aux colonies depuis un siècle', *Annales médico-psychologiques*, 1 (1943), 356–78, at 361.

18 On patient transfers across the Mediterranean, see N.S. Studer, *The Hidden Patients: North African Women in French Colonial Psychiatry* (Vienna, Cologne andWeimar: Böhlau, 2015), 108–11.

19 See Anon., 'Extrait du rapport du directeur, médecin en chef, de l'asile d'aliénés d'Aix (Bouches-du-Rhône)', in *Impressions. Projets de lois, propositions, rapports, etc. Sénat. Session Ordinaire de 1887*, vol. 1 (Paris: P. Mouillot, Imprimeur du Sénat, 1887), 163–6, at 164.

20 The psychiatrist Abel-Joseph Meilhon, for example, mentioned in 1896 that alcoholism was becoming more and more frequent among his Muslim patients at the Montperrin asylum in Aix-en-Provence. Meilhon, 'Aliénation mentale', 34.

21 The first French colonial psychiatrists who were born in Algeria, like Robert Susini and Jean Sutter, worked in the psychiatric institutions established in the 1930s. See R. Susini, 'Aspects cliniques de l'hystérie chez l'indigène nord-africain (en milieu militaire)' (medical thesis, University of Algiers, 1947), title page; Sutter, 'Épilepsie mentale', title page. In the 1940s and 1950s the first wave of French-trained North African psychiatrists, like Jacques Azoulay and Suzanne Taïeb in Algeria and Sleïm Ammar in Tunisia, started to work in these institutions. See A. Cherki, *Frantz Fanon, portrait* (Paris: Seuil, 2000), 74; S. Taïeb, 'Les idées d'influence dans la pathologie mentale de l'indigène nord-africain: Le rôle des superstitions' (medical thesis, University of Algiers, 1939), title page; Keller, *Colonial Madness*, 171.

22 C.A. Chopin, 'Embodying "the new white race": colonial doctors and settler society in Algeria, 1878–1911', *Social History of Medicine*, 29, no. 1 (2016), 1–20.

23 C. Bardenat, 'Criminalité et délinquance dans l'aliénation mentale chez les indigènes algériens', *Annales médico-psychologiques*, 2 (1948), 317–33, 468–80, at 318. On the establishment of Blida-Joinville and the development of the patient population, see also Studer, *The Hidden Patients*, 121f.

24 Desruelles and Bersot, 'Assistance', 591. See also 'Réceptions et excursions', in P. Combemale (ed.), *Congrès des médecins aliénistes et neurologistes de France et des pays de langue française* (Paris: Masson et Cie, Éditeurs, 1938), 381–7, at 383, https://archive.org/details/BIUSante_110817x1938/mode/2up (accessed 20 August 2021).

25 Desruelles and Bersot, 'Assistance', 593.

26 See A. Porot, 'Les services hospitaliers de psychiatrie dans l'Afrique du Nord (Algérie et Tunisie)', *Annales médico-psychologiques*, 1 (1936), 793–803, at 796, https://archive.org/details/BIUSante_90152x1936x01/mode/2up (accessed 20 August 2021).

27 A. Porot and J. Sutter, 'Le "primitivisme" des indigènes Nord-Africains: Ses incidences en pathologie mentale', *Sud médical et chirurgical*, 15 April1939, 226–41. On criticism of this theory of a North African 'primitivism', see Cherki, *Frantz Fanon*, 96f.

28 F. Fanon. *Les damnés de la terre* (Paris: Éditions La Découverte/Poche, 2002), 290. See also Cherki, *Frantz Fanon*, 112; R. Berthelier. 'Fanon, psychiatre encore et toujours', *VST – Vie sociale et traitements*, 89 (2006), 76–84, at 77; M.A. Bencharif and B. Ridouh, 'Docteur Fanon, à votre arrive à la psychiatrie ... ?', *VST – Vie sociale et traitements*, 89 (2006), 30–6, at 33.

29 M. Porot and J. Gentile, 'Alcoolisme et troubles mentaux chez l'indigène musulman algérien', *Bulletin sanitaire de l'Algérie*, 522 (May 1941), 125–30, https://gallica.bnf.fr/ark:/12148/bpt6k9535252t/f1.item (accessed 20 August 2021). Maurice Porot also headed one of the four departments in Blida-Joinville in 1943. The others were headed by Jean Sutter, Charles Bardenat and Jean Olry. Porot, 'Œuvre psychiatrique', 364.

30 Porot and Gentile, 'Alcoolisme et troubles mentaux', 129. On the same page of their article, Porot and Gentile argued that, in their opinion, the numbers for alcohol consumption among institutionalised psychiatric patients were greatly above the corresponding numbers among the general population: 'we do not have the impression that half of the Muslims in Algeria consume alcohol'.

31 Porot, 'Œuvre psychiatrique', 376.

32 Porot and Gentile, 'Alcoolisme et troubles mentaux'.

33 G.A. Manceaux, J.M. Sutter and Y. Pélicier, 'Les états mélancoliques chez l'indigène nord africain: à propos de cent nouvelles observations', in P. Cossa (ed.), *Congrès des médecins aliénistes et neurologistes de France et des pays de langue française* (Paris: G. Masson, 1954), 270–3, at 271.

34 The psychiatrist André Donnadieu combined both these aspects in an article on alcoholism in Morocco: 'Moroccan women also provide their share [of psychiatric patients suffering from alcoholism], but almost exclusively in the category of prostitutes or servants.' A. Donnadieu, 'L'alcoolisme mental dans la population indigène du Maroc', *Maroc médical*, 214 (November–December 1940), 163–5, at 164. Case studies of female alcoholics are very rare in the source material, but can be found in Pierre Pinaud's and Suzanne Taïeb's dissertations. Pinaud, 'Alcoolisme', 31; Taïeb, 'Idées d'influence', 92, 118.

35 Porot and Gentile, 'Alcoolisme', 126f.

36 The lack of statistical evidence in psychiatric publications was partly due to the absence of psychiatric institutions before the 1930s in

Algeria which could have collected data. I studied this curious lack of statistical evidence in publications by French colonial psychiatrists in detail in the sub-chapter 'French Colonial Statistics as a Historical Source' of my PhD. See Studer, *The Hidden Patients*, 136–42. This is in stark contrast to the situation in Chile and Brazil in the late nineteenth century, as discussed by Rebolledo Chapter 3 of this book, in which he describes the development of statistical evidence as an important aid in the establishment of the authority of psychiatry.

37 Alcoholism was often described as a problem that affected only non-French settlers in Algeria. In 1867, for example, the Frenchman Henri Lierre had written that 'Cases of alcoholism, which were never very numerous in Algeria, have almost disappeared and are observed only among some Maltese or Spaniards.' H. Lierre, *La question de l'absinthe* (Paris: Imprimerie Vallée, 1867), 62, https://gallica.bnf.fr/ark:/12148/bpt6k6456605j?rk=21459;2 (accessed 20 August 2021). More generally, French and European settlers in Algeria were often portrayed as lacking moderation in their alcohol consumption and were criticised for this by the mainland French. The idea that European settlers consumed dangerously excessive amounts of alcohol in Algeria had been discussed since the 1840s and was often specifically linked to the consumption of absinthe. In 1862, for example, the French doctor Louis Figuier exclaimed: 'Our African army and our settlers make a deplorable abuse of the *green poison*.' L. Figuier, 'Sur les effets pernicieux de la liqueur d'absinthe', *L'année scientifique et industrielle*, 6 (1862), 336–46, at 336, https://gallica.bnf.fr/ark:/12148/bpt6k7324x.r (accessed 20 August 2021). After the prohibition of absinthe in 1915, the excessive consumption of alcohol by European settlers in Algeria as a whole became the principal point of criticism.

38 R. Vadon, 'L'assistance médicale des psychopathes en Tunisie' (medical thesis, University of Marseille, 1935), 44.

39 N.E. Gallagher, *Medicine and Power in Tunisia, 1780–1900* (New York: Cambridge University Press, 1983), 95.

40 Foley, 'Aperçu', 301.

41 This was discussed in 1940 by the psychiatrist André Donnadieu for the Moroccan context. He stated that alcoholism was most common among former Moroccan soldiers, adding: 'After the military come the urban workers and particularly the drivers, waiters in cafés, cooks, labourers.' Donnadieu, 'Alcoolisme mental', 164.

42 J. Sutter, M. Porot and Y. Pélicier, 'Aspects algériens de la pathologie mentale', *Algérie médicale*, 63, no. 9 (1959), 891–6, at 894. A similar sentiment about this strict, geographic divide in drinking habits can be

found in Antoine Porot and Don Côme Arrii, who stated: 'The wise precepts of the Qur'an about fermented beverages are no longer respected except in the countryside; yet still on some agricultural sites, on payday evenings, regrettable scenes of drunkenness take place. In the city, wine, but especially anisette – this Algerian scourge – wreaks increasingly appalling havoc.' Porot and Arrii, 'Impulsivité criminelle', 599. On alcohol consumption in the cities, see also Pinaud, 'Alcoolisme', 27f.; Sutter, 'Épilepsie mentale', 83f. It is likely, though, that alcohol consumption in the countryside was better hidden from the eyes of the curious French observers, as Algerians in the countryside often drank in secret and often consumed traditional, locally produced forms of alcohol and not imported liquors. On the allegedly lower alcohol consumption in the countryside, see Porot and Gentile, 'Alcoolisme', 126, 129; Donnadieu, 'Alcoolisme mental', 164.

43 I. Al-Issa, 'Culture and mental illness in Algeria', in I. Al-Issa (ed.), *Al-Junūn: Mental Illness in the Islamic World* (Madison: International Universities Press, 2000), 101–19, at 109.

44 Anon., 'L'alcoolisme au Maroc', *La lanterne*, 13306 (26 September 1913), 1, https://gallica.bnf.fr/ark:/12148/bpt6k75184653 (accessed 20 August 2021).

45 R. Collignon, 'La construction du sujet colonial: le cas particulier des malades mentaux: Difficultés d'une psychiatrie en terre africaine', in M. Kail and G. Vermès (eds), *La psychologie des peuples et ses dérives* (Paris: Centre National de Documentation Pédagogique, 1999), 165–81, at 166f. For other colonial contexts, see A. Conklin, *A Mission to Civilize: The Republican Idea of Empire in France and West Africa, 1895–1930* (Stanford: Stanford University Press, 1997), 6.

46 P.M.E. Lorcin, *Imperial Identities: Stereotyping, Prejudice, and Race in Colonial Algeria* (London: I.B.Tauris, 1995), 171.

47 There was a nineteenth-century tradition of 'humorous' anecdotes about 'assimilated', 'half-civilised' Muslims in Western clothes, who proudly tried to show their level of assimilation – in the eyes of the European observers – by drinking aperitifs in the European cafés of the cities. See for example W.G. Windham, *Notes in North Africa: Being a Guide to the Sportsman and Tourist in Algeria and Tunisia* (London: Ward and Lock, 1862), 47; L. Vignon, *La France en Algérie* (Paris: Hachette et Cie, 1893), 409f, https://gallica.bnf.fr/ark:/12148/bpt6k5829613z?rk=21459;2 (accessed 20 August 2021); P. Lapie, *Les civilisations tunisiennes (musulmans, israélites, européens): étude de psychologie sociale* (Paris: F. Alcan, 1898), 63f, https://gallica.bnf.fr/ark:/12148/bpt6k71505r?rk=171674;4 (accessed 20 August 2021).

48 See for example R.F. Betts, *Assimilation and Association in French Colonial Theory, 1890–1914* (New York and London: Columbia University Press, 1961), 59. While the majority of French authors were convinced that Algerians could never be assimilated, there were also voices in the twentieth century that held assimilationist positions. Many left-wing politicians in France in the 1920s and 1930s, for example, were generally anti-colonial and against France's further colonial expansion, while still assimilationist in the context of the existing colonies. See W.B. Cohen, 'The colonial policy of the Popular Front', *French Historical Studies*, 7, no. 3 (1972), 368–93, at 374; F. Tostain, 'The Popular Front and the Blum–Viollette Plan, 1936–37', in T. Chafer and A. Sackur (eds), *French Colonial Empire and the Popular Front: Hope and Disillusion* (London and New York: Palgrave, 1999), 218–29, at 218f.
49 Lorcin, *Imperial Identities*, 213.
50 Pinaud, 'Alcoolisme', 10.
51 M. Soualah. *La société indigène de l'Afrique du Nord (Algérie, Tunisie, Maroc, Sahara)* (Algiers: Imprimerie la Typo-litho et de J. Carbonel réunies, 1937), vol. 3, 334.
52 Pinaud stated in 1933: 'From the moment that he [the Arab] decided to violate the sacred precepts [i.e. the prohibition of alcohol in the Qur'an], there is no more question of keeping the slightest measure …; he must make the most of this foray into secular habits.' Pinaud, 'Alcoolisme', 12.
53 Porot and Gentile, 'Alcoolisme', 129. Emphasis in the original. This same formulation was taken up by Maurice Porot, Jean Sutter and Yves Pélicier: 'The Muslim who drinks does not drink moderately: the minute proportion of light drinkers is quite remarkable and the percentage of heavy drinkers outweighs that of moderate drinkers.' Sutter et al., 'Aspects algériens', 894.
54 Porot, 'Notes', 383f.; Porot and Arrii, 'Impulsivité criminelle', 599f.
55 Porot, 'Œuvre psychiatrique', 375.
56 On this movement in France, see T. Fillaut. 'La lutte contre l'alcoolisme dans l'armée pendant la Grande Guerre. Principes, méthodes et résultats', in L. Guignard, H. Guillemain and S. Tison (eds), *Expériences de la folie. Criminels, soldats, patients en psychiatrie (XIXe–XXe siècles)* (Rennes: Presses universitaires de Rennes, 2013), 141–52.
57 P.E. Prestwich. 'Female alcoholism in Paris, 1870–1920: the response of psychiatrists and of families', *History of Psychiatry*, 14, no. 3 (2003), 321–36, at 324.
58 Porot and Sutter, 'Primitivisme', 226–41.

59 Porot and Arrii, 'Impulsivité criminelle', 600. A very similar sentiment can be found in Sutter: 'the daily aperitif appears to be most often insufficient to these new enthusiasts of the ethyl poison: they must, every time, go to the end of their physical or financial capacity; they do not stop on the road of drunkenness'. Sutter, 'Épilepsie mentale', 84.

60 N. Znaien, 'Drinking and production patterns of wine in North Africa during French colonisation, *c.* 1830–1956', in W. Ernst (ed.), *Alcohol Flows across Cultures: Drinking Cultures in Transnational and Comparative Perspective* (London: Routledge, 2020), 44–60, at 47ff.

61 Pinaud, 'Alcoolisme', 21.

62 Ibid., 27f. See also four case studies on alcoholism stemming from an over-consumption of anisettes, with one of them concerning a patient who drank a bottle of anisette each day: ibid., 25, 29, 30, 31.

63 Ibid., 33.

64 Ibid., 21.

65 There was a long tradition of framing Maghrebi Muslims as extreme and of comparing the behaviour of the colonised with that of addicts. The psychiatrist Pierre Maréschal, for example, argued that Tunisian Muslims over-consumed everything, from hashish to tea, from alcohol to opium, and then added: 'There are indeed, between the mentality of the Arab and that of the addict, some strong analogies: a taste for day-dreaming, for inaction, contempt for the concept of time, the very relative importance given to truth, this very particular conception of the native for whom to buy on credit is to buy for free, to be conditionally condemned is to be acquitted, and, in this way, finally, to live "the short week" [i.e. to have a long weekend] seem to be common features in Arabs and addicts.' P. Maréschal, 'L'héroïnomanie en Tunisie', in Combemale (ed.), *Congrès des médecins aliénistes et neurologistes de France et des pays de langue française* (1937), 255–9, at 255, https://archive.org/details/BIUSante_110817x1937/mode/2up (accessed 20 August 2021).

66 Pinaud, 'Alcoolisme', 11. See also n. 55 above.

67 D. Lachenmeier, D. Nathan-Maister, T. Breaux, J.-P. Luauté and J. Emmert, 'Absinthe, absinthism and thujone: New insight into the spirit's impact on public health', *Open Addiction Journal*, 3 (2010), 32–8, at 34; P. Prestwich. *Drink and the Politics of Social Reform: Anti-Alcoholism in France since 1870* (Palo Alto: Society for the Promotion of Science and Scholarship, 1988), 1, 19f.

68 Pinaud, 'Alcoolisme', 21. Pinaud mentioned this number in his text. However, in the affiliated case studies, he described four Algerian Muslim men drinking three to four litres of wine each day, i.e. less than five to six litres. Ibid., 22–4.

69 Casimir Frégier, for example, discussed the dangers posed by the 'essential oils' in absinthe in his study on 'absinthism'. C. Frégier, *Études législatives et judiciaires sur l'Algérie: l'absinthisme en face de la loi* (Algiers: Typographie de L. Marle, 1863), 15f, https://gallica.bnf.fr/ark:/12148/bpt6k5600716q.r (accessed 20 August 2021).

70 Pinaud, 'Alcoolisme', 27. See also Sutter, who wondered whether 'these violent manifestations of alcoholism in Algeria borrow, in part, their character of brutality to the particular virulence of the essences of anise and of star anise, which are the bases of the "anisette", a veritable national liquor'. Sutter, 'Épilepsie mentale', 84.

71 R. Matthee, 'Alcohol in the Islamic Middle East: ambivalence and ambiguity', *Past and Present*, supplement 9 (2014), 100–25, at 103. Like Pinaud, Matthee explained this through the fact of Muslim drinkers being aware that their habit broke societal and religious rules.

72 Keller, *Colonial Madness*, 143f.

73 Ibid. See also ibid., 208; D. Macey, 'The Algerian with the knife', *Parallax*, 4, no. 2 (1998), 159–67.

74 P. Dunwoodie, 'Assimilation, cultural identity and permissible deviance in Francophone Algerian writing of the interwar years', in P. Lorcin (ed.), *Algeria and France 1800–2000: Identity, Memory, Nostalgia* (Syracuse: Syracuse University Press, 2006), 63–83, at 67. Colonial psychiatrists also referred to reports on the criminal acts committed by free-roaming 'lunatics' in Algeria. Henry Reboul and Emmanuel Régis, for example, stated: 'the press reports every day on the attacks of all kinds committed by lunatics at liberty'. H. Reboul and E. Régis, 'L'assistance des aliénés aux colonies', in H. Reboul and E. Regis (eds), *Congrès des médecins aliénistes et neurologistes de France et des pays de langue française* (Paris: Masson et Cie, Éditeurs, 1912), 78, https://archive.org/details/BIUSante_110817x1912x03/mode/2up (accessed 20 August 2021).

75 Keller, *Colonial Madness*, 208. In 1959 Sutter et al. even claimed that in Algeria the inherent 'impulsiveness of the Algerian [male] Muslim' drove the colonised particularly often to violent reactions or, in their words, to 'violence and murder'. Sutter et al., 'Aspects algériens', p. 895.

76 Pinaud, 'Alcoolisme', 27.

77 C. Mejda, E. Feten, Z. Anis, L. Afef and A. Hedi, 'Histoire de la stigmatisation des malades mentaux en Tunisie', *L'information psychiatrique*, 83, no. 8 (2007), 689–94, at 693. See also Berthelier, 'À la recherche', 133.

78 Porot and Sutter, 'Primitivisme', p. 237. See also Porot, 'Œuvre psychiatrique', 376.

79 Soualah, *Société indigène*, vol. 3, 334.
80 Sutter, 'Épilepsie mentale', 83f. See also D. Arrii, 'De l'impulsivité criminelle chez l'indigène algérien' (medical thesis, University of Algiers, 1926), 15; Porot and Gentile, 'Alcoolisme', 130.
81 A. Porot, 'Alcoolisme chronique', in A. Porot (ed.), *Manuel alphabétique de psychiatrie clinique et thérapeutique* (Paris: Presse universitaire de France, 1952), 14–19, at 19.
82 The fear of alcohol damaging the offspring of drinkers is particularly obvious in the discussion of the effects of absinthe in the nineteenth century, both in France and in Algeria. The French doctor Victor Anselmier, for example, remarked in 1862: 'Considered from the point of view of the individual and the species, absinthe is redoubtable: the father imparts the special character of his suffering to his progeny; the most varied troubles of functions, an irregular development of the body, epilepsy and idiocy, this is the only legacy that the absinthe drinker bequeaths to his children.' V. Anselmier, *De l'empoisonnement par l'absinthe* (Paris: Imprimerie de J. Claye, 1862), 11f, https://gallica.bnf.fr/ark:/12148/bpt6k6464352t?rk=42918;4 (accessed 20 August 2021.
83 E. Aubert, *L'alcoolisation de la France: pour que la France vive* (Paris: Bossard, 1920), 37, https://gallica.bnf.fr/ark:/12148/bpt6k54849542 (accessed 20 August 2021).
84 D. Pick, *Faces of Degeneration: A European Disorder, c. 1848–c. 1918* (Cambridge: Cambridge University Press, 1989), 21, 92. During the nineteenth century, France had been particularly concerned about depopulation. See P. Prestwich. 'Temperance in France: the curious case of absinth', *Historical Reflections/Réflexions historiques*, 6, no. 2 (1979), 301–19, at 307; M. Huisman, J. Brug and J. Mackenbach. 'Absinthe: is its history relevant for current public health?', *International Journal of Epidemiology*, 36 (2007), 738–44, at 740.
85 I. Dowbiggin, *Inheriting Madness: Professionalization and Psychiatric Knowledge in Nineteenth-Century France* (Berkeley, Los Angeles and Oxford: University of California Press, 1991), 162. See also I. Dowbiggin, 'Back to the future: Valentin Magnan, French psychiatry, and the classification of mental diseases, 1885–1925', *Social History of Medicine*, 9, no. 3 (1996), 383–408, at 383f.
86 Pinaud, 'Alcoolisme', 40.
87 Keller, 'Pinel in the Maghreb', 467f.; Keller, *Colonial Madness*, 41. See also J.P. Boddy, *Civilizing Women: British Crusaders in Colonial Sudan* (Princeton and Oxford: Princeton University Press, 2007), 32; M. Rodinson, *Europe and the Mystique of Islam* (London: I.B. Tauris & Co, 1988), 60.

88 On the role of French colonial doctors in the shaping of settler opinions in Algeria, see Chopin, 'Embodying "the new white race"'.
89 Pinaud, 'Alcoolisme', 11f.
90 Ibid., 40.

9

Alcoholism, family and society in post-World War II Japan

Akira Hashimoto

This chapter explores the treatment of alcoholism in post-World War II Japan, focusing on drug treatment, rehabilitation programmes and self-help groups. It looks at hospital-centred medical approaches as well as patients' and their families' initiatives in dealing with alcohol-related problems, such as Alcoholics Anonymous (AA), and Japanese-style treatments such as Danshukai and Naikan.

Alcoholism does not appear to have drawn much government and medical attention until the second half of the twentieth century, despite the fact that early Christian missionaries had brought temperance ideas to Japan during the early 1880s within the context of the modernisation drives of the Meiji period (1868–1912), followed by short-lived Buddhist temperance initiatives.[1] Only a small number of patients with alcoholism were reported in official records before World War II. Sakaki Hajime, who had studied psychiatry in Berlin from 1882 to 1886 and became the first university professor of psychiatry in Japan, talked about the state of psychiatry in his homeland at a conference in Berlin in 1884. He held the view that alcoholism was 'relatively little known' and that the Japanese 'in general can tolerate little alcohol, and that's why they take little'.[2] He thought that this was due to racial differences in biological sensitivity to ethanol. Most Japanese people and other Asians lack the enzyme related to alcohol metabolism, which makes for low alcohol tolerance.[3] His contention seemed to be validated by the annual reports of one of the oldest public mental hospitals in Japan. In Matsuzawa Hospital in Tokyo, alcoholism was diagnosed in only 1 per cent of cases from 1920 to 1924.[4]

Other pre-World War II reports also indicated that the number of patients diagnosed with alcoholism was very low.[5] Whether alcoholism was a factor among patients with other diagnoses is difficult to ascertain. The situation changed when alcohol consumption increased markedly after World War II, in tandem with economic growth, a rise in national income and changes in lifestyle. More attention came to be paid to alcohol use disorders across the country, within the context of wider anxieties about the family during this period.[6] The traditional large Japanese family was supplanted by small nuclear families, which played a major role in rapid post-war economic growth, and new eugenic legislation, introduced by government to stem population growth, led to a declining birth rate.[7] Alcoholism was seen to jeopardise the stability of the new nuclear family structure, which had come to consist of a working man, his housekeeping wife and their children. Alcoholism emerged not just as an individual illness, but as a family malady and as a symptom of social anxieties.

The Drunkenness Prevention Act, 1961

In post-World War II Japan, drinking and alcoholism were deeply embedded in the Japanese family and gender structure and were sometimes accompanied by poverty and violence. More attention was paid to the issue of alcoholism after a murder that occurred in Tokyo in 1958. According to a newspaper article, two young daughters, thirteen and sixteen years old, strangled their alcoholic father on Fathers' Day.[8] They lived in a slum in the Adachi area. The article stated that the father was frequently inebriated and often hit his wife, and that he was unemployed and used any money earned by his family for liquor. His wife was a day labourer, the elder daughter worked at a *sōzaiya* or Japanese delicatessen, and the younger daughter worked illegally as a housemaid (this was illegal because she was still required to be in compulsory education). There were three sons in this family, but they had run away from home. On 14 June the mother left home and did not return, saying that she was disgusted with her husband. According to the article, the daughters decided to kill their father in order to save the family.

Tragedies such as this directly influenced activists who were fighting to improve the position of women and children in Japanese society. Kōro Mitsu, a woman elected to the National Diet (Assembly) in 1946 – at the first general election since women's suffrage was granted – attempted to introduce legislation for the prevention of similar cases.[9] In 1961 Kōro and twenty-three other Diet members, mainly women, submitted a bill on the regulation of disruptive acts and violence to the general public caused by drunkenness (the Drunkenness Prevention Act). At the committee meeting in the Diet she explained the rationale underlying the suggested legislation:

> Since the end of World War II, it has been said that Japan is a drunkard's paradise: Japanese society is very tolerant of drunken people. Domestic and foreign experts point out that there are no countries where as many drunken people are seen in public places as in Japan.[10] ... family tragedies due to alcohol abuse continue to occur. It is true that drunken people could be controlled by laws that already exist. But if Japan wishes to clear its notorious reputation as a drunkard's paradise and become a civilised nation in international society, it is not enough. We must bear in mind that the Olympic Games will be held in Tokyo in 1964.[11]

One of the concerns discussed was that Article 6 of the bill allowed the police to enter the homes of alcoholics who tried to assault their family members. Kōro explained that the aim was to prevent a drunken husband or father from causing pain to the family at home. Adding to her explanation, Kashiwamura Nobuo, Commissioner General of the National Police Agency, stated, 'although we do not like the fact that the police will enter private houses, we hope that Article 6 will become a warning for all men'.[12] Some Diet members held that Article 6 was unnecessary, for the Police Duties Execution Act of 1948 had already stipulated that the police could enter houses to protect personal life and property. But Kōro asserted that including Article 6 in this new law on drunkenness and increasing public awareness of alcoholism would make alcoholics themselves reflect on their drinking habits and the occurrence of family tragedies would be reduced.[13] The Drunkenness Prevention Act was enacted on 1 July 1961. The law was aimed at the protection, punishment and treatment of alcoholics. An additional resolution of this law by the National Diet stipulated that the government should take budgetary measures for establishing institutions to treat alcoholism as soon as possible.

National Kurihama Hospital

As a result, in 1963 the government began to build a special men's ward with forty beds for alcoholic patients in National Kurihama Hospital, located on the coast in the suburb of Yokosuka near Tokyo.[14] It was the first national facility for the psychiatric treatment of alcoholism. The hospital in Kurihama had originally been established in 1941 as a branch of Yokosuka Kaigun Byōin (Yokosuka Naval Hospital). After World War II it was mainly used for tuberculosis patients under the administration of the Ministry of Health and Welfare, but when the number of those patients decreased, it was converted to a psychiatric ward.

The patients participated in a three-month rehabilitation-oriented programme based on group activities such as meetings, occupational therapy and *kōgun* or long-distance walking. These therapies were strictly controlled, being incorporated into the patients' daily, weekly or monthly routines. A *jichikai*, or patients' autonomous organisation, was established in the ward. This programme, called the 'Kurihama method', was new to psychiatrists at the time and was taken as the model for the treatment of hospitalised alcoholics in Japan.[15] The psychiatrist and essayist Nada Inada (real name Horiuchi Shigeru), who had worked at 'Tōroku' or Ward East 6, dedicated to alcoholic patients since it opened, described the previous treatment regime: it was thought that there was no effective therapy for alcoholism, and alcoholic patients were accommodated in closed wards together with patients with other mental illnesses.[16] But it should be noted that even after the 'Kurihama method' became famous around the country, the treatment of alcoholics remained underdeveloped in other mental hospitals. For instance, a newspaper article from 17 June 1969 reported that thirty-four alcoholic patients escaped from the closed ward of a mental hospital in Hachiōji in Tokyo after negotiations with the hospital staff to improve treatment had broken down.[17]

Nada was appointed as a ward doctor at Tōroku in 1963 (although the ward was still under construction). Shortly afterwards he went to Europe for a year in order to gain more knowledge of alcoholism, and experienced first-hand the extent to which the background and treatment of alcoholism varied from country to country. He was conducting research in order to find a treatment model that could be suitable for the new ward established at Kurihama. Despite learning much about group therapy in Great Britain and northern Europe, he was unable to identify an appropriate model that could be transferred to Japan. He concluded that he would need to start from scratch, and in 1964 he returned to Japan and began to develop a treatment programme together with another psychiatrist, Kōno Hiroaki: the 'Kurihama method'.[18]

This new approach was based on the medical management of alcoholic patients in a hospital setting. Nada and Kōno agreed that it was crucial that patients continued to live soberly after leaving the hospital. Given the need for supportive rehabilitation measures for recovering alcoholics, they decided to collaborate with the self-help group Danshukai, as discussed below. The underlying premise was that 'the only way to recover from alcoholism is to continue complete abstinence'.[19]

It is clear that the debates surrounding the new legislation resulting from the Drunkenness Prevention Act drew on the image of an idealised family, composed of a working man, his housekeeping wife and their well-educated children, during a period of high economic growth in the 1960s. Within this context, a family that consisted of an alcoholic man, and a wife and children abused by him, was recognised as a social problem. The ward in Kurihama was expected, as a national institution, to have a social (and national) role of changing a problematic family to the ideal image of a family by isolating an alcoholic man from his family, giving him a variety of therapies and discharging him from the hospital back to his home within three months. Hospitalised patients originated from a variety of social backgrounds. Many of those who had caused family conflicts wished for the 'normalisation' of the family and not just for their own successful recovery. For example, the 'Tōroku elegy', which is said to have been sung for a long time by hospitalised patients in the Tōroku ward, expresses patients' regret and deep attachment to their families. Some of the lyrics are as follows: 'On account of alcohol, I am isolated for three months in the hospital at Kurihama, the place people don't like. My lovely wife must be lonely.' Or: 'I had a dream about my child, who wished me to do my best. Then I awoke and heard the waves from the coast. Suddenly tears sprang from my eyes.'[20]

As the 'Tōroku elegy' indicates, patients did not only harbour regrets about ending up hospitalised but were also hopeful for their lives after leaving hospital. After discharge, many were involved in self-help groups to maintain recovery and assist rehabilitation.

Medical approaches to alcoholism: pharmacotherapy

Shortly after the end of World War II, pharmacotherapy for alcoholism was practised in Japan for the first time by Geshi Takamaro, a pioneering psychiatrist who was actively committed to the medical treatment of alcoholism. Born in 1914 in Kōchi, Shikoku, in south-west Japan, he studied medicine at Okayama Medical College, where he specialised in psychiatry and physiology, and became medical director at Seikaen Mental Hospital in his home town in 1947. He founded Geshi Hospital in 1959. His understanding of the reported rise of alcoholism was that:

> The chaos after World War II dramatically increased the number of alcoholic people. Kōchi Prefecture, where I live, was well known for many alcoholic people even before the war, but now this trend seems to have expanded nationwide.[21]

Because earlier treatments for alcoholism, such as persuasion, confinement in mental hospitals and electroconvulsive therapy, had little effect, he began to use emetine and disulfiram (trade name Antabuse). Although at the time it was difficult for doctors in Japan to obtain these drugs, Geshi was able to get emetine from the US military. He also asked a Japanese pharmaceutical company to produce a sample of disulfiram.[22]

The emetic drug emetine was used as a stimulus to produce an aversion to alcoholic beverages. This Pavlov-style 'conditioned-reflex' treatment for chronic alcoholics had first been applied by Walter Voegtlin and his colleagues in a sanatorium in Seattle, Washington, during the 1930s.[23] Voegtlin found the secret of success to be proper timing. The onset of nausea from emetine had to occur at the same time as the alcoholic drinks were consumed. As was shown in an article by Voegtlin and William Broz in 1949, over a period of ten and a half years conditioning procedures caused 85 per cent of the 3,125 of patients diagnosed as chronic alcoholics at the institution to remain abstinent for six months or longer; 70 per cent remained abstinent for over one year.[24]

Geshi knew about and referred to Voegtlin and Broz's article and practised emetine aversion treatment with 343 alcoholic patients between 1950 and 1951.[25] According to Geshi, the approximate dosage was 0.04 grams of emetine per *san shaku masu* (a wooden cup for sake, which has a capacity of about 54.1 ml). The drug was given once a day after a meal for ten consecutive days. It seems that the patients did not know that the alcohol they drank contained emetine; most of them vomited within thirty minutes. Geshi reported the results of the treatment of 261 patients and concluded that more than half of the patients avoided alcohol for some time following emetine therapy. Geshi also practised disulfiram therapy on 154 patients and evaluated it positively.[26] When he presented the effects of pharmacotherapy (using emetine and disulfiram) at a medical conference in Kōchi in 1950, the event was reported in the mass media and brought to public attention.

Disulfiram was the first medicine for the treatment of alcoholism that made use of the action of alcohol metabolism. It was invented in 1948 by the Danish physician Erik Jacobsen and his colleagues in their laboratory in Copenhagen.[27] Disulfiram produces unpleasant effects when taken with alcohol because the drug inhibits the oxidation process of alcohol. In the 1950s medicines for alcoholism such as Temposil and Cyanamide were developed, and they had similar effects to Antabuse. Temposil was developed in North America, while in Japan, Cyanamide was the drug of choice, having mainly been developed by Japanese doctors.

Despite their apparent success, from the 1950s onwards Geshi came to believe that there were limits to the usefulness of drug treatments in alcoholism cases unless they were accompanied by further interventions.[28] During this time Geshi met an alcoholic patient, Matsumura Harushige.[29] Matsumura was born in 1905 as the second son to a family working in agriculture and forestry in an economically deprived village in Kōchi Prefecture. In his twenties he served as head of *seinendan*, a local young men's association that existed in almost every rural community before World War II. He was also involved in a socialist group in Kōchi until it was made illegal under the wartime regime. Then, in 1939, he went to Pusan in Korea, which was under Japanese rule at the time, and worked at a shipping company, where he developed what was then described as alcoholism.[30] After the war he returned to Kōchi and became an active member of the Socialist Party, but he was severely dependent on alcohol and was hospitalised repeatedly. His doctor, Geshi, treated him with emetine therapy, but it was all in vain, and Geshi gave up on him as a completely hopeless case upon his fifth hospitalisation. However, at that moment, when Matsumura saw his doctor's face full of empathy and despair, he realised for himself that he should stop drinking alcohol.

On the basis of his encounter with Matsumura, Geshi began to attend the regular meetings of Danshukai in Tokyo, a self-help group of patients suffering from alcoholism. Geshi had realised that there was a need for the continued support of patients and for rehabilitation measures after their discharge from hospital.

Nihon Kinshu Dōmei, Alcoholics Anonymous and the rise of Danshukai

Danshukai was modelled on AA. AA was first introduced to Japan by the temperance association Nihon Kinshu Dōmei, which was established in 1898 and aimed at ridding society of alcohol.[31] One of its leaders, Yamamuro Buho, was seemingly the first Japanese person to participate in an alcoholism treatment workshop held at Yale University in 1952. In the same year, Ōtsuji Kimiko was sent to the USA as an abstinence ambassador by Nihon Kinshu Dōmei and visited the head office of AA. AA describes itself as 'a fellowship of men and women who share their experience, strength and hope with each other that they may solve their common problem and help others to recover from alcoholism'.[32] It dates back to the 1935 encounter in Akron, Ohio, between two people then experiencing alcoholism: the surgeon Bob Smith and the stockbroker and entrepreneur Bill Wilson.

In 1953 Nihon Kinshu Dōmei formed an AA group, but it closed after about four years. It is assumed that the failure of AA at this time was due to problems associated with the cultural transfer of an American-bred model as well as organisational problems.[33] The reappearance of AA had to wait until 1975, when, as a result of interaction with AA members within a US military base in Japan, an AA meeting was held at a Christian church in Kamata, Tokyo.[34] Shortly before this, Tanaka Michio, the Japanese priest of the church, who himself was an alcoholic, had met John Meaney, the American priest of Maryknoll Mission in Japan, who was an active AA member. The latter had become an alcoholic during his stay in Japan, had been treated in the USA and subsequently returned to Japan with the aim of helping others experiencing alcoholism. In the early years, many of the AA members in Tokyo came from the US military base. Later, meetings also began to be held in other parts of Japan. Unlike Danshukai, which will be discussed below, AA was thought to be useful for alcoholics who lived alone, away from their families. From the 1980s to the 1990s, when AA groups spread nationwide, it was common for hospital and welfare staff in the Tokyo area to refer individuals who received public assistance and lived alone to AA. AA Japan General Service estimates that in 2018 there were more than 600 AA groups and over 5,700 members in Japan.[35]

Danshukai became active in the late 1950s as a new organisation, using AA as a model. Geshi Takamaro often visited the Danshukai meetings in Tokyo and was impressed by them. As at AA meetings, individuals who had been formerly diagnosed with alcoholism talked about their experiences. Geshi lent his support to this non-directive approach to group psychotherapy. Unlike temperance groups, Danshukai did not aim at a wholly sober society, but simply supported those who had experienced and were experiencing alcoholism in their quest to abstain from drinking completely. In 1957 Geshi visited the USA for three weeks as a member of a mental hospital inspection team from Japan.[36] This inspection was significant for him, as he had previously been interested in American group psychotherapy, and he tried to position Danshukai as such. He was impressed by the fact that patients with alcoholism were well treated in the state mental hospitals he visited, and by the recreational and group activities. The inspection visit convinced Geshi of the effectiveness of Danshukai. He started collecting information on AA and the treatment of alcoholism with the help of Sawamura Eiichi, an English literary scholar at Kōchi University, who had previously won a Fulbright Scholarship in the USA.[37]

In January 1958 Geshi encouraged his patient Matsumura to establish a Danshukai group in Kōchi in order to help others to deal with their alcoholism.[38] In November 1958, inspired by an earlier lecture by Koshio Kanji, a leader of Nihon Kinshu Dōmei, Geshi and Matsumura founded Danshukai (Kōchi-ken Danshu Shinseikai).[39] The organisation gradually expanded nationwide. In 1963, at the fifth anniversary meeting held in Kōchi, Danshukai in Kōchi and Tokyo cooperated to set up a national organisation of Danshukai called Zen Nihon Danshu Renmei (Zendanren).[40] Matsumura was appointed first president of Zendanren. By the end of the twentieth century, it had grown into Japan's largest self-help organisation for alcoholism, with more than 10,000 members.[41]

The feasibility of abstinence rather than moderation in drinking became a major issue of debate. Complete abstinence from drinking seems to have been the aim for the treatment of alcoholism shared by Danshukai and medical doctors at the time. For example, Erik Jacobsen, the above-mentioned pioneer of pharmacotherapy, spoke about the ideal and the reality of the treatment of alcoholism as a guest speaker at the fifteenth General Assembly of the Japanese Association of Medical Sciences held in Tokyo in 1959:

> The rational treatment of alcoholism would be a cure which could bring the patients to control their alcohol consumption, that is, to make them drink like 'other people'. This is the dream of every alcoholic, but unfortunately such a treatment is not yet known. ... Today the only possible treatment of an alcoholic is to make him

> abstinent and to keep him abstinent for the rest of his life. For this reason, we never say that an alcoholic has been 'cured'.[42]

However, there were some who thought that complete abstinence was not the only possible approach to alcoholism. For example, the psychiatrist Mukasa Hiroshi, who founded the mental hospital in Nakatsu, Ōita, doubted the practicability of complete abstinence and opposed Jacobsen's view. He contended that:

> everyone knows well how difficult it is for alcoholic patients to stop drinking alcohol. Yet, if they were allowed to drink like ordinary people, they would be satisfied. For that, the most reasonable way is to reduce the amount of alcohol they can drink.[43]

Mukasa had developed Cyanamide, an alcohol-deterrent drug, and insisted that it would be possible to moderate drinking by means of pharmacotherapy. On the basis of the results of 200 individuals with alcoholism, he observed that it was better for them to maintain their social lives by drinking a little than to abstain from alcohol completely. Mukasa's favourable view of the use of drugs contrasts with that of Geshi, who focused on the Danshukai approach rather than pharmacotherapy.

Like Mukasa, Tsukue Ichirō, the director of a private mental hospital in Hiroshima, regretted that many psychiatrists did not expect pharmacotherapy to be efficacious and that they had become predominantly interested in Danshukai, with its emphasis on the social adaptability of alcoholics who would commit to abstinence, exchange their experiences with other Danshukai members and maintain a sober life. Tsukue believed that there was still much room to conduct research into the pharmacotherapy of alcoholism, both in Japan and in the West.[44] As in Western countries, so too in Japan, psycho-pharmaceuticals were used widely from the 1950s onwards in the treatment of alcoholism and mental illness.[45] But, despite the possibilities of pharmacotherapy envisaged by authors such as Mukasa and Tsukue, and because many others held the view that it would be impossible for individuals to control or moderate their drinking, the treatment of alcoholism was (and still is now) based predominantly on the principle of complete abstinence.[46] Danshukai was widely thought to be indispensable for the care of alcoholics within the community, as its regular meetings were believed to help them remain sober outside hospital.[47] At the beginning of each Danshukai meeting, members declared their pledge to remain abstinent. They were expected to speak of their own experiences regarding their alcohol-related problems, share their feelings with members and deepen their insights into the disease (see Figure 9.1).

Although Danshukai was inspired by AA, there are notable differences.[48] While the abstinence pledges and the 'Twelve Steps' (a set of guiding principles for recovery from alcoholism) are similar, AA refers to God or a greater power in the recovery process. In contrast, Danshukai does not invoke any religious notions. As Chenhall and Oka have suggested, it is thought that AA's Christian principles 'do not correspond with Japanese understandings of recovery from alcoholism'.[49] Another important difference is that, unlike AA,

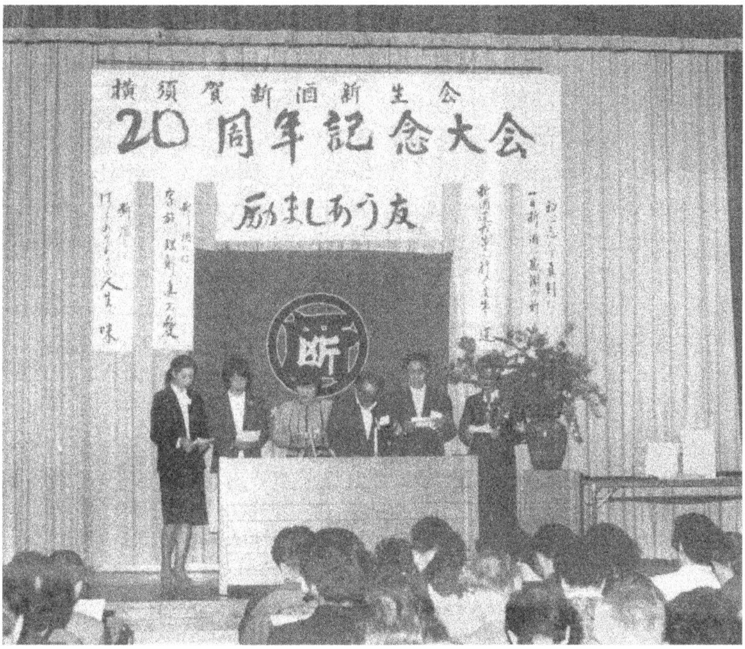

Figure 9.1 The twentieth anniversary meeting of Yokosuka Danshukai, held in 1987

Danshukai is based on the non-anonymity of its members.[50] While AA has a horizontal organisational structure, Danshukai is 'top-down' and all relationships are vertically organised. What is more,

> the constitution of membership in Danshukai reflects various social norms related to gender and the family. ... The typical model for a family entering Danshukai is an alcoholic man with his supporting non-alcoholic wife. ... Compared to AA, where family members do not attend meetings, ... families are encouraged to participate in Danshukai. Wives, mothers, fathers, and children of alcoholics participate in meetings.[51]

Chenhall and Oka note that in Danshukai 'recovery is not an individual journey but is inclusive of the family in the therapeutic process'.[52]

In order for Danshukai to gain wider acceptance in Japan, some principles, such as compatibility with existing Japanese family and gender structures and values, had to come to the fore. This focus was not limited to Danshukai. It had also been important in regard to the kind of treatment pursued at Kurihama and had been a vital aspect of the discussions of the murder case in the lead-up to the Drunkenness Prevention Act. It is therefore vital to explore the changing relationship between alcohol problems and the Japanese family and gender structure. Ideas about alcoholism in post-World War II Japan typically appeared at first in the guise of narratives that tended to focus on a drunken and violent husband who was to be punished, and an abused wife and children who were to be rescued. However, the premise of such a narrative about alcoholics and their families changed once the idea of 'alcoholism as a family disease' spread more widely, by the 1980s at the latest.

The psychiatrist Saitō Satoru, who had worked in Kurihama, asserted in his 1985 book that when a person developed alcoholism they were, in his words, 'born' as part of a family problem, and the stress produced by the 'birth' of that person would make the problems even worse.[53] This suggestion had some affinity with Joan Jackson's studies of the mid-1950s, conducted on the partners of AA members and excessive drinkers in Seattle.[54] Saitō explored the complex relationship between the recovery process from alcoholism and the changing family roles of husbands and wives. He pointed out that the husband's recovery from the disease and his subsequent resumption of the traditional role as the head of the household could threaten the stability of the family and even lead to the wife becoming mentally ill. In the text used during the 1980s for the family education programme on alcoholism at Tokyo Toritsu Seishin'eisei Sentā (Tokyo Metropolitan Mental Health Centre), in which Saitō was referred to, the notion of 'alcoholism as a family disease' was emphasised.[55] The assumption was that when a husband developed alcoholism, the family dynamics changed, with the wife taking on the husband's previous domestic and social roles. The wife, according to this model, depended on the children (especially the eldest) to support her in this like a husband. Children who took on these responsibilities were, it was thought, forced to grow up too fast. Mental health guidance recommended that the family should not let itself be ruled by the person with alcoholism, but should return responsibilities to him and focus on their own recovery.

Because Danshukai kept a close relationship with medical institutions, it took on board the idea of alcoholism as a family disease. This is demonstrated in the newsletter of a Tokyo Danshukai group.[56] A woman wrote a short essay about her memories of when her alcoholic husband was hospitalised in January 1983. When the doctor said to her, 'You are also an alcoholic, or an alcoholic patient who never drinks', she was puzzled. However, following the doctor's advice, she joined Danshukai in the Setagaya area and attended the regular meetings. At first, she was not interested in what other people attending the meeting said, as she was strongly conscious that she herself was not experiencing an alcohol dependency. But, as time passed, she noticed that her efforts to help her husband not only were in vain but were exacerbating his condition. She gave her essay the title 'A silly wife and mother'. Thanks to her involvement with Danshukai, she realised that her role as 'rescuer' had maintained undesirable family dynamics and encouraged her husband's continued role as that of the 'patient'. She asserted that changing her own role in the family led to her husband's recovery.

With the aim of spreading the idea of alcoholism as a family disease, Danshukai published a booklet for the wives of those with alcoholism titled 'Madam, there is something you can do!'[57] According to the booklet, alcoholism involved the whole family, and therefore all family members were implicated in the patient's and the family's recovery process. Attendance at Danshukai meetings was important not only for alcoholic husbands but also for their wives. Once the husband had recovered, it was expected that the role as the head of the family (*shujin*), which the wife had assumed during his illness, must be returned to him as soon as possible. As the booklet shows, in the context of Danshukai alcoholism as a family disease seems to be narrowly defined as occurring only in marital settings.[58]

It is however important to keep in mind that the phrase 'alcoholism is a family disease' makes sense only if the family is not yet broken. Danshukai in Tokyo published an essay written by a member who had joined the group after his family's collapse.[59] This individual, who worked as a cartoonist and had drunk heavily for twenty years from his twenties onwards, had been hospitalised repeatedly, presenting with hallucinations and delusions. He eventually lost his family and his job. After the last hospitalisation, in 1986, he began to attend a Danshukai meeting. The extent to which the concept of 'a family disease' was relevant to his recovery is difficult to ascertain. However, in his essay, he still expressed his regrets to his divorced wife and children and his hopes for a continued sober life.

While recent studies have shown that a considerable number successfully recover from alcoholism by attending Danshukai meetings together with their spouses, there has been a decline in the number of Danshukai groups.[60] According to Zendanren, the umbrella organisation of Danshukai, the total number of members continues to decrease, having fallen to around 8,500 in 2012.[61] Despite an increased alcohol intake among women in the general population, the number of female members has not increased. Furthermore, Danshukai is little known to the younger generation.[62] The members are ageing, and in 2012 the proportion of existing members over the age of sixty was close to 60 per cent.[63] Moreover, the proportion of members who were over sixty when they entered Danshukai reached 25 per cent in the same year.[64] Zendanren suggests that these trends are due to the fact that the treatment of alcoholism has tended to depend more and more on medical institutions and, as a result, the age when people enter Danshukai has increased. The organisation is concerned that its treatment, which it considers vital for maintaining continued abstinence, is no longer taken up in the earlier stages of life.

Shimmitsu Setsuko points out that Danshukai's activities have stagnated despite the fact that its views on the treatment of alcoholism have continued to develop in tandem with changing medical approaches in institutional settings.[65] However, she notes that Danshukai does not favour abstinence that relies exclusively on medical treatment. It considers its comprehensive approach indispensable for the 'real' and sustained recovery of alcoholics. There is currently no agreement among those involved in the treatment of alcoholism on the extent to which medical staff and Danshukai members should work in unison. Sometimes these two parties even compete against each other.

Danshukai is similar to the 'Hudolin model' or the Club of Treated Alcoholics developed in Communist Yugoslavia, which is discussed in this volume by Mat Savelli (see Chapter 10). In both approaches, family participation is thought to be of immeasurable value in establishing and maintaining abstinence.[66] However, in the Hudolin model professional involvement is much stronger. Moreover, while Geshi Takamaro was influenced by foreign trends such as American AA and group therapy, he is unlikely to have had contact with ideas of preventive and social psychiatry which influenced Yugoslavian psychiatrists in the United Kingdom. There is also no evidence that Geshi and other Danshukai leaders had direct or indirect contact with colleagues in Yugoslavia.

Focusing on individual change: Naikan

Separate from group-oriented treatments, such as Danshukai and AA, an individual psychotherapy called Naikan also gained prominence in Japan. The Japanese word *Naikan*, if literally translated, means 'looking inwards'. It was founded as a form of psychotherapy by Yoshimoto Ishin in the 1940s. Yoshimoto was born in Nara in 1916 as the third son of a farmer.[67] Under his mother's influence he became deeply interested in the teachings of Jōdo Shinshū, a Buddhist sect. In the process of religious practice, Yoshimoto experienced *mishirabe* (looking into oneself thoroughly). According to Jōdo's teaching, *mishirabe* leads to the conviction that a peaceful death is guaranteed. Yoshimoto adapted the practice and applied it to a popular technique of psychotherapy, in which one looks back on one's relationships with others. The religious scholar Shimazono Susumu explains the essence of Naikan practice:

> A participant stays in a one-metre square space created by screen partitions for one week, engaged in focused introspection on the subject of his or her past relationship with others. The participant sits and meditates in this small space from 5:30 a.m. to 9:00 p.m., with breaks for meals, baths, and interviews with a [spiritual or therapeutic] guide. ... The principal purpose of Naikan ... is to ask 'What he/she did for me', 'What I did for him/her in return', and 'What troubles I caused him/her'.[68]

Some psychiatrists were interested in Naikan and applied it to the treatment of alcoholism from the end of the 1960s onwards. In 1967 the psychiatrist Suwaki Hiroshi visited Yoshimoto's *dojo* (space or centre for immersive teaching or meditation) and participated in the Naikan training.[69] Suwaki was convinced that, since those experiencing alcoholism clearly caused their families worry, Naikan would motivate individuals to deal with their disease and remain abstinent. He introduced Naikan as a psychotherapy in some psychiatric institutions in Okayama.

Another example is the psychiatrist Takemoto Takahiro, who was based at Kagoshima Kenritsu Seishin'eisei Sentā (Kagoshima Prefectural Mental Health Centre) and became involved in the treatment of alcoholism in 1970.[70] Staff at Kagoshima had become increasingly concerned about patients with alcoholism because there was almost no medical treatment available for them at the time. Takemoto first set up a Danshukai group in 1971 and held its regular meetings in the health centre. However, many members withdrew from Danshukai and only few of them remained abstinent. Takemoto felt a necessity for a special ward for the treatment of alcoholism, modelled on the one at the National Kurihama Hospital. He proposed the idea to the director of the centre, but it was rejected. Takemoto therefore founded the Ibusuki-Takemoto Hospital for alcoholism. Initially the treatment was unsuccessful. Takemoto concluded that it was not enough to rely on the methods of Danshukai; crucially, for him, the failure of Danshukai methods was related to how members engaged with their past. Therefore Takemoto visited Yoshimoto in 1975 to undergo Naikan training. Since then, Naikan has been used as one of the psychotherapy programmes available at his hospital.

In 1978 Takemoto became a founding member, alongside others involved in psychiatry and psychology, and with Yoshimoto Ishin as an advisor, of the Japan Naikan Association, an academic society promoting Naikan therapy. According to the programmes of recent annual meetings, reports of research undertaken by domestic and international speakers – as well as clinical case studies – are presented, and Naikan training sessions held.[71] Today, about twenty Naikan *dojos* have been established around Japan, and Naikan extends to Europe, the USA, South Korea and China.[72] But seen in relation to the general trend of the treatment of alcoholism in recent years in Japan, Naikan does not necessarily surpass Danshukai. Takemoto's preference for Naikan was based on his critical view of the group-oriented approach practised by self-help groups such as Danshukai, in which the participants were expected to talk about their experiences without specific focus on their past behaviour and its impact on their families and friends.[73] He was convinced that as a systematic individual therapy Naikan would lead to spiritual growth and behavioural change, and that it should therefore be applied more widely in the treatment of alcoholism. However, according to Miki Yoshihiko, a clinical psychologist and one of the founding members of the Japan Naikan Association, Takemoto also recognised the limitations of Naikan.[74] First, a one-week programme of Naikan is time-consuming for both the therapist and the patient. Second, Naikan tends to be misunderstood as religion, and some patients avoid it for that reason. Third, some people are averse to looking back on relationships with others that involve a sense of guilt, which constitutes the core principle of Naikan. Miki Yoshihiko suggests that these issues need to be addressed if Naikan is to flourish.

Conclusion

The mainstream treatment of alcoholism in post-World War II Japan consisted of pharmacotherapy, rehabilitation programmes in mental health hospitals and self-help groups. These treatments complemented each other, and practitioners across all three shared the understanding that the best treatment for alcoholics was to encourage them to become abstinent and remain abstinent for the rest of their lives, as the Danish physician Erik Jacobsen had declared before a Japanese audience in 1959. During the period of post-war chaos, views on alcoholism focused on its connection to family and gender dynamics, which were closely linked to poverty, violence and family tragedies. Early activists, who intended to improve the position of women and children, were involved in the passing of legislation that was aimed at the control of alcohol consumption and the treatment of alcoholics. The 1961 Drunkenness Prevention Act led to the establishment of a centre for alcoholism at the National Kurihama Hospital, where the first rehabilitation programme for alcoholic patients (the 'Kurihama method') was implemented. This was a place where married men experiencing alcohol dependency were isolated from their wives and children in order to take part in a variety of therapies before being sent home within three months.

Apart from medical programmes in psychiatric institutions, a variety of approaches to alcoholism such as AA, Danshukai and Naikan were available. The former two developed as group therapies and the latter as an approach that focused on the individual. These approaches, while being influenced by Western psychotherapeutic practices, developed alongside modernisation, Westernisation and social change during a period of rapid economic recovery in Japan after the war. The Japanese traditional family structure that supported industrial society and high economic growth also played a decisive role in the emergence and management of Danshukai. Danshukai, the most popular self-help group in Japan, was originally inspired by AA and group therapy in America, which emphasised a horizontal relationship between the participants. However, conforming to the Japanese socio-cultural context,

Danshukai was based on vertical relationships between members and on the power structure of traditional family gender politics between husbands and wives. On the other hand, the Sapporo psychiatrist Saitō Toshikazu evaluated Danshukai's wider societal and political influence in positive terms.[75] According to him, its close connection with the Nihon Kinshu Dōmei (Japan Temperance Union) and its power as a social movement facilitated the passing of important legislation, such as the Basic Act on Measures against Alcohol-Related Harm to Health in 2013.

Increasingly, some groups of psychiatrists began to pay attention to approaches that focused on the individual, such as Naikan. Naikan had been invented in the 1940s and applied to the treatment of alcoholism from the end of the 1960s onwards, but in the context of the recent worldwide boom of mindfulness, some authors refer to the similarities between these approaches.[76] A common goal is said to be to strengthen self-affirmation through self-insight. It is very probable that the current trend emphasising individual insight over group dynamics has influenced Danshukai's loss of appeal, leading to its decline. The emphasis on individuals over groups is also seen in the change of medical programmes in the National Kurihama Hospital.[77] With the increase of patients who are not amenable to group activities, the focus of its rehabilitation programme has changed from the use of group dynamics to the treatment of individuals by means of cognitive behavioural therapy, for example.

Japan's alcohol consumption peaked in the mid-1990s and since then has continued to decrease gradually.[78] However, according to estimates by the Ministry of Health, Labour and Welfare, the number of alcoholics treated both within medical institutions and in the community over the past thirty years has been stable, at around 40,000.[79] With Japan's rapidly ageing population and changes to the family structure, such as an increasing number of single-person households, the approach to alcoholism has changed. Moreover, the worldwide upsurge in pharmacotherapy, in particular in the shape of Nalmefene, may make moderate alcohol consumption possible and change the focus on complete abstinence that has been so prominent among Japanese therapists and self-help groups.[80]

Notes

1 The Japanese temperance movement was deeply influenced by Christian missionaries from the USA. The 1886 visit to Japan by Mary Clement Leavitt as the first round-the-world missionary for the Woman's Christian Temperance Union (WCTU) inspired the foundation of the temperance organisation for women by Yajima Kajiko, an educator and Christian activist. In 1890 Andō Tarō, the former Consul-General of Japan in Hawaii, and Nemoto Shō, who later became a member of the National Diet (Assembly), established the temperance organisation Tokyo Kinshukai (later developed into the national organisation Nihon Kinshu Dōmei) shortly after Jessie Ackermann, the second round-the-world missionary for the WCTU, visited Japan. See http://nippon-kinshu-doumei.fd531.com/a-ayumi-01.html (accessed 20 August 2018). Buddhists, on the other hand, felt a sense of crisis on account of the Christian expansion in the country and founded a temperance organisation against Christianity. Students studying at a Buddhist school attached to Nishihonganji Temple in Kyoto organised the reform group Hanseikai in 1886 and began to publish a journal the following year to promote their temperance movement and reform the 'old' Buddhism in order to gather more believers. But Hanseikai's activities continued for only a short time. See Nihon Bukkyō Shakaifukushi Gakkai (ed.), *Bukkyō shakaifukushi jiten* [The Dictionary of Buddhist Social Welfare] (Kyoto: Hōzōkan, 2006), 252.

2 H. Sakaki, 'Ueber das Irrenwesen in Japan', *Allgemeine Zeitschrift für Psychiatrie und psychisch-gerichtliche Medizin*, 42 (1886), 144–53. Translations are by the author except where otherwise stated.

3 In the oxidation process from ethanol via acetaldehyde to acetic acid, two enzymes, alcohol dehydrogenase (ADH) and aldehyde dehydrogenase (ALDH), play a crucial role. The intermediate structures, acetaldehyde, can be toxic, and general 'hangover' symptoms appear. It is said that the ALDH deficiency of most Japanese people and other Asians is manifested by slow acetaldehyde removal and, as a result, low alcohol tolerance, which leads to a relatively low frequency of alcoholism. See D.W. Crabb et al., 'Overview of the role of alcohol dehydrogenase and aldehyde dehydrogenase and their variants in the genesis of alcohol-related pathology', *Proceedings of the Nutrition Society*, 63 (2004), 49–63; Y. Yamada, 'Nihonjin no arukōru taishakōso no identeki takei to inshu kōdō oyobi inshu niyoru kenkōshōgai no kankei' [Association of genetic polymorphisms in alcohol-metabolizing enzymes in Japanese

with their drinking behaviors and the consequent health hazards], *Journal of Kanazawa Medical University*, 30 (2005), 448–55.

4 Tokyo Furitsu Matsuzawa Byōin, *Tokyo Furitsu Matsuzawa Byōin nenpō* [Annual Reports of Tokyo Furitsu Matsuzawa Byōin from 1921 to 1924] (Tokyo: Tokyo Furitsu Matsuzawa Byōin, 1928), 75 (the annual reports do not have admission diagnoses, only discharge diagnoses). The occurrence of Dementia praecox (schizophrenia) among discharged patients was 48 per cent during the same period.

5 For instance, see K. Kubo and N. Hikaru, 'Mansei shusei chūdokusha no kenkyū' [A study of chronic alcoholics], *Shinkeigaku zasshi*, 33, no. 4 (1931), 237–85.

6 T. Hirayama, 'Arukōru no kenkō eikyō' [The influence of alcohol on health], in H. Kōno and F. Ōtani (eds), *Wagakuni no arukōru kanren-mondai no genjō* [The Present State of Alcohol-Related Problems in Japan] (Tokyo: Kōken shuppan, 1993), 5–41.

7 M. Iwata, *Shakai hukushi no toposu* [Themes of Social Welfare] (Tokyo: Yūhikaku, 2016), 138–40.

8 'Sake to mazushisa: Chichi no hi no higeki' [Alcohol and poverty: a tragedy on Father's Day], *Asahi Shinbun*, 16 June 1958, 7.

9 www.city.anan.tokushima.jp/docs/2013062600031/ (accessed 2 September 2018).

10 After this part of Kōro's statement in 1961, some authors reported on the Japanese tolerance of drunken behaviour. For example, David Pittman constructs four cultural positions in reference to attitudes about drinking: an abstinent culture, an ambivalent culture, a permissive culture and an over-permissive culture. Spain, Portugal and Japan are permissive cultures, 'in which the prevailing attitude is positive toward the use of alcoholic beverages'. See D.J. Pittman, 'International overview: social and cultural factors in drinking patterns, pathological and nonpathological', in D.J. Pittman (ed.), *Alcoholism* (New York, Evanston and London: Harper & Row, 1967), 3–20. In addition, Harry Kitano explored the differences in norms in regard to alcohol consumption among Japanese people in Japan, Hawaii and California. They found that Japanese people in Japan held the most tolerant views of heavier drinking for men, whereas Japanese-Americans were more tolerant of female drinking than the Japanese. The differences were explained by enculturation and acculturation. See H.H. Kitano et al., 'Norms and alcohol consumption: Japanese in Japan, Hawaii and California', *Journal of Studies on Alcohol*, 53, no. 1 (1992), 33–9.

11 Minutes of the Local Administrative Committee of the House of Councillors, no. 15 (18 April 1961).

12 Minutes of the Local Administrative Committee of the House of Representatives, no. 31 (18 May 1961).
13 Minutes of the Local Administrative Committee of the House of Representatives, no. 32 (19 May 1961).
14 Kōseishō [Ministry of Health and Welfare] (ed.), *Kokuritsu ryōyōjo shi seishin hen* [History of National Hospitals: Psychiatric Hospitals] (Tokyo: Kōseimondai kenkyūkai, 1976), 64–7.
15 T. Saitō, 'Arukōru kanren shōgai shindan gainen to chiryō no hensen' [A history of the diagnosis concept and treatment of alcohol-related disorders], *Frontiers in Alcoholism*, 3, no. 2 (2015), 198–202.
16 I. Nada, *Arukōru chūdoku monogatarifū* [A Tale of Alcoholism] (Tokyo: Gogatsu shobō, 1996), 15–16.
17 'Aruchū 34 nin dassō' [34 alcoholic patients escaped], *Asahi Shinbun*, 17 June 1969, 16.
18 Nada, *Arukōru chūdoku monogatarifū*, 22–5.
19 *Nyūin sareru minasama e* [Guidebook for Hospitalised Patients] (Kurihama: Kokuritsu ryōyōjo Kurihama byōin Tōroku byōtō, n.d.).
20 M. Suwa, 'Tadaima nyūinkanja 36 mei: Kokuritsu Kurihama Byōin higashi rokugō byōtō no kaigo to kibō' [36 patients are hospitalised now: regret and hope in Ward East 6 of National Kurihama Hospital], *Zaikai tenbō*, special issue 26, no. 9 (2006), 194–200.
21 Takamaro Geshi, 'Mansei shuseichūdokushō no chiryō' [Treatment of chronic alcoholism], *Shin'yaku to rinshō*, 1, no. 7 (1952), 379–401. Kōchi has a reputation, whether deserved or not, for having many heavy drinkers, and its culture is one of a close relationship between tolerating alcohol and alcohol-related problems. See Y. Mozue and Y. Sudō, 'Nihon seishin'igaku shin fudoki Kōchi ken' [Psychiatric culture and geography in Kōchi Prefecture], *Rinshō seishin'igaku*, 37, no. 10 (2008), 1379–84.
22 Geshi, 'Mansei shuseichūdokushō no chiryō'.
23 W.L. Voegtlin and W.R. Broz, 'The conditioned reflex treatment of chronic alcoholism, X: an analysis of 3125 admissions over a period of ten and a half years', *Annals of Internal Medicine*, 30, no. 3 (1949), 580–97.
24 Ibid., 596.
25 Geshi, 'Mansei shuseichūdokushō no chiryō'.
26 Ibid.
27 H. Kazamatsuri, 'Nihon kindai kōseishin'yaku ryōhō shi (9): Kōtenkan'yaku, suimin'yaku, kōpākinson'yaku, kōshuyaku nado' [A history of psychotropic drugs in modern Japan 9: anti-epileptic drugs,

hypnotics, anti-Parkinson medication, anti-alcohol drugs and so on], *Rinshō seishin'igaku*, 35, no. 11 (2006), 1583–9.

28 According to his son Geshi Takayuki, his father Takamaro was frustrated that he was unable to cure alcoholic and mental health patients. He had been involved in medical research in cooperation with the Japanese military before the end of World War II; from the 1950s he was keen to provide for his patients the kind of medical care introduced from the West that was then considered as advanced, such as electroconvulsive therapy and lobotomy. But he did not see the desired effects. See Takayuki Geshi, *Danshukai ni yorisotte: Geshi Takamaro den* [Biography of Geshi Takamaro] (Kōchi: Livre shuppan, 2018), 102–4.

29 Unless otherwise stated, evidence provided in this paragraph is based on T. Kobayashi, 'Kaisei eno dōhyō: Danshukai no sōshisha Matsumura Harushige ryakuden' [Road to recovery: a brief biography of the Danshukai founder Matsumura Harushige], in S. Saitō (ed.), *Gendai no esupuri: arukohorikusu no monogatari* [The spirit of today: stories of alcoholic patients] (Tokyo: Shibundō, 1988), 97–105.

30 In Japan the term 'alcoholism' is thought to have appeared first in 1876 in the textbook of psychiatry *Sheishinbyō yakusetsu* by Kanbe Bunsai, the medical officer of Kyoto Prefecture. His textbook was a Japanese translation from the English text 'Insanity' by Henry Maudsley, which was included in the three-volume *System of Medicine*, edited in 1872 by Russell Reynolds. See Y. Okada, *Nihon seishinka iryōshi* [The History of Psychiatry in Japan] (Tokyo: Igakushoin, 2002), 150.

31 www.dansyu-renmei.or.jp/zendanren/rekishi_1.html (accessed 21 December 2019).

32 AA Grapevine, 'A.A. Preamble', 15 May 2013, www.aa.org/assets/en_US/smf-92_en.pdf (accessed 2 September 2018).

33 www.dansyu-renmei.or.jp/zendanren/rekishi_1.html (accessed 21 December 2019).

34 S. Fujita, 'Jijo gurūpu' [Selp-help group], in Kōno and Ōtani (eds), *Wagakuni no arukōru kanren mondai no genjō*, 283–301. For Maryknoll Mission in Japan, see http://maryknoll-in-japan.blogspot.com/ (accessed 16 December 2019).

35 AA Japan General Service, http://aajapan.org/introduction/ (accessed 2 September 2018).

36 For Geshi's trip to the USA, see Takayuki Geshi, *Danshukai ni yorisotte*, 79–81, 101–2, and N. Tani, Takamaro Geshi et al., 'Amerika no seishi eisei no genjō wo shisatsu shite' [Survey of the present state of mental hygiene in America], *Kōchi seishin eisei*, 2 (1957), 1–2.

37 Takayuki Geshi, *Danshukai ni yorisotte*, 178.

38 Takamaro Geshi, 'Danshukai hasshō kara no sokuseki' [A history of Danshukai], *Nihon arukōru seishin'igaku zasshi*, 11, no. 1 (2004), 63–70.

39 Ibid.

40 Ibid.

41 Kōseirōdōshō (Ministry of Health, Labour and Welfare), 'Zendanren sono genkyō' [The present state of Zendanren], www.mhlw.go.jp (accessed 2 September 2018).

42 E. Jacobsen, 'The treatment of alcoholism in Denmark', in Japanese Association of Medical Sciences, Fifteenth General Assembly (ed.), *Nihon igakukai sōkai gakujutsu shūkai kiroku dai 15 kai dai 5 kan* [The Fifteenth General Assembly of the Japanese Medical Congress: The Records of the Academic Meetings] (Tokyo: Japanese Association of Medical Sciences, 1959), vol. 5, 1031–8.

43 H. Mukasa, 'Cyanamide (H_2NCN) no seitai arukōru han'nō ni oyobosu eikyō narabini chiryōteki ōyō' [Studies on the physiological anti-alcohol effects of Cyanamide and its clinical application], *Seishin shinkeigaku zasshi*, 64, no. 5 (1962), 469–91.

44 I. Tsukue, 'Arukōru chūdoku tokuni arukōru shihekisha no chiryō narabini mondaiten' [Treatment and problems of alcoholics], *Hiroshima igaku*, 22, no. 9 (1969), 794–802.

45 T. Kawano and K. Inada, 'Wagakuni no seishinka chiryōyaku no tazai tairyō chōki shohō no genjō to kadai' [The current situation and issues of multi-drug, high-dose, long-term prescription of psychiatric drugs in Japan], *Yakkyoku*, 69, no. 9 (2018), 2812–16.

46 S. Shimmitsu, 'Arukōru izonshō to iryōka' [Alcoholism and medicalisation], in Y. Morita and Y. Shindō (eds), *Iryōka no poritikusu: Kindai iryō no chihei o tou* [The Politics of Medicalization: The Horizon of Modern Medicine] (Tokyo: Gakubunsha, 2006), 115–27.

47 T. Noda et al., 'Long-term outcome in 306 males with alcoholism', *Psychiatry and Clinical Neurosciences*, 55 (2001), 579–86.

48 R.D. Chenhall and T. Oka, 'An initial view of self-help groups for Japanese alcoholics: Danshukai in its historical, social, and cultural contexts', *International Journal of Self Help and Self Care*, 5, no. 2 (2006–07), 111–52.

49 Ibid., 121.

50 According to Chenhall and Oka, 'An initial view of self-help groups for Japanese alcoholics', one Danshukai member told them that a samurai used to shout his name before his enemy and that Danshukai members should likewise announce their own names in meetings, suggesting that to hide one's true identity in Danshukai would be shameful.

51 Ibid., 126. According to research on Danshukai members in Okayama Prefecture in 1978, 202 research participants (of a total of 290 members) were men, 81.7 per cent of whom were living with their wives. In addition, 82.7 per cent attended regular meetings with a companion; 83.2 per cent of these companions were their wives. See S. Takahashi et al., 'Okayamaken ni okeru Danshukai kaiin no jittai chōsa' [A survey of Danshukai members in Okayama Prefecture], *Okayama igakukai zasshi*, 93, nos 7–8 (1981), 729–38.

52 Chenhall and Oka, 'An initial view of self-help groups for Japanese alcoholics', 144.

53 S. Saitō, *Arukōru izonshō no seishinbyōri* [Psychopathology of Alcoholism] (Tokyo: Kongō shuppan, 1985), 55–69.

54 J.K. Jackson, 'The adjustment of the family to the crisis of alcoholism', *Quarterly Journal of Studies on Alcohol*, 15, no. 4 (1954), 562–86.

55 Tokyo Toritsu Seishin'eisei Sentā, *Arukōru kazoku kyōiku puroguramu tekisuto* [The Text of the Family Education Programme on Alcoholism], 2nd edn (Tokyo: Tokyo Toritsu Seishin'eisei Sentā, 1987).

56 'Gusai gubo' [A silly wife and mother], *Tokyo Danshu*, 215 (20 March 1987), 10–11.

57 Tokyo Danshu Shinseikai, *Okusan, anata nimo dekiru koto ga arimasu!* [Madam, there is something you can do!] (undated, but used in the 1980s).

58 Identified alcoholics have been predominantly male. However, the habit of drinking alcohol became firmly established among women by the 1980s. A government survey of the drinkers found that 19 per cent of adult women drank alcohol in 1968, a proportion that increased to 43.2 per cent in 1987. For men the figures for these years were 68 per cent and 73.6 per cent respectively. See K. Takano and K. Nakamura, 'Josei no inshu shūkan no henka to arukōru kanrenmondai' [Changes in women's drinking habits and alcohol-related problems], in Kōno and Ōtani (eds), *Wagakuni no arukōru kanrenmondai no genjō*, 81–9. Danshukai did not ignore the problems of women alcoholics. Its national organisation Zendanren held its first Women's Alcohol Abuse Awareness Meetings in 1986 and 1987, both in Kyūshū, in the most southern part of Japan. In one of the meetings, a woman reflected on her own experience of turning into an alcoholic after her divorce and eventually deciding to abstain for the sake of her children. In the 1980s, the word *Kicchin dorinkā* (kitchen drinker), which referred to ordinary housewives suffering from alcoholism, became popular in the media. 'Josei shugai taisaku Nagasaki taikai hiraku' [Women's Alcohol Abuse Awareness Meeting was held in Nagasaki], *Kagaribi*, 20 (1 July 1987), 3.

59 'Kazoku hōkai' [Family collapse], *Tokyo Danshu*, 217 (20 May 1987), 5–6; 218 (20 June 1987), 2–3.
60 For instance, see M. Kodawara and K. Ishihara, 'Arukōru izonshōsha to kazoku no Danshukai sanka ni yoru ishiki no henka ni kansuru kenkyū' [Study of the change of consciousness of alcoholic patients and their families after participating in Danshukai], *Nihon seishinka kango gakkaishi*, 52, no. 2 (2009), 228–32, and S. Maeda, 'Fūfu mensetsu kara erareta arukōru izonshōsha no kaifuku no purosesu: Danshukai ni kayou fūfu o taishō toshita shitsuteki kenkyū' [Recovery process of alcoholic patients that we learned from interviews with couples: qualitative research based on interviews with alcoholic husbands and their wives who attend the Danshukai meetings], *Nihon kangogakkai ronbunshū seishinkango*, 42 (2012), 230–2.
61 Kōseirōdōshō, 'Zendanren sono genkyō'.
62 M. Masaki, 'Nihongata jijo soshiki Danshukai no tanjō to sono yakuwari' [On the establishment of Danshukai, a Japanese self-help group for alcoholics], *Bulletin of the Faculty of Education, Hokkaido University*, 119 (2013), 167–76.
63 Kōseirōdōshō, 'Zendanren sono genkyō'.
64 Ibid.
65 Shimmitsu, 'Arukōru izonshō to iryōka]'.
66 Z. Zoričić et al., 'Importance of the club of treated alcoholics', *Alcoholism*, 42, no. 1 (2006), 35–42.
67 H. Suwaki, 'Naikan ryōhō' [Naikan therapy], in K. Ōhara and S. Watanabe (eds), *Seishinka chiryō no hakken* [Discovery of psychiatric treatments] (Tokyo: Seiwa shoten, 1988), 31–44.
68 S. Shimazono, 'From salvation to healing: Yoshimoto Naikan therapy and its religious origins', in C. Harding et al. (eds), *Religion and Psychotherapy in Modern Japan* (London and New York: Routledge, 2015), 154.
69 Suwaki, 'Naikan ryōhō'.
70 T. Takemoto, 'Arukōru izonshō chiryō no rekishi o furikaeru' [Transition and history in the treatment of alcoholism], *Frontiers in Alcoholism*, 2, no. 1 (2014), 76–81. Further details cited in this paragraph come from the same source unless otherwise indicated.
71 The Japan Naikan Association, www.jpnaikan.jp/meetings/index.html (accessed 2 September 2018).
72 Y. Miki, 'Naikan ryōhō no genzai oyobi kongo no tenkai to kadai' [Naikan therapy: current situation, future challenges and development], *Seishin ryōhō*, 40, no. 1 (2014), 92–6.
73 T. Takemoto, 'Arukōru izonshō chiryō no rekishi o furikaeru'.

74 Y. Miki, 'Naikan ryōhō no genzai oyobi kongo no tenkai to kadai'.

75 T. Saitō, 'Jijo gurūpu no rekishi to hensen' [The history and development of self-help groups]', *Frontiers in Alcoholism*, 4, no. 2 (2016), 105–9.

76 For instance, see M. Takahashi, 'Maindofurunesu ga shinriryōhō ni motarasumono: Naikan ryōhō tono kanren kara' [What kind of impact does mindfulness have on psychotherapy in Japan? From the relationship with Naikan therapy], *Seishin ryōhō*, 42, no. 4 (2016), 483–90, and T. Maeshiro, 'Naikan ryōhō kara mita maindofurunesu' [Mindfulness seen from the viewpoint of Naikan therapy], *Seishin igaku*, 61, no. 6 (2019), 693–701.

77 M. Miyoshi, 'Nihon ni okeru serufu herupu gurūpu eno kitai to mondai no genjō' [The expectations and the present conditions of problems to the self-help groups in Japan], *Bungaku kenkyū ronshū (Meiji University)*, 42 (2015), 51–69.

78 Kokuzeichō (National Tax Agency), 'Sake repōto heisei 30 nen 3 gatsu' [Alcohol report, March 2018], www.nta.go.jp/ (accessed 2 September 2018).

79 www.mhlw.go.jp/toukei/saikin/hw/kanja/10syoubyo/ (accessed 9 December 2019).

80 K. Amano, 'Arukōru izonshō chiryō no rekishi wo furikaeru' [History of the treatment of alcoholism], *Frontiers in Alcoholism*, 3, no. 1 (2015), 66–71.

10

'May it last, such peace and life': treating alcoholism in Tito's Yugoslavia, 1948–1991

Mat Savelli

In 1971 a remarkable album was released by Jugoton, Yugoslavia's premier record label. Normally associated with rock stars, pop acts and folk singers, the record represented Jugoton's foray into an entirely new domain. Formally known by its catalogue number LPY 50908, *Alkoholizam u riječi i pjesmi* (Alcoholism in Word and Song) was jointly credited to Vladimir Hudolin and Ruža Vešligaj.[1] Vešligaj, who handled the music and lyrics, had herself entered into treatment for alcoholism in 1965, later transitioning to provide counselling and musicotherapy to fellow alcoholics. Hudolin's main contribution to the LP, meanwhile, consisted of recorded lectures about the causes, nature and treatment of alcoholism. A psychiatrist and the country's leading alcohologist (the term Yugoslavs sometimes used to describe specialists in alcoholism treatment), he was undoubtedly well positioned to provide such an education, having already been regularly offering courses on alcoholism to families and patients within his clinic in Zagreb. Perhaps most significantly, vocals on the album's eight musical tracks were performed by the Vocal Octet of the Zagreb Club of Treated Alcoholics, a group of patients who, like Vešligaj, had graduated through Hudolin's innovative treatment programme housed on the rather ironically titled Vinogradska Cesta (Vineyard Road). The LP, which found its way into homes and treatment centres across Yugoslavia, was emblematic of Hudolin's signature approach to alcoholism, combining public education about the illness with social opportunities for his patients. This chapter details what came to be internationally known as the 'Hudolin method', highlighting the essential components of Yugoslavia's most significant form of alcoholism treatment and charting its evolution and expansion from the Vinogradska clinic to dozens of countries across the world. It demonstrates that the Yugoslav approach to managing alcoholism both was shaped by and contributed to the global social psychiatry movement. As such, it offers historians a less-researched example of how treatment methods for alcoholism proliferated globally throughout the twentieth century.

By the early 1960s, it had already become apparent that the modernisation programme launched after World War II by the new Communist authorities could not necessarily solve all of the problems facing Yugoslav citizens. Gains had been made in several key economic and social indicators, especially after Yugoslavia's 1948 break from the Soviet sphere of influence, but the large-scale changes brought about by Yugoslavia's unique self-managing socialism model shed light on several emerging social problems.[2] One of the most significant issues facing the new Yugoslavia, in terms of both health and social costs, was alcoholism. Throughout the 1950s and 1960s, psychiatric researchers raised alarms about the increasing rates of alcohol abuse, noting that consumption was rising among traditional drinkers (agricultural and industrial workers) as well as among segments of the population that had historically eschewed drinking, including women and the country's sizeable Muslim population.[3] Researchers' concerns soon transformed into panic, with Hudolin and others warning that hundreds of thousands of alcoholics remained hidden, beyond the reach of the country's small number of psychiatric practitioners.[4] With these numbers in mind, physicians warned that alcoholism represented 'one of the most difficult problems of contemporary social medicine' and the single most significant national problem facing Yugoslavia.[5]

In their efforts to explain the explosion of alcoholism, researchers were generally split between those who assumed a change in the real rates of alcoholism and those who believed that increased prevalence rates were primarily related to changing conceptions of problem drinking and better education of both the public and practitioners. Those who favoured the latter perspective largely blamed the country's high alcoholism rates on holdovers from the past, such as peasant drinking traditions and alcohol's traditional pre-eminence in rural medical treatment.[6] Those who favoured the idea that rates of problem drinking were really increasing, on the other hand, instead pointed to modernisation itself as the crux of the issue. In the first decades of Communist rule, urbanisation and industrialisation proceeded at a comparatively rapid pace. Researchers highlighted the way in which rural workers became disconnected from family structures through migration to the cities, finding solace in pubs and bars.[7] Others focused on the fact that industrialisation not only increased the opportunities for drinking (through mechanised production and subsequently lower prices), but also involved working conditions that themselves prompted drinking, either for self-medication or because of the workplace's professional culture.[8] However one framed things, it was apparent to practitioners across Yugoslavia that the problem with alcoholism not only was widespread, but was also threatening the country's future. If the climate of optimism and sense of progress that marked Yugoslavia in the late 1950s and the 1960s were to be maintained, finding a way to tackle the problem of alcoholism was paramount.

Yugoslav responses to alcoholism

Against a backdrop of professional (and to a lesser extent popular) panic over alcoholism, the country's mental healthcare providers were inspired to theorise and test novel forms of treatment, eager to come up with something that could stem the rising tide of problem drinking. Many of Yugoslavia's clinicians read and travelled widely, which provided them with opportunities to test the varied forms of treatment being discussed within European psychiatry. For example, like their colleagues elsewhere, many Yugoslav practitioners experimented with psycho-pharmaceuticals, albeit with limited results. The only medication to gain traction was disulfiram (Antabuse), which researchers noted had the ability to help to prepare patients for more meaningful psychotherapeutic treatment.[9] In Slovenia, meanwhile, the Ljubljana-based practitioner Janez Rugelj (notorious for his authoritarian temperament) crafted an unorthodox therapeutic intervention that aimed to raise the level of culture and masculinity of his patients. Deeming his treatment programme 'the most difficult in the world', he demanded that his patients participate in regular eight-kilometre running sessions and alpine mountain climbs. He compiled mandatory reading lists that drew from both the fictional and non-fictional worlds and insisted that patients raise their intellectual and cultural awareness if they were to remain in the programme, which he insisted had a success rate of 95 per cent.[10] Others, such as Marko Trbović of Sarajevo, continued to apply more traditional forms of individually focused treatment, with psychodynamic psychotherapy in particular enjoying some success.[11]

On the whole, however, the most significant new form of treatment drew heavily on the principles of social psychiatry, an emerging approach that was finding traction across the psychiatric world in the 1960s. Whether in Belgrade (at the Institute for Mental Health) or at Zagreb's Stojanović University Hospital, the most significant forms of alcoholism treatment would look beyond the individual to their wider social milieu. These practitioners acknowledged the alcoholic as a problematic individual, but stressed that wider social networks – families, social groups and workplaces – were themselves integral in prompting and supporting alcoholism, described by one expert as a 'social-infectious disease'.[12] Moreover, they looked to society more broadly, locating the roots of alcoholism in the economic demands of the drinks industry, the peasant tradition of home distillation and even Yugoslavia's abundant population of plum trees (from which the favoured local spirit šljivovica was made).[13] Put simply, for leading Yugoslav theorists, alcoholism was fundamentally better understood as a social illness than as a disease of the individual.

The person most responsible for applying social psychiatry to the problem of alcoholism was Vladimir Hudolin, who dedicated his career to developing a treatment modality capable of reducing the enormous social, economic and health burden of alcoholism that he saw as a threat to both Yugoslavia and the wider world. As early as 1960, he articulated the notion that responding to the country's mass alcoholism problem would necessarily involve an entirely new approach, one that required novel forms of intervention both inside and outside the clinic.[14] By the 1980s, he had become so convinced by his experiments with alcoholism treatment that he began calling for a full-on social psychiatric revolution within the profession as a whole, seeing the lessons he had learned in treating alcoholics as applicable to wider groups of the mentally ill.[15]

Although what would eventually become internationally known as the 'Hudolin method' was a product of Yugoslavia, its roots can be traced to the UK. In 1959, as he was assuming the position of chief psychiatrist at the Stojanović University Hospital in Zagreb (otherwise known as the Vinogradska clinic), Hudolin was one of several Yugoslav clinicians to visit the UK for advanced training.[16] Although he met a number of practitioners during his sojourn, he came to be particularly influenced by the work of Maxwell Jones and Joshua Bierer, controversial figures whose work challenged the tenets of mainstream psychiatry. At the Belmont Hospital, Jones had spent the 1950s testing a form of 'social therapy', which would eventually blossom into the concept of the 'therapeutic community'.[17] Although therapeutic communities would spread widely and diversify over the years, Jones's initial desire was rooted in the notion that more democratic, egalitarian and group-minded forms of treatment would be ultimately beneficial to patients. Hudolin and others would follow Jones's unusual career as he travelled the globe seeking to inject social-mindedness into the psychiatric profession. Bierer, a progenitor of the social psychiatry movement, echoed Jones's desire for new forms of treatment that defied the traditional top-down, closed-door facility of the psychiatric hospital. Initiating one of the UK's first open-door facilities, the Marlborough Day Hospital, Bierer was also famous for the creation of social clubs whose membership included current and former patients, as well as staff.[18] Bierer adopted something of an evangelical zeal, dedicating a substantial portion of his life to bringing together like-minded practitioners in the International Association for Social Psychiatry. Although it is difficult to know exactly how much time Hudolin spent studying under these practitioners, they clearly left an impact; his work would continually reference Jones's research, and Hudolin was even responsible for having Bierer's autobiography published.

Shortly after his return to Yugoslavia, Hudolin laid out his vision for how the country ought to tackle the burgeoning alcoholism problem, devising a strategy to guide his fellow practitioners.[19] Firstly, he argued, it was necessary to take the struggle against alcoholism to society itself, engaging in widespread public education campaigns that would be led not only by physicians but also by treated alcoholics themselves. Given that central role that social structures played in supporting alcoholism, he encouraged the participation of other social actors (such as the Red Cross and temperance organisations) as well. Secondly, he strongly encouraged outpatient therapy when possible, anchoring treatment in various forms of psychotherapy. Although he believed that some individuals would require a short stay in hospital, it was important that they be returned to the community as quickly as possible. Thirdly, he insisted that family and the wider social environment of the patient be involved in the therapeutic process, seeing individually focused treatment as insufficient. Guided by the ideas of social psychiatry, he described alcoholism as an illness implicating the entire social network of the alcoholic; concentrating solely on the individual would be unlikely to result in significant improvement. His fourth and fifth pillars of alcoholism treatment – the therapeutic community as the organising principle for inpatient treatment and the formation of post-treatment social clubs of former alcoholics – clearly reflected the learning he had done in the UK. While these notions would evolve and be taken up somewhat differently by alcohologists across the country, this skeletal framework would guide thinking on alcoholism for decades.

For those patients who required hospital stays, whether in long-term open-door facilities or in day hospitals, socially oriented care would be the order of the day. It was important, Hudolin cautioned, that the principles of the therapeutic community guide all forms of inpatient care.[20] The community itself was consisted of patients, nurses, psychiatrists and social workers, all of whom were, theoretically at least, members of equal standing, able to cooperatively craft regulations for the community's management. Group-focused tasks made up the bulk of activity within the hospital, either through various types of therapy or in educative endeavours. Regular group psychotherapy, in which patients discussed their issues with their peers and staff, was a fixture of Hudolin's method, and individually focused treatment was comparatively frowned upon.[21] Group therapy was seen as important because, on the one hand, practitioners believed that problems in social relationships were often fundamental causes of alcoholism; learning to work out one's problems in the context of a social environment could only have positive consequences for patients with anti-social tendencies.[22] Given Yugoslavia's expertise in group psychotherapy, itself something partially forged through connections with London-based practitioners like Wilfred Bion and S.H. Foulkes, Hudolin's insistence that group psychotherapy form the backbone of treatment aligned with the capabilities of Yugoslav practitioners.[23] Clinicians hoped that the group orientation of the programme would provide patients with a forum in which they would learn to re-establish non-alcohol-dependent relationships.[24]

On the other hand, group treatment also offered the possibility of patients engaging in mutual assistance and care, something practitioners hoped would inculcate a sense of agency and capability among those being treated. The therapeutic community approach required patients to become more self-reliant than was expected in classical, top-down psychiatric approaches, and tasks such as cooking and recreational planning fell under the auspices of patients rather than staff. If successful, patients would regain belief in their own abilities and faculties. To further this goal, the therapeutic community also employed occupational therapy.[25] In Hudolin's clinic, the patients set up a carpentry shop to construct their own recreational area and remodel portions of the clinic itself. Others, meanwhile, operated a printing operation that published educational materials about alcoholism, as well as Hudolin's own alcoholism journal.[26] To further entrench a notion of sociality and self-confidence, decisions related to life within the community were to be democratically taken in large daily group meetings.[27] Such an approach aimed to stymie the development of a paternalistic relationship between staff and patient, using the principles of cooperative self-management to guide decision-making.[28] In this formulation, it was thus the responsibility of patients to overcome their drinking problem; physicians merely provided them with a social environment to bolster their likelihood of success.

To this end, clinicians were expected to encourage patients to take an active role in organising social life within the community. In a Belgrade-based therapeutic community, following Bierer's lead, patients organised parties on a regular basis, with each patient taking responsibility for specific tasks relating to the event.[29] Psychiatrists hoped to demonstrate that fun could be had without alcohol, and that this lesson would carry on beyond the patients' discharge from the clinic. Beyond parties, patients took charge of organising sports, games and various arts and crafts. Given Hudolin's sense that music was the best way to activate the emotional powers of the patient, regular hours were also set aside for singing and instrument playing, culminating in the release of *Alcoholism in Word and Song*, which Hudolin described as chronicling 'the greatest moments from the lives of alcoholics in musical composition and interpretation by alcoholics'.[30] In his view, the fact that patients wrote and recorded the material themselves was of crucial therapeutic importance, and musicotherapy enjoyed a prominent position within the world of alcoholism treatment.

Yet the LP, which was disseminated across Yugoslavia, formed only one portion of the educative component of the Hudolin approach. In reality, education about alcoholism took up much of the time in a patient's day, with therapists underscoring that patients could better deal with their illness if they understood the key psychiatric precepts behind it. Patients read widely on the illness and were expected to pass exams on the subject at various intervals in their treatment. Yet they were not the only individuals who needed to be educated; families, and in some cases even a patient's work colleagues, were also brought into the clinic to undergo education. Several practitioners held the conviction that wives (patients were overwhelmingly men) played a near-decisive factor in determining the success of treatment, so he saw their alcohology education as paramount for successful treatment.[31] In Belgrade, Branko Gačić was a pivotal figure in conducting family education on alcoholism, establishing a special programme for families at the Institute for Mental Health in 1973. Beyond the family, Gačić also felt it important to expand education about alcoholism into the patient's wider social circle, including friends and colleagues, who were also expected to take examinations on the topic of alcoholism.[32] In Zagreb, Hudolin offered lectures to family members on topics such as 'How to handle an alcoholic' and 'Family behaviour and alcoholism'.[33] Family members, especially wives, could then act as emissaries to transmit knowledge about alcoholism to the patient's wider social network.[34] In this way, Hudolin's groups were somewhat similar to the Danshukai self-help groups discussed by Akira

Hashimoto in this volume (see Chapter 9). In both instances, there was a clear understanding of alcoholism as an illness that struck the whole family, and thus the family as a whole could be brought into treatment. Abstinence, the stated goal of almost all Yugoslav alcoholism treatment, seemingly depended upon raising the level of knowledge and awareness within the patient's social circle and beyond into the wider community.

Yet families and friends were not only understood as potential facilitators of abstinence; they were sometimes described as incubators of alcoholism itself. For that reason, practitioners aimed not only to educate family members, but to actively treat them as well. At Belgrade's Institute for Mental Health, researchers emphasised that poor marriages were themselves important aetiological factors for alcoholism, with the passive-submissive personalities of some wives being singled out as problematic and thus in need of treatment.[35] Borislav Djukanović, based in Belgrade, argued in a monograph entitled *Alcoholism and the Family* that practitioners should consider the marriage itself alcoholic in nature, rather than simply the individual.[36] The roots of problem drinking were found in the way spouses related to each other, rather than simply within the drinker. Other practitioners, such as Belgrade's Slavka-Moric Petrović, looked into the past, highlighting deficiencies and flaws in the alcoholic's upbringing as integral to the development of problem drinking.[37] Unsurprisingly, parental abandonment, conflict and the father's own problems with drinking were all cited as evidence that families could act as 'alcoholic nurseries'.[38] For young alcoholics, parents could function as 'counter-alcoholics', in need of treatment themselves, if their child's alcoholism was to be truly addressed.[39] As Gačić summarised, 'The goal of our systemic treatment of alcoholism is not only the individual's abstinence … [o]ur major treatment goal is a process of change for the whole family which consists of a new life philosophy and a new and better lifestyle … .'[40] Beyond the family, experts described the drinking cultures and working conditions of certain workplaces as pathogenic in terms of alcoholism. In particular, those employed in manual labour (miners, steelworkers, railway workers and so on) were particularly threatened in this regard.[41] For this reason, practitioners extended treatment to include a whole host of 'co-alcoholics' in a problem drinker's life, including their 'friends, neighbours, colleagues, [and] bosses'.[42] To truly treat alcoholism in the Yugoslav fashion meant not only rehabilitating patients to deal with the outside world; it was also necessary to change the outside world by bringing a small part of it into treatment itself.

When a group of American psychiatrists visited Vinogradska in the early 1970s to learn about Hudolin's experimental methods, the importance of group therapy, the therapeutic community and the educative component of treatment could be seen in the clinic's daily schedule:

> 6.00–7.00: Grooming. Housekeeping.
> 7.00–7.45: Day patient arrival. Roll call. Calisthenics.
> 7.45–9.00: Breakfast. Drug therapy as needed. Meeting of group leaders.
> 9.00–10.00: Group meetings: psychotherapy and education.
> 10.00–11.45: Therapeutic Community meeting.
> 14.00–14.45: On alternate days; Lecture to all patients; Discussion of Lecture in groups; Experimental Club with social worker; Jolly Wednesday with family recreation.
> 15.00–15.45: Music Therapy, Experimental Clubs, Jolly Wednesday. Examinations. Free time.
> 16.30: Roll call for day patients, who go home except when their group is on call. Change of shifts for on call group. Visits by patients to clubs in Zagreb.[43]

Varied iterations of this schedule were probably common across much of Yugoslavia, and other accounts of the functioning of day hospitals and therapeutic-community-based approaches to alcoholism allude to the same sorts of activities.[44] Whether in day hospitals (which involved the patient attending treatment throughout the workday before returning to his family later) or in fully inpatient treatment, these interventions saw medical institutions as places to bring together alcoholics in the hope of resocialising them, offering opportunities to relearn how to form social relationships, lend one another mutual support and rediscover a sense of agency and capability. In this regard, institutions like Hudolin's Vinogradska clinic were putting Maxwell Jones's aims into action, hoping to fundamentally reshape the social landscape of the alcoholic.

Hudolin Clubs

To further this goal, Hudolin and others expended significant efforts elucidating a plan for people after their inpatient treatment had concluded. A fundamental flaw in most inpatient forms of alcoholism treatment, they argued, was that the individual must at some point leave the confines of hospital to re-engage with the 'real world'. Even those who had been through the confidence-building process of the therapeutic community would struggle upon returning to a society that, from Hudolin's perspective, was designed in such a way as to promote alcoholism. As a consequence, figuring out how to prevent relapse in the context of an alcohol-loving society was a primary concern.

In order to address these problems, Hudolin leaned upon Bierer's experiments with patient social clubs. Perhaps the therapeutic community, or at least its social atmosphere, could be 'extended' somehow beyond the end of official treatment. Known alternatively as Clubs of Treated Alcoholics, Sociotherapeutic Clubs or Alcohol Aftercare Clubs, the first of these groups began to appear in Yugoslavia during the late 1950s and early 1960s. In Belgrade, Dusan Petrović, who, like Hudolin, had spent part of 1959 in London studying the work of Maxwell Jones and Joshua Bierer, led efforts to set up 'Saturday Club at Six' (named to avoid stigmatising its members).[45] In Zagreb, meanwhile, Hudolin launched a group called 'Prepored' (Renaissance). The aim of these groups was to bring together former alcoholics, family members and at least one member of the medical community in a weekly meeting to offer mutual support against temptation and provide an alternative social environment so that the alcoholic could avoid 'drinking society'.[46] As with inpatient treatment, families, friends and colleagues of the alcoholic were central to the functioning of the club, reflecting the way in which Hudolin and colleagues positioned alcoholism as an illness of the patient's social ecology.

These clubs were not mere meeting places, and they often came to occupy a significant space in a person's life. Groups often published monthly newsletters, operated bars (selling only soft drinks), helped members find employment and engaged in wider community activities. In this regard, they were designed to magnify and prolong the confidence-building and socialising nature of the therapeutic community, providing a supportive arena and reminding members that they had agency in their lives. Another crucial function of the clubs was the continuation of patient education on the topic of alcoholism. For instance, after celebrating one year of club membership, former patients could undergo 'postgraduate' training in alcoholism which consisted of a one-week seminar course, after which time they would be included among the volunteer teachers and leaders of the club.[47]

As the popularity of these clubs spread (eventually reaching nearly 1,000 total clubs in Yugoslavia by the time of the country's dissolution in 1991) republic-level and federal-level meetings of club delegations were held to promote the public struggle against alcoholism (and frequently alcohol itself). One such federal meeting in Bosnia opened with the 'Anthem of Treated Alcoholics' (track 1 on the *Alcoholism in Word and Song* LP) and then continued with resolutions in favour of opening new chapters in rural areas, fighting 'disinformation' and 'malicious rumours' about the clubs' activities, pressuring the Yugoslav Lottery to donate funds to the club and finally proclaiming support for the decision to declare Comrade Tito a national hero (for the second time).[48] More generally, these large congregations allowed club members from across the region to share experiences, plot future possibilities for cooperation and hand out awards for long-term abstinence. Although published figures of membership numbers are not available, it is clear that tens of thousands of Yugoslavs participated in these clubs, with some of these organisations continuing to operate into the twenty-first century, well after the country's collapse.[49]

The spread of the Hudolin approach

On the surface, the Hudolin Clubs shared some characteristics with other alcoholism-oriented programmes built around mutual support, namely Alcoholics Anonymous (AA), and it might be tempting to conflate the two organisations. However, despite their shared interest in mutual self-help and creating new social possibilities for members, Yugoslavia's clubs of treated alcoholics differed in several important ways. Firstly, these groups were atheistic in tone, shunning the 'Twelve Steps' approach and its emphasis on giving oneself over to a higher power.[50] Secondly, as with Danshukai in Japan, the 'anonymous' aspect of AA was nowhere to be found in Yugoslavia, where any form of secret society was forbidden (in fact, Hudolin and the republican government of Croatia even kept an official register of treated alcoholics).[51] Far from claiming anonymity, members of these clubs often outed themselves by participating in public information activities and campaigns against alcoholism – an important facet of the Hudolin approach. Thirdly, the clubs typically required the participation of a healthcare professional (psychiatrist, nurse, social worker or similar), something that stands in sharp contrast to AA's lay-oriented approach. Finally, as a consequence of the ecological approach favoured by Yugoslavia's most important alcohology theorists, families and friends participated in Hudolin Clubs with great regularity, further separating the Hudolin approach from AA.

These differences may help to explain the remarkable fact that Hudolin Clubs did not remain confined to Yugoslavia, offering historians a comparatively rare example of East European medical expertise being exported globally. By the mid-1960s, Hudolin's personal connections to key members of the wider world of alcohology, ranging from Max Glatt and Archer Tongue in the UK to staff at the Rome Clinic in Italy, meant that the principles of his approach were being disseminated beyond Yugoslav borders.[52] Moreover, following in the footsteps of Bierer, Hudolin was very active in the emerging social psychiatry movement, which resisted the tendencies of both biological and Freudian schools of thought by underscoring that mental health problems were consequences of social environments (rather than simply individual deficiencies). Alongside figures such as Jules Masserman (USA), George Vassiliou (Greece), A. Guilherme Ferreira (Portugal), Jose Angel Bustamante (Cuba), Henri Collomb (Senegal) and others, Hudolin was an important early member of the International Association for Social Psychiatry (later renamed the World Association of Social Psychiatry), hosting the organisation's international congresses in

Zagreb on several occasions and being elected as the third president of the association in 1974. Moreover, he was a regular contributor to the journal founded by Bierer in 1955, the *International Journal of Social Psychiatry*, and served on the World Health Organization's expert committee on alcoholism from 1965 to 1992. In short, far from being isolated behind the Iron Curtain, as historians of science and medicine have sometimes been too quick to assume about those operating in Eastern Europe, Hudolin and Yugoslavia's other alcohologists were well connected to global networks of psychiatric knowledge.

These relationships, both personal and professional, acted as the seeds for the global spread of Hudolin Clubs towards the final decades of the twentieth century. Although Hudolin travelled widely, his efforts to spread this social psychiatric approach to alcoholism treatment were initially concentrated in Italy. In 1979, on the heels of the hospital closure reforms initiated by Franco Basaglia (with whom Hudolin maintained a long-term friendship), he helped to launch the first Italian club of treated alcoholics in Trieste, helping to cement the viability of outpatient treatment.[53] Over subsequent decades, Italy would play host to several thousand Hudolin Clubs, offering a significant alternative to AA, and the Hudolin name would be revered in Italy for many years to come.[54] Beyond Italy's borders, Hudolin-inspired clubs of treated alcoholics proliferated globally from the 1980s onwards, with groups operating in more than thirty countries across the world on four continents, ranging from Ecuador and Venezuela to Scandinavia, sub-Saharan Africa (Cameroon, Kenya) and South Asia (India, Sri Lanka). Although the proliferation of clubs involved some evolution of the original concepts, they still largely follow the fundamental principles laid out by Hudolin.

Conclusion

In the late 1980s, just a few years before the country's collapse, one researcher published a series of articles which succinctly depicted the contours of the decades-long struggle against alcoholism that Hudolin and others had waged. Publishing in the journal *Socijalna psihijatrija* (Social Psychiatry), one of the country's most prestigious medical journals (a sign of how deeply entrenched the ideas of social psychiatry had become), Dragoslav Nikolić highlighted what must have been a frustrating conundrum for the country's expanding community of alcohologists. On the one hand, practitioners like Hudolin and Gačić had been successful in convincing their fellow physicians that alcoholism was an issue worthy of psychiatric attention, and treatment capacity for alcoholism had increased substantially in the period between the 1960s and 1980s. At the same time, however, despite the substantial proliferation of both alcohologists and treatment possibilities, the country's alcoholism problem remained significant. By the mid-1980s, alcoholism was the seventh most commonly treated medical problem (it had been the seventeenth most common in in 1969), and every seventh patient in Yugoslav psychiatric hospitals was diagnosed with alcoholism.[55] Although some of the increase may be attributable to the fact that physicians and the public were much more educated and accepting of alcoholism in the 1980s than they had been in the 1960s, it is also quite possible that rates of problem drinking were truly accelerating despite the best efforts of the alcohologists.[56] Undoubtedly, practitioners hoped that continued public education and the spread of the social psychiatric approach would eventually allow them to bring down the country's soaring alcoholism rates, despite the social forces that propelled drinking.

Ultimately, the story of Yugoslavia's experimental approach to tackling alcoholism suffered from two deaths. The first was that of the country itself. In June 1991 Croatia and Slovenia declared their intention to leave the federation, with Bosnia and Macedonia following shortly thereafter. Several years of warfare marked by near-unimaginable brutality, itself often facilitated by drunken rages, consumed the Balkans throughout the 1990s and brought about a definitive end to Yugoslavia. Throughout the conflict, Hudolin-style clubs suffered greatly for a host of reasons – lack of funds, population movements and the deaths of members – and comparatively few continued to function after the war. The second death was that of Hudolin himself, who passed away in Zagreb in 1996, less than a year after the cessation of hostilities in Croatia. And although Hudolin's legacy endures into the twenty-first century, it is most significant in areas outside the former Yugoslavia, with the World Association of Clubs of Alcoholics in Treatment (WACAT) continuing to spread the Hudolin model around the globe.

Notes

1 The title of this chapter, 'May it last, such peace and life', is taken from the lyrics of the album's first track, 'Neka traje nam to', also referred to as the 'Anthem of treated alcoholics'. The song could often be heard at meetings of the Clubs of Treated Alcoholics.

2 Although Communist authorities initially attempted to replicate the Soviet model of economic management in the period immediately after World War II, they soon adopted a rather different approach under the banner of self-managing socialism, the brainchild of a party ideologist by the name of Edvard Kardelj. At the risk of oversimplification, these reforms included a greater degree of economic decentralisation and the inclusion of more market principles. For more on the Yugoslav economic model, see Vladimir Unkovski-Korica, *The Economic Struggle for Power in Tito's Yugoslavia: From World War II to Non-Alignment* (London: Bloomsbury Publishing, 2016).

3 V. Hudolin, 'Savremeni problem alkoholizma' [The contemporary problem of alcoholism], in N. Peršić (ed.), *Psihijatrija: simpozij o neurologije i psihijatriji* [Psychiatry: Symposium on Neurology and Psychiatry] (Ljubljana: Lek, 1969), 263–86; A. Despotović, J. Vesel anI D. Vranješević, 'Neke epidemiološke i demografske varijacije raširenosti alkoholima u sr srbiji' [Some epidemiological and demographic variations in alcohol prevalence in the Socialist Republic of Serbia], in *III kongres neurologa i psihijatara Jugoslavije* [Proceedings of the Third Congress of the Neurologists and Psychiatrists of Yugslavia] (Split: Udruženje Neuropsihijatara Jugoslavije, 1968), 125.

4 In Hudolin's work in the early 1960s, he estimated that Yugoslavia was home to about 300,000 alcoholics, roughly 1.5 per cent of the population. By the end of the decade, he warned that a full 10 per cent of Croatia's population might be suffering from alcoholism and alcohol-related mental disorders, with figures as high as 20–30 per cent in particular cohorts, like industrial workers. See Vladimir Hudolin, 'Prevencija alkoholizma, liječenje i rehabilitacija alkoholičara' [Prevention of alcoholism, treatment and rehabilitation of alcoholics], *Medicinski glasnik* [Medical Herald], 15 (1961), 76–80; Vladimir

Hudolin, 'Alcoholism in Croatia', *International Journal of Social Psychiatry*, 15 (1969), 85–91. For a more detailed account of the panic over alcoholism, see Mat Savelli, 'Diseased, Depraved, or Just Drunk: The Psychiatric Panic over Alcoholism in Communist Yugoslavia', *Social History of Medicine*, 25, no. 2 (2012), 462–80.

5 Vladimir Hudolin, *Jugoslavenska bibliografija alkoholizma* [Yugoslav Bibliography of Alcoholism] (Zagreb: Pliva, 1964), ix; I. Milaković, 'Alkoholizam – Sve alkuelniji' [Alcoholism: ever more relevant], *Život i zdravlje* [Life and Health] (1976), 1–2. Translations are by the author except where otherwise stated.

6 M. Mičev, 'Psihosocijalni korenovi alkoholizma u SR Makedoniji' [Psychosocial roots of alcoholism in the Republic of Macedonia], in *III Kongres neurologa i psihijatara Jugoslavije* [Proceedings of the Third Congress of the Neurologists and Psychiatrists of Yugoslavia] (Split: Udruženje Neuropsihijatara Jugoslavije, 1968), 126; K. Vujoselić and G. Kapor, 'Oblici alkoholizma i premorbidna ličnost alkoholičara u armiji' [Types of alcoholism and premorbid personality of alcoholics in the army], *Vojno-sanitetski pregled* [Military Medical Review], 21, no. 2 (1964), 771–4.

7 V. Rogina, 'Suvremene tendencije u zbrinjavanju psihijatriskih bolesnika' [Contemporary tendencies in the care of psychaitric patients], in K. Korbar, K. Pospišil-Završki, S. Triva and R. Turčin (eds), *Civilno-pravni status ii problemi zastite psihijatrijskih bolesnika, II savjetovanje o forenzičkoj psihijatari* [Civil Law Status and Problems in the Protection of Psychiatric Patients: Second Conference on Forensic Psychiatry] (Zagreb: Medicinska Naklada, 1967), 21–36; D. Gavrilović, Z. Grujić and M. Mladenović, 'Alkoholizam u Sokolcu – Socijalno-ekonomske poslijedice' [Alcoholism in Sokolac: socio-economic consequences], in Geza Čeh (ed.), *Zbornik radova: Prvi Bosansko-hercegovački simpozijum o alkoholizmu i narkomanijama* [Proceedings of the First Bosnian-Hercegovinian Symposium on Alcoholism and Narcomania] (Zenica: n.pub., 1972), 370–3.

8 J. Poleksić, A. Despotović and D. Milovanović, 'Kritične profesije i alkoholizam' [Critical professions and alcoholism], in *III kongres neurologa i psihijatara Jugoslavije* [Proceedings of the Third Congress of the Neurologists and Psychaitrists of Yugoslavia] (Split: Udruženje Neuropsihijatara Jugoslavije, 1968), 128; J. Poleksić, *Učestalost, uzroci i socijalno-medicinske posledice alkoholizma u rudara Kolubarskog Basena* [Frequency, Causes and Socio-Medical Consequences of Alcoholism among the Miners of the Kolubara Basin] (Belgrade: Naucna Knjiga, 1976).

9 Disulfiram, often known by the trade name Antabuse, was widely used in other parts of the world. See S. Betlheim, D. Blazević and N. Persić, 'The influence of barbiturates on chronic alcoholic patients', *Acta medica iugoslavica*, 8, no. 3 (1954), 82–4; V. Hudolin and V. Muacević, 'Psihofarmakologija i psihoterapija alkoholizma' [Psychopharmacology and psychotherapy of alcoholism], in N. Bohaček (ed.), *Prva Jugoslavenska psihofarmakološka simpozija* [First Yugoslav Psycho-Pharmaceutical Symposium] (Zagreb: Medicinska Naklada, 1968), 154–61; A. Despotović, 'Psihofarmakoterapija alkoholizma', in N. Bohaček (ed.), *Prva Jugoslavenska psihofarmakološka simpozija* [First Yugoslav Psycho-Pharmaceutical Symposium] (Zagreb: Medicinska Naklada, 1968), 251–7.

10 See Janez Rugelj, *Dolga Pot* [The Long Path] (Ljubljana: Republiški odbor Rdečega križa Slovenije, 1977) and L. Bennett, 'Treating alcoholism in a Yugoslav fashion', *East European Quarterly*, 18, no. 4 (1985), 495–519.

11 Trbović started publishing about his psychodynamic approach to alcoholism in the 1970s, publishing the results of a ten-year study of alcoholics in the pages of *Socijalna psihijatrija* (Social Psychiatry) in the 1980s. See, for example, M. Trbović, 'Paranoidno impotentni oblik alkoholizma' [Paranoid impotent type of alcoholism], *Socijalna psihijatrija*, 11, no. 1 (1983), 17–24; M. Trbović, 'Infantilno maternalni oblik alkoholizma' [Infantile maternal type of alcoholism], *Socijalna psihijatrija*, 11, no. 1 (1983), 25–36; M. Trbović, 'Mazohisticko depresvni oblik alkoholizma' [Masochistic depressive type of alcoholism], *Socijalna psihijatrija*, 11, no. 2 (1983), 133–42; M. Trbović, 'Animatorno klaunski oblik alkoholizma' [Animatory clown type of alcoholism], *Socijalna psihijatrija*, 11, no. 4 (1983), 239–46.

12 V. Hudolin, 'Rehabilitacija alkoholičara i narkomana' [Rehabilitation of alcoholics and drug addicts], in S. Mahkota (ed.), *Zbornik: III kongresa lekara Jugosljavije* [Proceedings of the Third Congress of Yugoslav Physicians] (Ljubljana: Savez Lekarskih Društava Jugosljavije, 1971), 172–95.

13 Hudolin, 'Alcoholism in Croatia'; V. Hudolin, 'Organizacija naučno-istrazivačkog rada na području alkoholizma' [The organisation of scientific research in the field of alcoholism], *Anali bolnice Dr. M. Stojanović* [Annals of Dr M. Stojanović Hospital], 4, no. 3 (1965), 191–6; C. Vasev, 'Proizvodni potencijali alkoholnih pića na području BiH – Faktor porasta alkoholizma' [The production potential of alcoholic drinks in Bosnia: a factor in the rise of alcoholism], in Geza

Čeh (ed.), *Zbornik radova: Prvi Bosansko-hercegovački simpozijum o alkoholizmu i narkomanijama* [Proceedings of the First Bosnian-Hercegovinian Symposium on Alcoholism and Narcomania] (Zenica: n.pub., 1972), 335–9.

14 Vladimir Hudolin, 'Prevencija alkoholizma, liječenje i rehabilitacija alkoholičara' [Prevention of alcoholism, treatment and rehabilitation of alcoholics], *Liječnicki vjesnik* [Medical Herald], 82, no. 6 (1960), 473–85.

15 Vladimir Hudolin, 'Social psychiatry today', in Vladimir Hudolin (ed.), *Social Psychiatry: Proceedings of the Eighth World Congress of Social Psychiatry* (New York: Springer Science, 1981), 1–8.

16 Other visitors to London at this time, such as the Belgrade-based Dusan Petrović, implemented treatment programmes that closely echoed that made famous by Hudolin.

17 See Catherine Fussinger, '"Therapeutic community", psychiatry's reformers and antipsychiatrists: reconsidering changes in the field of psychiatry after World War II', *History of Psychiatry*, 22, no. 2 (2011), 146–63; Maxwell Jones, *Social Psychiatry in Practice: The Idea of the Therapeutic Community* (Harmondsworth: Penguin, 1968).

18 Liam Clarke, 'Joshua Bierer: Striving for power', *History of Psychiatry*, 8, no. 31 (1997), 319–32; J. Bierer and F.P. Haldane, 'A self-governed patients' social club in a public mental hospital', *Journal of Mental Science*, 87, no. 368 (1941), 419–26.

19 Hudolin, 'Prevencija alkoholizma, liječenje i rehabilitacija alkoholičara' (1960).

20 Hudolin, 'Prevencija alkoholizma, liječenje i rehabilitacija alkoholičara' (1960).

21 Vladimir Hudolin, 'The day hospitals in the treatment of alcoholics', *British Journal of Addiction*, 61, nos 1–2 (1965), 29–33, at 31.

22 Hudolin, 'Alcoholism in Croatia', 86–8; Hudolin, 'Rehabilitacija alkoholičara i narkomana', 173.

23 For more on group therapy in Yugoslavia, see Mat Savelli, '"Peace and happiness await us": psychotherapy in Yugoslavia, 1945–85', *History of the Human Sciences*, 31, no. 4 (2018), 38–57.

24 Apparently, the patients even played a role in determining whether fellow alcoholics were ready to be discharged from the hospital. See B. Sikic, R.D. Walker and R.D. Peterson, 'An evaluation of a program for the treatment of alcoholism in Croatia', *International Journal of Social Psychiatry*, 18, no. 3 (1972), 171–81, at 159–60.

25 S. Morić-Petrović et al., *Metodi lečenja i rehabilitacije alkoholičara* [Method of Treatment and Rehabilitation of Alcoholics] (Belgrade: Zavod za Mentalno Zdravlje, 1973), 15.

26 Sikic, Walker and Peterson, 'An evaluation of a program for the treatment of alcoholism in Croatia', 160–2.
27 Bennett, 'Treating alcoholism in a Yugoslav fashion'.
28 Although it is tempting to assume that the focus on self-management and patient-driven decision-making might be reflective of Yugoslavia's wider practice of self-managing socialism (in which firms and enterprises were also partially self-governed by workers), it is striking that Hudolin and others never made reference to this wider practice. The omission is all the more notable because it might have been an easy way to build goodwill and attract favour from governing authorities. Yet rather than paying homage to this component of the country's ideological platform, clinicians justified the organisation of the clinic instead through frequent reference to Maxwell Jones's writings on the therapeutic community.
29 V. Djordjević-Banković and T. Sedmak, 'Odeljenjski praznik kao dopunski socijalno psihijatrijski metod u lečenju alkoholizma' [Party on the ward as an additional social psychiatric method in the treatment of alcoholism], in Aleksandar Ilić (ed.), *Zbornik radova: Internacionalni simpozijum o rehabilitacije u psihijatriji* [International Symposium on the Rehabilitation of Psychiatry] (Belgrade: n.pub., 1972), 339–46.
30 V. Hudolin et al., 'Health education of patients in the field of social psychiatry, notably alcoholics', *International Journal of Social Psychiatry*, 18, no. 3 (1972). 22–5.
31 B Gačić et al., 'Komunikacije bračnih partnera u toku intesivne porodične terapije alkoholizma' [Spousal communication in the course of intensive family therapy for alcoholism], *Psihijatrija danas* [Psychiatry Today], 9, no. 1 (1977), 109–20; V. Fridman, M. Fligić and D. Petrović, 'Uloga supruge u nastavku pozitivne motivacije za lečenje' [The role of the wife in the maintenance of positive motivation for treatment], *Socijalna psihijatrija* [Social Psychiatry], 4, no. 3 (1976), 301–8.
32 Gačić proposed that five to ten people around the alcoholic should be intimately involved in his therapy, including bosses and work colleagues. B. Gačić, 'Petnaest godina porodične terapije alkoholizma – Rezultati i implikacije' [Fifteen years of family treatment for alcoholism: results and implications], *Psihijatrija danas* [Psychiatry Today], 21, no. 1 (1989), 89. He was by no means alone in advocating such extensive measures to reach the patient's extended social environment. See also A. Haasz, I. Haasz and S. Ćuk, 'Rehabilitarcija alkoholičara I socijalna sredina' [The rehabilitation of alcoholics and the social environment], in Aleksandar Ilić (ed.), *Zbornik radova: Internacionalni simpozijum o*

rehabilitacije u psihijatriji [Proceedings of the International Symposium on Rehabilitation in Psychiatry] (Belgrade: n.pub., 1972), 149–52; J. Bamburac and J. Zimonja-Krisković, 'Utjećaj radne sredine na resocijalizaciju liječenog alkoholičara' [The influence of the work environment on the resocialization of the treated alcoholic], in Aleksandar Ilić (ed.), *Zbornik radova: Internacionalni simpozijum o rehabilitacije u psihijatriji* [Proceedings of the International Symposium on Rehabilitation in Psychiatry] (Belgrade: n.pub., 1972), 153–8; P. Kastel, T. Sedmak and R. Grcić-Micović, 'Osobenosti velike grupe alkoholičara' [Features of a large group of alcoholics], *Psihijatrija danas* [Psychiatry Today], 14, no. 1 (1982), 79–90.

33 Sikic, Walker and Peterson, 'An evaluation of a program for the treatment of alcoholism in Croatia'.

34 Sikic, Walker and Peterson, 'An evaluation of a program for the treatment of alcoholism in Croatia'.

35 A. Despotović, S. Stojilković and F. Petrović, 'Analiza socijalne strukture lečenih alkoholičara' [Analysis of social structure of treated alcoholics], *Anali bolnice Dr. M. Stojanović* [Annals of Dr M. Stojanović Hospital], 5, no. 1 (1966), 287–300;' Morić-Petrović et al., *Metodi lečenja i rehabilitacije alkoholičara.*

36 B. Djukanović, *Alkoholizam i porodica* [Alcoholism and the Family] (Belgrade: Republika Zajednica Nauke SR Srbije, 1979).

37 Morić-Petrović et al., *Metodi lečenja i rehabilitacije alkoholičara.*

38 Morić-Petrović et al., *Metodi lečenja i rehabilitacije alkoholičara.*

39 T. Sedmak and V. Djordjević-Banković, 'Primarne porodice i mladih hospitalizovanih alkoholičara' [The bind between family of origin and young treated alcoholics], in Aleksandar Ilić (ed.), *Zbornik radova: Internacionalni simpozijum o rehabilitacije u psihijatriji* [Proceedings of the International Symposium on Rehabilitation in Psychiatry] (Belgrade: n.pub., 1972), 347–54.

40 B. Gačić, 'Belgrade Systemic Approach to the treatment of alcoholism: principles and interventions', *Journal of Family Therapy*, 14, no. 2 (1992), 103–22, at p. 107.

41 Poleksić, Despotović and Milovanović, 'Kritične profesije i alkoholizam', 128; Poleksić, *Učestalost, uzroci i socijalno-medicinske posledice alkoholizma u rudara Kolubarskog Basena* ; J. Poleksić, 'Alkoholizam u industriji' [Alcoholism in industry], *Engrami*, 7, no. 4 (1985), 55–76.

42 Gačić, 'Belgrade Systemic Approach to the treatment of alcoholism', 106. In this article, in which Gačić reviewed the therapeutic system that he had developed in Belgrade during the 1970s, he speculated that

the ability to bring a person's co-workers and managers in for treatment was probably possible only in the context of Yugoslav socialism, acknowledging that it might seem strange to Western readers.

43 'Jolly Wednesday' referred to the fact that extra time was set aside for recreational activities on Wednesdays. See Sikic, Walker and Peterson, 'An evaluation of a program for the treatment of alcoholism in Croatia', 160.

44 Examples of other therapeutic communities used to treat alcoholism are dIscribed in Morić-Petrović et al., *Metodi lečenja i rehabilitacije alkoholičara;* T. Sedmak, 'Terapijska zajednica alkoholičara' [A therapeutic community of alcoholics], in S. Morić-Petrović (ed.), *Socioterapija u psihijatriji* [Sociotherapy in Psychiatry] (Belgrade: Zavod za Mentalno Zdravlje, 1973), 135–44; E. Kapetanović and S. Ivković, 'Prva iskustva u liječenju alkoholičara metodom terapeutske zajednice' [First experiences of using a therapeutic community in the treatment of alcoholics], *Medicinski zbornik* [Medical Proceedings], 3, no. 3 (1968), 121–4.

45 For brief histories of the movement of alcoholic aftercare clubs in Yugoslavia, see B. Lang and J. Srdar, 'Therapeutic communities and aftercare clubs in Yugoslavia', in H. Klingemann, Jukka-Pekka Takala and Geoffrey Hunt (eds), *Cure, Care, or Control: Alcoholism Treatment in Sixteen Countries* (New York: SUNY Press, 1992), 53–63; and J. Potrebić, 'Dvadesetpet godina rada Socioterapijskog Kluba Lečenih Alkoholičara Instituta za Mentalno Zdravlje u Beogradu' [Twenty years of work in the Sociotherapeutic Club of Treated Alcoholics at the Institute for Mental Health in Belgrade], *Psihijatrija danas* [Psychiatry Today], 21, no. 4 (1989), 397–402.

46 S. Ivković, 'Šta je Klub Liječenih Alkoholičara?' [What is a Club of Treated Alcoholics?], *Život i zdravlje* [Life and Health] (1976), 3–4.

47 Hudolin et al., 'Health education of patients in the field of social psychiatry, notably alcoholics'.

48 Exactly what sort of rumours or disinformation the clubs were concerned about is unclear, and I have not been able to find any sources that speak to this issue. Udruženja Klubova Liječenih Alkoholičara [Association of Clubs of Treated Alcoholics], 'Plenarni sastanak' [Plenary meeting], in Geza Čeh (ed.), *Zbornik radova*: *Prvi Bosanskohercegovački simpozijum o alkoholizmu i narkomanijama* [Proceedings of the First Bosnian-Hercegovinian Symposium on Alcoholism and Narcomania] (Zenica: n.pub., 1972), 498–518.

49 According to the Croatian Union of Clubs of Treated Alcoholics, clubs continue to function across the country (www.hskla.hr/index.html).

The same seems to be true in Serbia, according to the Association of Clubs of Treated Alcoholics of Serbia (https://zklas.org/).

50 The twelve steps outlined in the group's foundational text include several that are overtly religious, including the third step ('Made a decision to turn our will and our lives over to the care of God as we understood Him'), the sixth step ('Were entirely ready to have God remove all of these defects of character'), and eleventh step ('Sought through prayer and meditation to improve our conscious contact with God as we understood God, praying only for knowledge of God's will for us and the power to carry that out). See Alcoholics Anonymous, *The Story of How Many Thousands of Men and Women Have Recovered from Alcoholism* (New York, Alcoholics Anonymous World Services, 2001), 59.

51 Anon., 'Republicki registar alkoholicara' [Republic registar of alcoholics], *Socijalna psihijatrija* [Social Psychiatry], 3, no. 1 (1975), 75.

52 V. Hudolin, 'Uvod' [Introduction], *Anali bolnice Dr. M Stojanović* [Annals of Dr M. Stojanović Hospital], 5, no. 1 (1966), 3–6.

53 V. Patussi, E. Tumino and F. Poldrugo, 'The development of the Alcoholic Treatment Club system in Italy: fifteen years of experience', *Contemporary Drug Problems*, 23, no. 1 (1996), 29–42.

54 O. Curzio, A. Tilli, L. Mezzasalma, M. Scalese, L. Fortunato, R. Potente, G. Guidoni and S. Molinaro, 'Characteristics of alcoholics attending "clubs of alcoholics in treatment" in Italy: a national survey', *Alcohol and Alcoholism*, 47, no. 3 (2012), 317–21. Such was the reverence for Hudolin that the town of Loreto Aprutino, in the province of Pescara, renamed a street in his honour (via Vladimir Hudolin).

55 D. Nikolić, 'Primary health care and alcoholism in Yugoslavia', *Socijalna psihijatrija* [Social Psychiatry], 15, no. 3 (1987), 273; D. Nikolić, 'Stanje i problemi psihijatriskih bolnici u SFR Jugoslaviji' [Status and problems of psychiatric patients in the Socialist Federal Republic of Yugoslavia], *Socijalna psihijatrija* [Social Psychiatry], 16, no. 2 (1988), 168.

56 D. Nikolić, 'Kretanje broja alkoholičara u SFR Jugoslaviji i preventivna zaštita' [Trends in the number of alcoholics in the Socialist Federal Republic of Yugoslavia and preventative care], *Socijalna psihijatrija* [Social Psychiatry], 13, no. 4 (1985), 283–4.

11

A cradle of psychotherapy: treatment of alcohol addiction in Communist Czechoslovakia, *c.* 1948–1989

Adéla Gjuričová

In 1957 the eminent Czech poet František Hrubín, who had inspired the patriotic Czech public on the eve of World War II, as well as subsequent generations, wrote in the foreword to a textbook on alcoholism:

> Long weeks, day by day, hour by hour, I was a careful participant-observer of the doctor and his team's work at a clinic for alcoholics. Theirs is a highly creative activity. They aim at a great and precious target: to return dignity to ruined human beings with shattered souls.[1]

Hrubín had first-hand experience of treatment at an alcohol treatment facility. He was an alcoholic and was treated in Communist Czechoslovakia in the early 1950s. He described his frame of mind after the treatment: 'A man who had doubts about himself, a man who had been doubted by the whole world, once again feels the desire of his entire being to live and to create his life again.'[2]

Rather than representing a typical description of psychiatric care in Stalinist Czechoslovakia, Hrubín's observations highlight an important paradox. In spite of drastic political limitations imposed on socially and psychologically oriented approaches to health, and despite the marginalisation of psychiatric and psychological conditions in most socialist countries, the treatment of alcohol addiction experienced dynamic development within the field of socialist medical care from the late 1940s. Legislation targeted at alcohol addiction introduced compulsory treatment, *addictology* was established as a prominent medical sub-discipline, and extensive public resources were invested into a number of treatment centres and campaigns. These were spaces where shattered souls like Hrubín could be restored to health in a dignified way.

This chapter examines the generally conservative and repressive context of psychiatric care in Czechoslovakia and complicates this picture with examples of psychiatrists who managed to practise alternative approaches within the system of public healthcare. In this sense, it represents an important complement to Christian Werkmeister's chapter on Soviet treatment in this book (see Chapter 12). It also explores the context within which different approaches to alcoholism emerged, and their theoretical backgrounds, political backing and actual practices. Emphasis is on the assessment of the therapeutic approach followed by Jaroslav Skála and colleagues. It will be argued that these psychiatrists employed particular strategies in order to channel public health resources into the kind of care they considered useful for clients, and which were, in some instances, subversive of the authoritarian Communist system of healthcare as well as Communist governance in general. The treatment of alcohol abuse will also be contextualised as an example of institutionalised expert environments that have recently been described as key to understanding the dynamics of communist rule and its dissolution.[3]

Hitherto research of psychiatry in communist countries has largely focused on the abuse of psychiatry by communist police and judiciary authorities.[4] In contrast, this chapter presents the kinds of professional, intellectual and moral dilemmas medical staff were faced with in an authoritarian context. It directly links the medical with the political history of Czechoslovakia.

Pavlovism and 'active therapy'

As in many other spheres, the treatment of mental illnesses in Czechoslovakia was subject to centralised policies endorsed by the Communist state since its foundation in 1948. The campaign against psychoanalysis was a key aspect of such policy. For example, the removal of the memorial plaque commemorating Sigmund Freud from the house of his birth in the northern Moravian town of Příbor shortly after Communist government was established in Czechoslovakia in 1948 was just one manifestation of the anti-psychoanalysis operations initiated by the Communist authorities.[5] (Ironically, a first such plaque had been destroyed by the Nazis when Příbor became part of Germany in 1938.[6]) This anti-psychiatry campaign forced practitioners and prominent authors of psychoanalysis to either engage in other approaches or to practise illegally.[7] The theoretical basis for building a new 'socialist' psychiatry included Pavlovism, an approach based on I.P. Pavlov's reflex theory. It was based on an understanding of all social relations as external stimuli that created conditioned reflexes in people and influenced their behaviour. Since this approach held that Western psychotherapy individualised social problems, thereby concealing and sustaining their real causes such as economic inequality and class-specific exploitation, communism was believed to have erased these underlying causes. Pavlovism aimed to integrate the theories of physiology, biology, psychiatry, psychology and pedagogy. The earlier pre-communist psychological perspective was replaced with an exclusive focus on 'higher nervous activity'.[8]

Within this guiding framework, the human mind was considered to be part of the biological organism. Any mental-health-related problems were framed as diseases, deviations and disorders. People suffering from mental illnesses were called 'patients' and had a right to treatment. This treatment was required to be scientific and measurable, and was meant to directly address the biological aspect of the mind. Psycho-pharmaceuticals, which had been invented and tested since the mid-twentieth century, were favoured over other treatments. The methods applied were often highly invasive and turned patients into passive objects of 'active therapy'. This was particularly so when treatments were tested on people, and their effects were unknown or not well understood. One example was insulin coma therapy, which was widely applied across the Soviet Union and in other communist nations, as well as in Western and other countries around the globe.[9] The number of active therapies provided in a given psychiatric facility was interpreted as a gauge of its excellence.[10]

Nevertheless, there was more ambiguity and heterogeneity than the general ideological guidelines and the rhetoric of a state-run healthcare service would suggest. This was especially true in the clinical sector, an area to which many resorted from the heavily surveilled sectors of medical education and academic research. Although de-Stalinisation in the Czechoslovak political sphere from the mid-1950s onwards was largely non-existent, this was also the period when psychology and psychiatry adopted, formulated and developed various unorthodox approaches. As Sarah Marks remarked in *Psychiatry in Communist Europe*,

> as medicine was afforded more autonomy than many other fields of intellectual endeavour, a remarkable level of plurality was able to flourish in spite of this even as early as 1957, when the Communist elites were still strongly resisting the tide of destalinisation which was occurring in the Soviet Union and other countries of the Warsaw Pact.[11]

Marks focused on the example of Oldřich Starý's integrative human ecology, which considered the impact of working and urban environments of patients as important factors in the prevention of mental illness. Other examples of approaches that did not follow the official Party line include that of Ferdinand Knobloch and Jiřina Knoblochová, who experimented with group psychotherapy in a number of public facilities (namely the previously private estates that had been nationalised after World War II, such as a farm in Doksany, a country house in Lniště and the Lobeč chateau near Mšeno). They developed so-called 'integrated psychotherapy' for the treatment of neuroses and ran psychotherapy training courses for professionals.[12] Along with many other talented practitioners, the Knoblochs left Czechoslovakia after the military invasion in 1968. Before that, in the 1960s, they introduced 'psycho-gymnastics' at Lobeč, an original mime-based therapy method that was later developed further by the psychoanalytically trained social worker Hana Junová.[13] Other alternative styles of therapy that contested official practices were explored by Eva Syřišťová, who introduced approaches based on mutual understanding and acceptance into treatment, along with respect for client imagination. Syřišťová summarised her understanding of schizophrenia in *The Imaginary World*, a book directed at the wider public.[14] Similarly, Stanislav Kratochvíl developed a community-based method of treatment at the psychiatric hospital in Kroměříž, where he had worked since the late 1950s.[15] Ondrej Kondáš formulated learning theory applications, and Petr Boš practised and taught family therapy at the Children's Psychiatric Hospital in Dubí near Teplice.[16] Clinical practice in institutions was usually accompanied by research, including unconventional experiments, such as those by Milan Hausner, who carried out research on the effects of LSD therapy in the treatment of psychiatric disorders at the clinic at Sadská from the early 1960s to the mid-1970s.[17]

While the focus on 'positive deviations' certainly tends to create a picture that does not fit in with common representations of communist countries as authoritarian and oppressive, the majority of hospitals did follow the official guidelines. Sarah Marks's depiction therefore does not quite reflect the situation in regard to more widely accessible psychiatric treatments. Jaromír Rubeš, the manager of several large psychiatric clinics from the 1950s to 1968 and later one of the founding fathers of the first psychotherapy training programme, described his experience at official psychiatric meetings and committees in his memoirs in 1991:

> These psychiatric gatherings always opened with a statement about how lucky our psychiatry was that it did not subscribe to speculative and unempirical directions, such as psychoanalysis or dynamic psychotherapy. Instead, it remained true to medicine, biology and natural sciences.[18]

Rubeš remarked that he had realised that 'what essentially accounts for "biological" psychiatry, does not, in fact, fall under the heading of psychiatry at all. It should fall under internal medicine or somewhere else, but not psychiatry.'[19]

Rubeš's memoirs also include numerous descriptions of the conditions in psychiatric hospitals, namely a lack of organisation, unethical attitudes to patients, the terror of electroshocks, erratic medication and so forth. For example, when he first entered the Dobřany Psychiatric Hospital near Pilsen as a young psychiatrist and as the new director, he noted 'chaos and nineteenth-century conditions', with patients tied up and an omnipotent rule of 'cliques of nurses and Communist cadres'.[20] Rubeš became famous for having managed to successfully turn this neglected facility into a treatment centre run on the basis of modern concepts. He restructured Dobřany hospital and established specialist departments, as well as one dedicated to internal medicine. Patients with alcohol addictions were placed in a separate building; this was meant to facilitate their detoxification and longer abstention.

From the mid-1950s onwards, psychiatric care in Communist Czechoslovakia was organised in secluded establishments. Despite the obvious flaws of what were, in the context of Western countries, described as impermeable institutions, their closed doors provided at the same time an opportunity for several leading open-minded psychiatrists to practise a surprising variety of approaches and methods. Nevertheless, as in Western countries, the closed-door system meant that patients were isolated from the outside world and rarely had a chance to influence their own treatment, and the segregation of patients from wider society encouraged the tabooisation of psychiatric conditions. Notwithstanding some notable exceptions, in the majority of state-run institutions the treatment prescribed by medical specialists was subject to political and ideological intrusion.

Alcohol abuse in a communist state

The approach to alcohol consumption and addiction adopted by the Czechoslovak Communist government contained a fundamental contradiction. It was argued that alcoholism was an issue inherent to capitalism and caused by its exploitative nature. At the same time heavy alcohol consumption was a common phenomenon not only among the former bourgeois elites and the Party leadership but also among the working class – a social group on which the rhetoric of the state relied for its legitimacy. When the psychiatrist Skála published the first book specialising on alcoholism in Communist Czechoslovakia in 1957, he concluded:

> Although in Czechoslovakia many of the economic causes (fear of unemployment, destitution, old age) which lead to alcoholism in capitalist countries have been eliminated, it cannot be said that the problem of alcoholism has thereby been solved.[21]

Although the government introduced extensive legislation, starting with the Law on Elimination of Alcoholism of 1948,[22] the consumption of alcoholic beverages kept rising dramatically throughout the Communist era: from 2.9 litres of pure alcohol per capita in 1949 to 9.2 litres in 1984.[23] To conceal the contradiction, cultural aspects of drinking and the fact that it was part of local tradition were downplayed, while the economic effects on collective prosperity were emphasised. Skála argued that alcohol consumption 'particularly stains a socialist society where one relies on the productive contribution of individuals and where reduced work performance or loss of work on the part of any citizen involved in the productive process must be made up by others'.[24] Furthermore, in Skála's view, alcohol consumption was responsible for the rising rates of crime, car accidents, divorce and other social problems, and hence it had to be combated.

Official discourse was hesitant to accept any cultural or sociological interpretations of the increased rate of alcohol consumption. Even as late as the period of *perestroika* (political and economic restructuring) in the late 1980s, the Slovak sociologist Martin Bútora struggled to have his book *It Can Never Happen to Me: On the Sociology of Alcoholism* published.[25] It summarised his professional experience, which he had acquired in counselling centres for alcohol addictions. Bútora offered a sociological interpretation and pointed out regional differences in the pattern of alcohol abuse, namely the high rates of alcohol addiction in Slovakia in contrast to the Czech region. As the book touched on a number of communist taboos, the authorities repeatedly rejected and delayed its publication.

It could be argued that the continued medicalisation of overconsumption of alcohol across the globe after World War II provided a convenient rationale for communist states because alcoholism became projected as an issue that had to be addressed medically rather than as a problem woven into the social fabric of a state. The framing of alcoholism as a disorder that required medical rather than social treatment and intervention was not new in post-war Czechoslovakia, for experiments with apomorphine therapy had been undertaken from the mid-1920s.[26] Apomorphine induced vomiting and other side-effects among some patients if taken together with alcohol. Although clinics practising this treatment were closed down by the Nazis in 1939, a similar type of treatment was re-introduced in Prague in 1947 and involved thousands of patients.[27] From the outset it was connected with Jaroslav Skála.

Skála's innovations and the role of the Apolinář

When Skála joined the psychiatric clinic of Prague University Hospital as a young psychiatrist in the late 1940s, his first contact with alcoholics was during experiments with emetine in the so-called *blinkačky* (vomit) cycles. Injecting the substance and allowing the client to consume alcohol created a psychological connection between the nausea and vomiting triggered by emetine and drinking. The therapy perfectly fitted the Pavlovian orthodoxy, as it built aversive reflex to alcohol: its smell and taste. In 1950 Antabuse therapy was introduced. Its major advantage was that the medication could be administered in the form of pills.[28] And yet when Skála had the first ever substantial monograph, *Alkoholismus* (Alcoholism), published by the State Healthcare Publishing House in 1957, he presented a much more complex picture. The foreword (quoted at the beginning of this chapter) was written by one of his patients, the well-known poet František Hrubín, who publicly revealed his own alcohol problem therein. What is more, the book proposed a system of treatment that evidently involved psychotherapy and the role of a therapeutic community. Neither psychotherapy nor therapeutic communities were meant to exist in public institutions, as they contradicted the state's healthcare ideology. Skála explained his shift away from the pure pharmacotherapy of addictions he was expected to perform at the clinic: 'I felt there was something missing in what I was doing.'[29]

Although state policy suggested that alcoholism was a medical, physiological problem, in reality many classical psychiatrists tended to rely on psychotherapy-oriented approaches in their practical work with alcoholics. Commenting on his career in the above-mentioned 'nineteenth-century-style' Dobřany hospital, Jaromír Rubeš said: 'I didn't have a clue about psychotherapy then, yet the place made me realise the extent of the issue of alcohol. When emetine therapy appeared, I immediately had the feeling that the problem was too complicated to be simply cured by emetine.'[30] Václav Hyrman, a follower of Ferdinand Knobloch's integrated psychotherapy, worked in the alcohol clinic in the North Bohemian city of Liberec until 1968 before he left for Canada. He recalled his first years in Liberec: 'Indoctrination and triggering the vomit reflexes to alcohol were the main treatments at the time. Yet psychotherapy and organised work could prove far more effective.'[31]

As early as 1948, Jaroslav Skála was promoted to head of the Alcoholism Treatment Centre in a detached building within the hospital compound. A building next to St Apollinaris Church, the so-called Apolinář, became home to a new system of alcoholism treatment and to Jaroslav Skála. The system of treatment he introduced to the centre combined the previous approaches of detailed medical examination, regular checks and pharmacotherapy with a characteristic strict 'regime' and a number of highly progressive psychotherapeutic methods.[32] Under the regime schedule, every hour of the day, starting at 5.45 a.m. and ending at 10 p.m., was used for an activity, be it therapy, exercise, work, jogging, relaxation, reading newspapers, cleaning, writing progress reports or walking in the garden. The treatment was the same for everyone, and patients had no say in it. Points were assigned or deducted on a behaviour chart that mapped patients' efforts. In popular understanding, Skála – whose name means 'rock' in Czech – became a synonym for a kind of boot-camp discipline and asceticism.

At the same time, the strict regime was complemented by a wide range of psychotherapeutic methods, including group therapy, diary keeping and reflections on the previous week in open discussions as well as art therapy, composition of motivational songs and theatre plays. There were lectures for the patients ('didactotherapy') and two-week sports camps in the countryside. Skála did not leave the Apolinář centre, where he lived in a small studio in the same building. In fact, he joined in all the patients' activities. This led him to the idea that only abstainers can help alcoholics overcome addiction, and that therapists should share the treatment process with their patients. This was a revolutionary idea in the paternalistic medical and educational system that was characteristic of the country. Success rates were impressive, with 60 per cent of patients remaining abstinent for at least one year after treatment.[33]

In Skála's view, leaving the programme after a successful four-month treatment in hospital was only the beginning of a possible long abstention. He set up a follow-up club for abstinent ex-patients at the Apolinář, where they benefited from a supportive peer community as well as expert advice.[34]

Skála managed to acquire a number of other state-owned buildings, mostly rural estates, which the Communist government had repossessed from nobility and religious orders after the Communist coup in 1948. For example, a new alcoholism treatment facility was set up at the Chateau Lojovice in 1958.[35] In 1971 Skála founded here the first department for women alcoholics and a rehabilitation centre for patients who had completed their programme at the Apolinář. Staff even invited the relatives of alcoholics to stay on the premises, and experimented with including patients, their partners and their children in the therapeutic process.[36] In a sports and recreation centre in Dobronice, South Bohemia, the Apolinář organised a summer camp each year, in which previous patients were joined by therapists from other facilities to experience the unusual mix of clients and staff and learn from the core team.

The original Apolinář programme became the blueprint for alcohol treatment departments set up at most psychiatric hospitals. Riesel suggests that contemporary authors who wrote about alcoholism treatment considered Skála's system to be the foundational model for inpatient treatment in Czechoslovakia.[37] Self-help publications and instruction booklets for teachers, healthcare staff and social workers, which were published by local administrations (the so-called National Committees), also relied on Skála's system.[38]

Skála's system also had a wider impact on the public administration of provision for alcoholics. A procedure for locating alcohol addicts within the population had been set up by the Law on Elimination of Alcoholism in 1948 and further developed by the Law on the Fight against Alcoholism in 1962.[39] Both laws required police or local National Committees to refer addicts they had identified or were informed about to local anti-alcohol counselling centres or, in the case of more serious 'anti-social behaviour', to compulsory inpatient treatment facilities. A network of specialised counselling and advice centres emerged from the 1950s and by the late 1970s reached about 200, in which over 130,000 patients had been officially registered.[40]

Jaroslav Skála provided the impetus for another innovation in the public system, a development that was subsequently established worldwide. These were the renowned detoxification units or medically supervised sobering-up cells. They were called *protialkoholní záchytné stanice* (anti-alcohol detention stations) in Czech and were designed for people in a state of acute alcohol intoxication who needed to be hospitalised compulsorily for their own protection or that of the people surrounding them. The first unit with twelve beds was set up at the Apolinář in Prague in 1951, and seventeen more detoxification facilities were established in various parts of the country by 1955. Over fifty remained in place by the 1980s.[41] Patients were required to stay for at least eight hours and were forced to pay a fee for the time spent in the centre, and their local anti-alcohol advice bureau had to be informed.[42] As the leading Czech psychiatrist J. Dobiáš pointed out in 1986, after its foundation, the network of detoxification centres became an inspiration for many other countries.[43]

A cradle of psychotherapy

Last but not least, the Apolinář also became a semi-official centre for the dissemination of ideas on addiction treatment, psychiatry and medicine in general. Skála obtained permission to use the Prague Faculty Hospital's cyclostyle printer to produce a number of semi-*samizdat* publications under the hospital's auspices.[44] *Zápisy z Apolináře* (Apollinaris Records) was launched in 1951, and its several annual issues included working material to be used by patients and therapists alike: excerpts from patients' diaries, discussion minutes, short stories and poems, historical overviews, but also Skála's reports and impressions about conference visits abroad and translations of short texts by foreign specialists.[45] From 1979, the more academically and clinically focused *Psychoterapeutické sešity* (Psychotherapeutic Dossiers) were produced under the auspices of the Prague Faculty Hospital's psychiatric clinic.[46] They mostly offered translations of noteworthy international texts on psychotherapy, which could not be published officially at the time; this issue will be explored further in the final section of this chapter.

A Friday seminar series at the Apolinář was originally designed for healthcare professionals who worked at other institutions. The seminars were characterised by an open-minded and politically liberal atmosphere, and became an attraction for intellectuals from various backgrounds. In the mid-2010s, Jitka Vodňanská, a psychologist working in Skála's team at the Apolinář, recollected that she invited her husband-to-be, the musician Jan Vodňanský, to one of the seminars in 1974. The psychologist Ivan Douda, who later specialised in non-alcoholic addictions, gave a lecture on Arthur Janov's *The Primal Scream*, which had been inaccessible at the time in Czechoslovakia.

> Jan was sitting there with other strangers interested in the material. Skála was simply great in this respect. Anything was possible. Unrestrained freedom. Artists came to the academic hospital to listen. Václav [Havel, playwright, dissident, founder of Charter 77 and President from 1989 to 1992] also used to come. Today, in a free country, something like this would be unthinkable. They would not pass through the reception, because of not carrying the right passkey.[47]

All of these activities are key to the Czech context for a simple reason. Psychotherapy as an institutionalised autonomous discipline did not officially exist. In psychiatry, it was accepted as 'one of the techniques' that could be applied to patients. Yet the official discourse always considered it only a supplementary method – an accessory to more invasive biological treatment. Moreover, psychiatrists and psychologists were expected to somehow acquire the technique on their own initiative, since no training was provided within the medicine and psychology syllabuses. Skála's alcoholism treatment model and his training and outreach initiatives at the Apolinář became the cradle of psychotherapy in Czechoslovakia.

Without systematic psychotherapeutic training and supervision well into the 1980s, Skála and his two colleagues – the psychologist Eduard Urban and the aforementioned Jaromír Rubeš – decided to establish a semi-formal scheme of psychotherapy training courses:

the so-called SUR, an acronym created from the first letters of the founders' surnames. It started in 1969, after Skála had returned from the 1967 Lindauer Psychotherapiewoche (Lindau Psychotherapy Week) in West Germany, an annual event of workshops and lectures on the latest approaches in the field. He organised a similar event for doctors and social workers in Czechoslovakia, initiating a four-year training course. SUR remained unofficial and unsubsidised; nonetheless, the courses and meetings moved between state-run psychiatric facilities. In his own words, Skála 'offered his institutions at Lojovice, Červený Dvůr and Dobronice as venues'.[48] The training combined educational lectures on psychotherapy with practical group therapy sessions based on self-experience. The small groups, each led by its own therapist, provided a space in which individuals exchanged difficult-to-access literature with others and experienced a special atmosphere of trust, or even conspiracy. The combination of small-group therapy and reflection on this experience within a larger community was admired even among Western colleagues.[49] The lack of commercial interest and of business-oriented efficiency, typical of a communist economy, contributed to a setting in which the trainees could profit from enhanced educational opportunities as well as being allowed enough time for their slow personal growth and continuing professional development at no cost – something a democratic state based on a competitive market economy could hardly offer.

SUR was an extraordinary undertaking, especially during the two decades following the Prague Spring in 1968, when the Soviet Union suppressed reforms with the invasion of Czechoslovakia by 600,000 Warsaw Pact troops. According to Antonín Šimek, SUR trained over two thousand very loyal and devoted graduates, who became the main source of the belated psychotherapeutic boom in the 1990s.[50] Participants remembered the training as 'a veil under which you could meet and talk freely, engage in uncensored discussions'.[51] Šimek suggests that official academic publications mentioned the training only reluctantly in the late 1980s in order to downplay any semblance of a potential political threat.[52] In an interview in 2000, Skála contrasted the SUR circle with the psychoanalysts, who, he contended, 'were holed up, all scared, while we weren't'.[53] He used controversial rhetoric in relation to the 1970s and 1980s. While these decades were referred to as the period of

'Normalisation' by the Communist Party, they were characterised by political purges and intellectual oppression. Skála noted in 2001 that he and his colleagues 'did not really mind the Normalisation. On the contrary, we were able to benefit from it, I suppose.'[54] Skála's initiatives attracted many talented people from the medical and care professions precisely because, after the military invasion put an end to the Prague Spring of 1968, they were disillusioned with the prospect of unreformed state socialism and some were even unable to work in their chosen professional field.

The politics behind expert success

The success of an idea and of a professional career usually comes with a degree of power. This particularly applies to a discipline such as the treatment of alcoholism, where success is often dependent on conformity with prevailing social and political agendas, and hence backing from the powers that be is often required. The need for acquiescence to political requirements was much stronger, if not crucial, in the case of communist dictatorships in Eastern and Central Europe.[55] Therefore historical examination of the innovative niches within an otherwise blinkered Czechoslovak psychiatry requires an excursion into the country's political history. Public archives and the official press do not contain any first-hand records that could offer a direct insight into what was essentially to remain concealed. Research is therefore limited to other sources, such as academic journals and reports drawn up by the State Security, as well as memoirs and other, largely unreliable, material. Even if their interpretation is inevitably often intuitive, these sources are indispensable in any attempt to present the full picture.

Official academic journals, which were controlled centrally, offer the most immediate tool with which to approach the theme. *Československá psychiatrie* (Czechoslovak Psychiatry) and *Československá psychologie* (Czechoslovak Psychology) were the most respected, albeit carefully censored, journals of the two disciplines. Occasionally, they published articles that contained carefully worded and tactical references to unorthodox approaches and procedures common in Western countries. At the same time, they fully conformed to the requirement to publish contributions celebrating such anniversaries as 'the triumphant February 1948' (the date of the Communist coup in Czechoslovakia) or 'Thirty years of socialist psychiatry'.[56] Many of the authors were even prepared to celebrate the prevailing isolation of and restrictions in psychiatry as welcome measures. Such obsequiousness may have been intended to earn a permit to travel to congresses abroad. The psychiatrist Petr Příhoda tellingly commented on colleagues who managed to go abroad: 'They had to be such ace experts, or such bastards.'[57] Jaroslav Skála, too, was accomplished in balancing routine political tributes and elaborate challenges of the authorities. In his publications, he usually added a few paragraphs in each chapter about how a given method or tool was practised – successfully – in the Soviet Union.[58] In addition to the multitude of ground-breaking innovations in the treatment of alcoholism, his authority helped raise self-confidence among his colleagues vis-à-vis the Communist government. When the petition *Několik vět* (A Few Sentences) was circulated and signed at the Apolinář in 1989, Skála refused to report the petitioners.[59]

The balancing of kowtowing and resistance was a tool that people in Communist Czechoslovakia widely exploited in order to arrange or secure whatever they were striving for, be it a travel permit, scarce goods or officially unavailable services. People assumed different identities depending on the requirements of the context. The identities they adopted were manifold and intricately interwoven, with plural loyalties. Skála and his colleagues frequently utilised public resources, buildings, material and staff for professional and social, albeit non-official, purposes. A liberal-minded therapist might be a member of the Communist Party, participate in the management of a large healthcare facility and serve on an editorial board of an academic journal in order to protect other spheres of her or his professional activity.

This sophisticated exploitation of the complex combination of multiple and fluid identities and loyalties enabled leading psychiatrists to maximise the political chances of their professional survival, to secure funding for their projects and to shape their specialist fields, as was the case in the treatment of alcoholism. The experienced hospital manager Jaromír Rubeš once described the careful preparations for the first psychiatric congress in Czechoslovakia, which was planned to include international participants. It was held in the mid-1950s in Jeseník, a remote northern Moravian spa town. Rubeš, as the head of the psychiatric ward, invited an official who was responsible for authorising the event. In the evening, he plied his guest with drinks until he was completely inebriated and the next day obligingly arranged the necessary massage and wellness procedures. The congress was duly authorised once the official had recovered from his hangover.[60] Such strategies may also have been at play in regard to the acquisition of badly needed treatment premises or recreation facilities for anti-addiction projects.

Specialists such as Rubeš and Skála were able to channel substantial public resources to finance projects that steered clear of official control and offered innovative approaches to treatment. The medical and counselling institutions also provided a cover for people and for semi-official activities, such as the production of semi-*samizdat* publications. Institutions related to psychiatry served as shelters for reform-minded specialists who had openly endorsed the Prague Spring reforms. During the post-1968 political purges in the public sector, these professionals found it virtually impossible to find highly qualified jobs elsewhere. In the 1970s, the state built a vast network of counselling centres. Once expelled from the university in Brno, leading clinical psychologists and psychiatrists such as Stanislav Kratochvíl found refuge in these centres.[61] Those involved in the treatment of addictions describe their field as yet another realm where the scrutiny of political loyalty was much less consistent than in academia and in the education sector.[62]

The preserved secret service files kept on some of the alcohol therapists indicate merely cursory interest on the part of the Communist regime in their creative projects and innovative activities. The files show that the State Security was almost solely concerned about contacts with former Prague Spring activists, Western nationals and emigrants, and about international travels to conferences, hiring new staff in hospitals and possible intakes of patients – individuals seeking refuge from police persecution. There seems to be no trace of attempts by State Security to infiltrate the SUR weekend courses or the alcoholics' summer camps in different facilities.[63] Yet one can only offer a hypothesis drawing from the preserved fragments of files, as their current state prevents a more comprehensive analysis.[64]

The patchy and inconsistent interest coming from the security apparatus is even more surprising given that Skála's innovative approach to the treatment of alcoholism was based on both strict regimes and self-experience therapy, and implicitly challenged some of the key hierarchies of Communist dictatorship. A system of treatment where space and time were shared by medical personnel, patients and even their relatives greatly undermined the doctor–patient hierarchy and domination by specialists. Skála and his colleagues described their method as intuitive learning from experience.[65] Although there is no evidence to show that they were supportive of the Western anti-psychiatry movement, their approach was implicitly subversive of the Communist system in general. Despite the ubiquitous equality rhetoric, social hierarchies prevailed widely, including those between specialist disciplines, and between experts and their patients.[66]

Conclusion

Jaroslav Skála was a central figure within the field of psychiatry who pioneered ground-breaking treatment of alcoholism. Despite finding himself in an ideologically conservative arena, he eagerly explored unconventional ideas from the start of his career. He succeeded in integrating non-Pavlovian and non-biological approaches into the officially endorsed system of alcoholism treatment. Skála led a number of addiction treatment facilities and introduced detoxification units. The long-term treatment that he introduced at the Apolinář rapidly spread to other psychiatric hospitals in Czechoslovakia. He and his colleagues reflected on their work in semi-official publications. They established a formal, though unofficial, system of psychotherapy training courses at a time when psychotherapeutic training and practice were non-existent.

Reflection on how Skála and his colleagues balanced the compulsory Communist rhetoric with medical reasoning, and on how they engaged in political bargaining using the charismatic if not authoritarian leadership style of Skála, offers insights into daily life and medical practice under Communist rule. Their methods and approaches emerged through a combination of transfer of Western ideas and expertise, independent local reflection and internal debates. In some cases, local innovations were even of interest to Western experts.

The psychiatrists dedicated to the treatment of alcoholism were no direct stakeholders of power in state socialism. Despite this, they were able to profit amply from the state resources. However, this eventually became their weak spot. After the collapse of Communism in 1989, psychiatry and psychotherapy experienced a boom in private training and counselling. Nonetheless, some of the founding fathers of the treatment of alcoholism and of Czechoslovak psychotherapy never quite accepted the principle of fee-based psychotherapy treatment.[67] They were hardly able to conceal their disillusion. Skála, who had once admitted that his circle had benefited from the politically depressing decades of the 1970s and 1980s, was much more modest in the mid-1990s: 'We can only hope that the women's anti-addiction facility at the Chateau Lojovice survives the restitution of assets.'[68] The chateau now serves as a private stud farm. A number of other progressive facilities which had been founded under, or in spite of, the Communist state met similar fates or were closed down.

Notes

The author works at the Institute of Contemporary History of the Czech Academy of Sciences. The text was created with support for the long-term conceptual development of the research organisation, RVO no. 68378114.

1 F. Hrubín, foreword to J. Skála, *Alkoholismus: terminologie, diagnostika, léčba a prevence* [Alcoholism: Terminology, Diagnostics, Treatment and Prevention] (Prague: Státní zdravotnické nakladatelství, 1957), 7. All translations of Czech quotations are by the author.

2 Ibid., 8.

3 M. Kopeček (ed.), *Architekti dlouhé změny. Expertní kořeny postsocialismu v Československu* [The Architects of Long Change: The Expert Roots of Post-Socialism in Czechoslovakia] (Prague: Argo, 2019).

4 For the case of Czechoslovakia, see e.g. J. Tesař, *Zamlčená diagnóza* [Concealed Diagnosis] (Prague: Triáda, 2003); M. Kordíková, *Augustin Navrátil a jeho disidentská činnost* [Augustin Navrátil and his Dissident Activities] (Prague: FF UK, 2012), 38–64, 103–25, 139–62; V. Borecký, 'Psychoanalýza v ilegalitě: osudy Freudova učení v českých zemích' [Psychoanalysis going underground: the story of Freud's teachings in the Czech lands], *Dějiny a současnost* [*History and the Present*], 28, no. 4 (2006), 34–6.

5 Borecký, 'Psychoanalýza v ilegalitě', 34–6.

6 Ibid.

7 M. Mahler (ed.), *Psychoanalýza v Čechách* [Psychoanalysis in the Czech Lands] (Prague: Nakladatelství France Kafky, 1997).

8 J. Hoskovec and S. Hoskovcová, *Malé dějiny české a středoevropské psychologie* [Short History of Czech and Central European Psychology] (Prague: Portál, 2000), 24–5.

9 B. Zajicek, 'Insulin coma therapy and the construction of therapeutic effectiveness in Stalin's Soviet Union, 1936–1953', in M. Savelli and S. Marks (eds), *Psychiatry in Communist Europe* (Basingstoke: Palgrave Macmillan, 2015), 50–72.

10 Ibid., 55–6.

11 S. Marks, 'Ecology, humanism and mental health in Communist Czechoslovakia', in Savelli and Marks (eds), *Psychiatry in Communist Europe*, 134–52, at 135.

12 F. Knobloch and J. Knobloch, *Integrated Psychotherapy* (New York: Jason Aronson, 1979).

13 J. Hučín, *Hovory o psychoterapii. Péče o duši současného člověka* [Talks on Psychotherapy: Caring for the Soul of Contemporary Man] (Prague: Portál 2001), 50–73.

14 E. Syřišťová, *Imaginární svět* [The Imaginary World] (Prague: Mladá fronta, 1974).

15 J. Pavlov Praško, 'Stanislav Kratochvíl osmdesátiletý' [Stanislav Kratochvíl turns eighty], *Česká a slovenská psychiatrie* [Czech and Slovak Psychiatry], 108, no. 3 (2012), 149–51.

16 I. Veltrubská, 'Můj strom rodinné terapie' [My family therapy tree], www.ivavel.cz/texty/Muj_strom_rodinne_terapie.pdf (accessed 26 January 2021).

17 M. Hausner and E. Segal, *LSD: výzkum a klinická praxe za železnou oponou* [LSD: Research and Clinical Practice behind the Iron Curtain] (Prague: Triton, 2016). The project has recently been commemorated in the Czech Republic with some reservations among psychiatrists, yet also with a degree of nostalgia in the case of the participants in the

experiment. A number of artists and intellectuals who were among the volunteers used the research as an opportunity to access LSD. See, e.g., the documentary *LSD Made in ČSSR* (dir. P. Křemen, 2015).

18 J. Rubeš, 'Co se Vám tady bude zdát divný (První část vzpomínek, úvah, názorů a vyprávění)' [What you'll find kind of strange (recollections, reflections, views and tales], *Konfrontace* [Confrontation], 2, no. 4 (1991), 6–12, at 6–7. The memoirs were recorded in 1991.

19 Ibid., 7.

20 Cited in Z. Kovaříková, 'Říkalo se o mně, že umím vládnout. Rozhovor s Jaromírem Rubešem' [I was said to be a good commander: an interview with Jaromír Rubeš], *Psychoterapeutické sešity* [Psychotherapeutic Dossiers], 1, no. 1 (2000), 16–20, at 16.

21 Skála, *Alkoholismus*, 209.

22 Act no. 87/1948, Coll.

23 Committee report on draft Act on the Protection against Alcoholism and Other Drug Addictions of 1989, in *Společná česko–slovenská digitální parlamentní knihovna* [Common Digital Czecho–Slovak Parliamentary Library], Česká národní rada 1986–1990, Tisky, Print no. 101, www.psp.cz/eknih/1986cnr/tisky/t0101_00.htm (accessed 18 February 2022).

24 Skála, *Alkoholismus*, 209.

25 M. Bútora, *Mne sa to nemôže stať. Sociologické kapitoly z alkoholizmu* [It Can Never Happen to Me: On the Sociology of Alcoholism] (Martin: Osveta, 1989).

26 Skála, *Alkoholismus*, 100.

27 Ibid., 100–4; J. Dobiáš, '70 let doc. Skály' [Seventy years of Professor Skála], *Československá psychiatrie* [Czechoslovak Psychiatry], 82, no. 6 (1986), 420–1. Cf. J. Skála, *Lékařův maraton: ber a dávej* [Doctor's Marathon: Give and Take] (Prague: Český spisovatel, 1998), 183–4.

28 See also Christian Werkmeister's reference to the use of this therapy in parts of the Soviet Union (Chapter 12 in this volume).

29 Skála, *Lékařův maraton*, 43.

30 Kovaříková, 'Říkalo se o mně', 17.

31 V. Hyrman, 'Úvod', in F. Knobloch and J. Knoblochová, *Integrovaná psychoterapie v akci* [Integrated Psychotherapy in Action] (Prague: Grada, 1999), 11.

32 The details in this paragraph are based on Skála, *Lékařův maraton*, 161–9. Cf. 'Náplň léčebného režimu u Apolináře' [Programme of the therapeutic regime at the Apolinář] in Skála, *Alkoholismus*, 214–15.

33 K. Plaček, *Alkoholismus a jeho prevence. Příručka pro cyklickou průpravu vedoucích pracovníků 4. okruhu funkcí* [Alcohol Abuse and its Prevention: A Handbook for Preparation of Senior Staff at

the Czechoslovak Ministry of Industry] (Prague: Institut pro výchovu vedoucích pracovníků min. průmyslu ČSR, 1977), 26.

34 Skála, *Lékařův maraton*, 161–3. In contrast to the 'Hudolin clubs' in Yugoslavia, described by Mat Savelli (see Chapter 10 in this volume), Skála himself founded and headed the large association based at the Apolinář.

35 Skála, *Lékařův maraton*, 54–8.

36 This approach was very different from the alcoholics' self-help groups and networks that had spread in many other countries, including Japan. See Akira Hashimoto's account in Chapter 9 of this volume.

37 See e.g. P. Riesel, *Alkoholismus a jeho problematika na okrese Chomutov v letech 1961–68. Autoreferát dizertace k získání hodnosti kandidáta lékařských věd* [Alcohol Abuse and its Phenomenon in the District of Chomutov in 1961–68: Report on Dissertation by the Medical Sciences Candidate] (Vlašim: n.pub, 1990).

38 See e.g. I. Mandlová and J. Viewegh, *Jak mu pomoci? Pokyny a rady pro manželky a rodinné příslušníky alkoholika* [How to Help Him? Instructions and Advice for Wives and Relatives of an Alcohol Addict] (Prostějov: ONV, 1973); Plaček, *Alkoholismus a jeho prevence.*

39 Act no. 120/1962, Coll.

40 Plaček, *Alkoholismus a jeho prevence*, 24.

41 Ibid., 29.

42 Skála, *Alkoholismus*, 98.

43 Dobiáš, '70 let doc. Skály', 420–1.

44 The first issue of *Zápisy z Apolináře* was printed as *Člověk & alkohol: alkoholismus a protialkoholní boj* [The Man and Alcohol: Alcoholism and the Fight against It] (Prague: Protialkoholní oddělení Státní psych. kliniky prof. Myslivečka, 1951).

45 Vols 1–39 of *Zápisy z Apolináře: léčebná pomůcka* were published between 1951 and 1989. The number of cyclostyled copies reached 1,500 in the 1980s.

46 Issues 1–54 of *Psychoterapeutické sešity* were put together between 1979 and 1992.

47 J. Vodňanská, *Voda, která hoří* [Water that Burns] (Prague: Torst, 2018), 111.

48 Hučín, *Hovory o psychoterapii*, 41.

49 Hoskovec and Hoskovcová, *Malé dějiny české a středoevropské psychologie.*

50 A. Šimek, 'Tři rozhovory se zakladateli SURu' [Three interviews with the founders of SUR], *Psychoterapeutické sešity* [Psychotherapeutic Dossiers], 1, no. 1 (2000), 4–5.

51 Ibid.
52 Dobiáš, '70 let doc. Skály', 420.
53 Z. Kovaříková, 'Zkušenosti mají větší cenu než půl milionu: Rozhovor s Jaroslavem Skálou' [The experience is worth more than half a million: an interview with Jaroslav Skála], *Psychoterapeutické sešity* [Psychotherapeutic Dossiers], 1, no. 1 (2000), 6–9.
54 Hučín, *Hovory o psychoterapii*, 43.
55 Cf. Kopeček (ed.), *Architekti dlouhé změny*. This recent publication explores different specialist fields in Czechoslovakia between the 1960s and 1990s; it is a dynamic portrait of specialist contexts, including various aspects of continuity between socialism and post-1989 developments.
56 See e.g. M. Zapletálek, '30. výročí Února' [The thirtieth anniversary of February 1948], *Československá psychiatrie* [Czechoslovak Psychiatry], 74, no. 1 (1978), 1–2; 'Lékaři proti jaderné válce' [Physicians against nuclear war], *Československá psychiatrie*, 78, no. 1 (1982), 1; L. Dobiášová, 'Psychiatrie v 7. pětiletce' [Psychiatry in the seventh five-year plan], *Československá psychiatrie*, 79, no. 1 (1983), 1–2; M. Kodým and M. Langová, 'Čtyřicet let úsilí za angažovanou československou psychologii' [Forty years of striving for a committed Czechoslovak psychology], *Československá psychologie*, 29, no. 2 (1985), 105–10.
57 Quoted in Skála, *Lékařův maraton*, 95.
58 Skála, *Alkoholismus*, 20, 100.
59 Vodňanská, *Voda, která hoří*, 362. The petition requested the release of political prisoners and democratic reforms, but unlike earlier, isolated appeals, this one was signed by as many as 40,000 people, including a number of well-known actors and pop singers.
60 Kovaříková, 'Říkalo se o mně', 18. Similarly, although without drinking, Jaroslav Skála enjoyed telling adventurous stories about receiving travel permits for his conference trips; see e.g. Skála, *Lékařův maraton*, 94–100.
61 T. Novák and P. Šmolka, *Manželské a rodinné poradenství* [Marriage and Family Counselling] (Prague: Grada Publishing, 2016), 17.
62 Vodňanská, *Voda, která hoří*, 397–411.
63 Prague, Archiv bezpečnostních složek [Security Services Archive], coll. Svazky tajných spolupracovníků [Secret collaborators' files], TS–MV, arch. no. 601607 [Jaromír Rubeš]; ibid., coll. KR–MV, arch. no. 632686 [John Reeves].
64 For example, archival material refers to a prominent psychiatrist in a file kept on another individual on the basis that the former reportedly

boasted at a party about being in contact with the emigré psychiatrist Stanislav Grof in the USA. However, the file that evidenced possible collaboration of that person was destroyed by the State Security before 1989. Archiv bezpečnostních složek, coll. Object files, OBŽ–UL, reg. no. 378.

65 Skála, *Lékařův maraton*, 54; J. Růžička, 'Tři rozhovory: Skála, Urban, Rubeš' [Three interviews: Skála, Urban, Rubeš], *Psychoterapeutické sešity* [Psychotherapeutic Dossiers], 1, no. 1 (2000), 1–2.

66 For detailed analysis of this phenomenon see A. Gjuričová, 'Bohatství pod neviditelným pláštěm? K psychoterapii v Československu po roce 1968' [Wealth under an invisible cloak? On psychotherapy in Czechoslovakia after 1968], *Soudobé dějiny* [*Czech Journal of Contemporary History*], 25, no. 3 (2017), 311–34.

67 Kovaříková, 'Zkušenosti mají větší cenu', 9; Hučín, *Hovory o psychoterapii*, 57, 116.

68 Skála, *Lékařův maraton*, 58.

12

'A society that is sinking ever deeper into a state of chronic alcohol poisoning': medical and moral treatment of alcoholics in the Soviet Union, *c.* 1970–1991

Christian Werkmeister

This chapter evaluates the Soviet approach to the treatment of alcoholism during the last two Soviet decades. It will be shown how the particularities of Russian and Soviet drinking habits were tackled by propagandists, psychiatrists and the police, especially in the newly established field of narcology. 'Narcology', a term coined in the Soviet Union in the 1960s, refers to a branch of psychiatry that specialises in the study and treatment of drug and alcohol abuse. Comprehensive in approach, narcological treatments incorporated numerous societal actors, such as healthcare professionals, security personnel, employers, and families and friends of alcoholics. The punitive potential of such treatments was underlined by the deprecation of alcoholism, and the subsequent stigmatisation of alcoholics, in the Soviet context. Soviet treatments for alcoholism held the power to permanently exclude individuals from Soviet society, while simultaneously ensuring the exploitation of their cheap labour in the so-called 'labour treatment centres' or 'labour treatment prophilactoria' (LTPs).[1]

On both sides of the Iron Curtain much has been written by academics and in popular media on Soviet and Russian drinking.[2] It is therefore generally known that the late Soviet years witnessed a well-documented surge in alcohol consumption. 'Between 1960 and 1979 alone, alcohol sales nearly quadrupled [with] disposable household income spent on alcohol reaching 15–20%.'[3] In 1982 the USSR ranked among the top four alcohol-consuming countries in the world.[4] In the Soviet case eight of the total of fourteen litres of alcohol consumed per person annually were 'distilled spirits 80-proof and higher'.[5] However, alcohol consumption patterns varied, depending on local cultural traditions, and some regions, especially the Muslim republics (such as Tadzhikistan, Turkmenistan and Uzbekistan), were notably less open to drinking. The Baltic republics and the Slavic Soviet states, like Russia, Ukraine and Belarus, on the other hand, consumed twice as much alcohol per capita.[6] This chapter focuses on the Slavic republics, where problems related to alcohol consumption proved to be the most common and severe.

As Sandra Anderson has shown, the sale of alcohol substantially subsidised the Soviet economy: 'By 1985, the taxes on alcohol amounted to about 40 percent of all direct and indirect taxes paid by Soviet citizens and about 13 percent of the state's entire budget receipts.'[7] This illustrates the traditional importance of alcohol for the national economy and the heavy dependence of the Soviet system upon its people's continued alcohol consumption, a tradition that is documented as far back as the late fifteenth century.[8] The consequences of this tradition for heavy drinkers, their families and for society itself proved to be grave.

Daniel Tarschys has calculated the total annual death toll due to alcohol abuse during the late 1970s as ranging from 370,000 to 400,000.[9] It was not only people dying from alcohol-related conditions that aroused official concern; because of heavy drinking, fewer children were being born, and infant mortality had increased significantly, with rising numbers of female alcoholics in the two final Soviet decades.[10] These concerns were reflected in the continuously rising average amount of liquor, beer and wine consumed by the Soviet population.[11] What is more, everyday life was severely affected by excessive alcohol consumption. The Ministry of Internal Affairs complained from the 1970s onwards that absenteeism, poor work performance, accidents, violent crimes and vandalism were often caused by workplace intoxication.[12] In total, harm related to alcohol abuse cost the state an estimated 10 per cent of the national income.[13] It was not only economists and government officials who were alarmed. The general public were well aware of the dangers of heavy drinking, and media reports openly addressed the issue. In 1972 the future Nobel Peace Prize laureate Andreĭ Sakharov (1921–1989) wrote a concerned letter to Leonid Brezhnev (1906–1982): 'Drunkenness has assumed the dimensions of a national calamity. It is one of the symptoms of the moral degradation of a society that is sinking ever deeper into a state of chronic alcohol poisoning.'[14] The alarm of commentators is even more striking given their unawareness of official statistical data for certain medical and forensic trends such as suicide rates in the Soviet Union, which were considered 'sensitive' and hence strictly kept under lock and key.[15]

Although the negative impact of heavy drinking was commonly known, it seems that the general public were not overly concerned. One explanation for this indifference towards the effects of alcohol abuse is rooted in the drinking tradition that was prevalent in some regions, which has been described as a 'disturbed permissive culture'.[16] In such a setting, excessive alcohol consumption was socially acceptable, thus shielding heavy drinkers from criticism or peer intervention.[17] Biss argues that in the second half of the twentieth century, large parts of the population tolerated public drinking rituals, bingeing and alcohol-induced violence.[18] Standard vodka bottles were not even resealable, encouraging consumers to finish the bottle once it was opened.[19] Even violent episodes, continuous drinking sprees, abusive behaviour and other forms of damage were tolerated, as long as they did not prompt state interference.[20] The famous actor and singer Vladimir Vyso□tskiĭ (1938–1980) struggled for years with his own substance abuse, which eventually led to his untimely death in 1980. His song 'Nikakoĭ oshibki' (Flawless) addresses the fear of an official psychiatric diagnosis and of institutional treatment, which often involved punishment. A physician's diagnosis marked the watershed between generally accepted social drinking and alcohol substance abuse:

> I come from a strong line, I admit: my grandfather was blind, my father-in-law a drinker. But father-in-law – that's not the blood line! ... Doctor, now from face to face, answer quick: will there be a diagnosis, or rather a verdict?[21]

As long as a person's drinking did not result in official attention in the workplace or by the police, it was hardly ever addressed.

In private settings, heavy drinking was even considered an asset. This was especially true for men, who were encouraged to drink by their peers, thus making drinking 'a male activity'.[22] Masculinity was often expressed by excessive drinking, and alcohol consumption helped to establish hierarchies, for example at work.[23] Various different rites of initiation involved drinking large quantities of alcohol and were commonly expected by colleagues and society. A failure to perform according to these unspoken rules aroused suspicion and resulted in being marked as 'feminine'.[24] Drinking was part of the role performed by Soviet men, and even the official newspaper *Komsomol'ska□ia pravda* (The Komsomol Truth) once warned of the 'emasculation' of official festivities if the availability of alcohol was to be reduced.[25]

These positions undermined the already weak political efforts to curb public alcohol consumption, although the negative effects of excessive drinking were pronounced, especially among men. Male life expectancy rates were steadily decreasing.[26] Dutton suggests that this was due to a number of reasons, such as 'circulatory system diseases as causes of death; the probably increasing death rates from accidents, suicides, and poisonings'.[27] He also suspects that the recorded increase in alcohol consumption per capita between 1959 and 1977 highlights the connection between drinking and disease.

Research on the relationship between gender and alcohol abuse in the Soviet Russian case has shown that both consumption of vodka and displays of violent behaviour increased from the 1960s onwards and that this increase was closely linked to post-Stalinist ideas of masculinity.[28] Drinking was widely regarded as a regular pursuit in Soviet society, and it also provided a safety valve for dissent and discontent. It became the antagonist of the arranged normalcy.[29] Among the wider population no critical conscience about the negative effects of prolonged alcohol abuse developed, and heavy drinking at work or during state holidays was sometimes actively encouraged by senior professionals or communist activists.[30] These kinds of behaviour were considered normal – until an individual was stigmatised and shunned by the diagnostic verdict of 'alcoholic'.[31] Although alcoholism evolved into an ever-growing burden for Soviet society, it was not dealt with in a consistent manner, as the following analysis of alcohol treatment in the Soviet Union shows.

Ideology and official campaigns

The medical treatment of alcoholism in the Soviet context proved to be challenging, since the medical profession was subjected to political pressure. As in most societies, in the Soviet Union alcoholics were stigmatised as morally weak individuals. They were considered 'deviants' and treated like a political problem, because they presented a challenge to the Soviet narrative of societal progress and scientific rationality.[32] Complex and ambiguous social phenomena muddied the clear waters of state-projected societal development towards Communism. In this line of thinking, alcoholism was considered a 'legacy of the past' and progressive members of society were to abstain from drinking (see Figure 12.1).[33]

Similar responses can be identified in Western European countries when abstinence movements, medical scientists and political thinkers have linked alcoholism to irrational and moral degradation, as Jasmin Brötz has shown in relation to late nineteenth-century and early twentieth-century Germany in her contribution to this volume (see Chapter 6). Soviet treatment programmes featured a combination of repressive and educational measures in order to eradicate alcoholism from Soviet society. Because excessive drinking was often observed in combination with criminal behaviour, party officials frequently called for compulsive treatment of alcoholics.[34] Since alcoholism challenged state narratives, its treatment was to follow standardised procedures whenever state representatives voiced concerns. This prevented the establishment of low-level interventions, such as local or private initiatives to help alcoholics, and was in stark contrast to treatments in other Eastern European countries, such as Czechoslovakia and Yugoslavia.[35]

The Soviet Union preferred a behavioural explanation for alcoholism over the concept of alcoholism as a disease. Therefore alcohol therapy focused on the de-conditioning of reflexes.[36] As in most fields of Soviet research, the principle of seniority led to a conservative research environment, where proponents of established

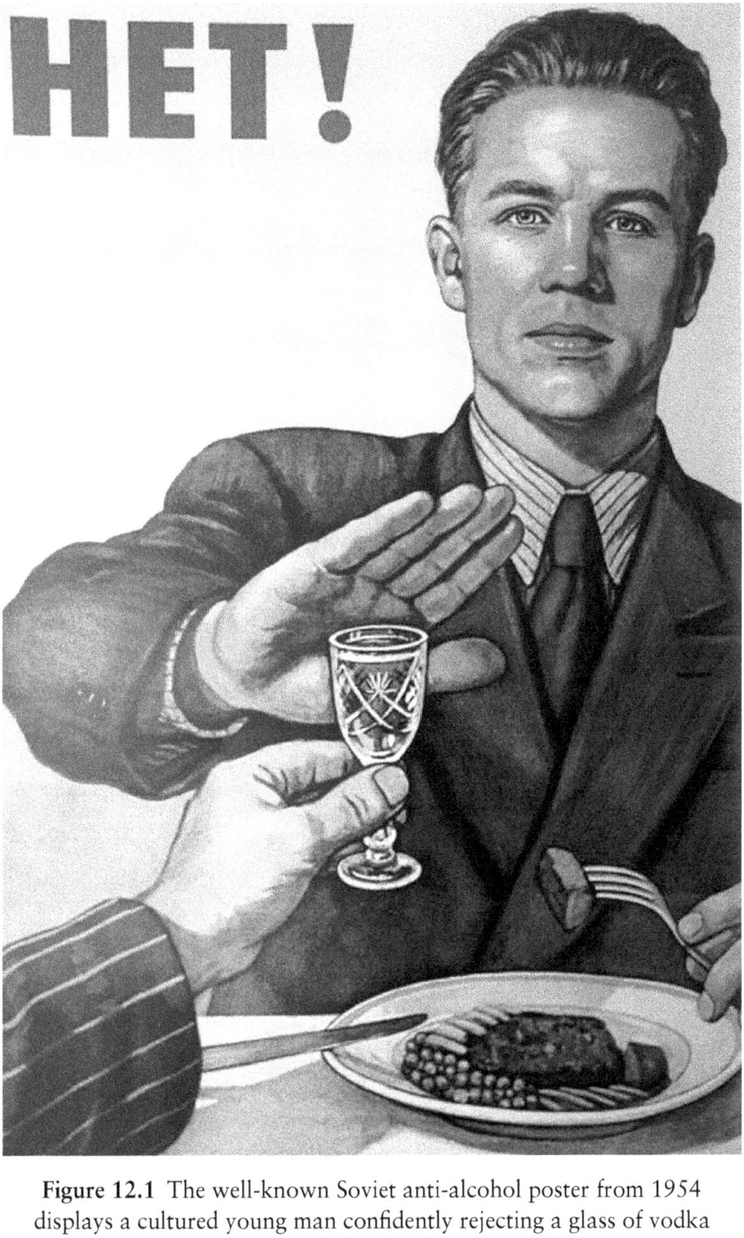

Figure 12.1 The well-known Soviet anti-alcohol poster from 1954 displays a cultured young man confidently rejecting a glass of vodka during a meal, with the simple command 'No!'

truths, such as the Pavlovians, held powerful roles.[37] This restrictive mindset dominated the scientific discourse on alcoholism and its treatment, as well as the administration of the health sector more generally.[38] Even so, some researchers were open to new ideas. For example, the Leningrad-based researcher Igor Sytinsky and Z.P. Gurevitch explained in a Western publication on the Soviet treatment of alcoholism in 1976: ‘Alcoholism is a very complex socio-psychological and medical problem ... a chronic and often recurring illness that has multiple causations including genetic, biological, psychological and sociological factors.’[39] But these conclusions were not sufficient to challenge the predominant ideological assumptions back in the Soviet Union.

The Communist Party and the Ministry of Health were officially in support of moderate drinking because, by itself, alcohol as a substance was not seen as the root of alcoholism. Although the decision of the Council of Ministers of the USSR in ‘O dopolnitel’nikh merakh po usileni□iu bor’by s p’□ianstvom i alkogolizmom’ (On additional measures for reinforcement of the struggle against drunkenness and alcoholism) of 1978 officially ‘intensified both the anti-alcoholic propaganda efficiency and the treatment of alcoholic patients’, it failed to reach its ambitious goal, ‘to eradicate alcoholism’.[40] As Sytinsky had pointed out only a few years earlier,

> the resolution of the Central Committee of the Communist Party of the Soviet Union, ‘On Measures to Enhance the Fight against Drunkenness and Alcoholism’, and the decree of the Presidium of the Supreme Soviet of the RSFSR dated June 9, 1972 issued on its base, have served as powerful stimuli for the elaboration of theoretical and practical aspects of alcoholism.[41]

The new official declarations were inapt when it came to alleviating the yoke of alcoholism; in this sense they were typical of late Soviet policies. As Anderson has pointed out, anti-alcohol campaigns were primarily ‘done by low-level Communist Party activists who have no medical knowledge’.[42] Their efficacy was therefore minimal.

However, there were political attempts to limit drinking in public and to reduce the negative effects of high alcohol consumption.

During Brezhnev's time as leader of the Soviet Union, prices of alcoholic beverages were raised in 1979 and 1981, and new political campaigns against heavy drinking were initiated on different political levels.[43] During the 1980 Summer Olympic Games in Moscow, the USSR even replicated the US policy of relocating alcoholics from urban centres to rural areas, thus removing them from the sight of international visitors.[44] Alcoholism therefore became a problem for officials in rural areas, and it was exacerbated by the fact that higher alcohol prices had revitalised the moonshining tradition of the Russian peasantry, namely the illicit private production and consumption of strong spirits.[45] Brezhnev's successor, Yuriĭ Andropov (1914–1984), intensified measures against alcohol abuse and even lowered alcohol prices in order to counter the negative consequences of private distilling and the abuse of low-grade alcohols. The less expensive legal brands of vodka introduced under Andropov, colloquially called 'Andropovka', also helped to alleviate fiscal losses.[46] This development did not indicate a turn in political intention, but appears to have been introduced as a matter of sheer necessity.

What was the main reason for the overall failure of repeated official attempts to tackle alcoholism? Since the general public lacked awareness of the dangers of alcohol abuse, official government campaigns were widely considered to be untrustworthy – a hallmark of late Soviet propaganda.[47] The government was well aware of its limited ability to re-educate a population that largely supported the common practice of excessive drinking.[48] The general population was accustomed to a discrepancy between official politics and the facts of everyday life, especially when it came to accepting shortages.[49] Consequently, alcohol, especially strong spirits, remained readily available. Consistent measures against drunkenness were not enforced, because the government was well aware of the great importance of alcohol as a means of substance-based escape from everyday life. The state depended upon fiscal revenues from alcohol sales and was not willing to jeopardise societal peace by taking away the soothing pastime of drinking. As long as the population was functional, namely worked hard and paid taxes on spirits, state control was assured.

Narcology: medical and political goals entwined

The greatest change in the Soviet treatment of alcoholics was the emergence of narcology in the 1960s.[50] This new psychiatric field was established for pragmatic reasons: most alcoholics had previously been treated in regular psychiatric hospitals, which could no longer keep up with the increasing number of patients with alcoholism. The overall number of alcoholic inpatients in Soviet psychiatric hospitals had tripled between 1965 and 1978,[51] and other psychiatric conditions increasingly could not be treated appropriately in the then woefully overcrowded institutions.[52]

By the mid-1980s, the profession of the psychiatrist-narcologist was established as an additional medical field in schools, university departments and research facilities.[53] But narcology was far from being an entirely new discipline. Most of its key elements had already become established decades earlier and merely merged 'into a coordinated and interlocking system' of coercion and medical treatment.[54] Unlike the Czechoslovak example, where local initiatives or interested professionals became trailblazers of successful alcoholism therapy, addiction treatment in the Soviet Union remained within the realm of psychiatric clinics and was policed by security institutions.[55] The fabric of the Soviet clinical regime was steeped in this repressive approach, as illustrated by the oath taken by Soviet doctors. Besides being duty-bound to preserve the 'noble traditions of national medicine', the Soviet physician was obliged to 'always obey and promote principles of Communist morality' and be ever-mindful of the honourable title of a 'Soviet physician ... always acting responsibly for the people and the Soviet state'.[56] Thus, aside from their role as physicians, medical personnel also fulfilled policing obligations.

One important innovation in the field of narcology was not related to alcoholism itself, but was connected to its administrative set-up. The Ministry of Health and the Ministry of Internal Affairs were jointly in charge of alcohol treatment, thus reflecting the Soviet view of alcoholism as both criminal offence and medical condition.[57] Official state publications openly called for 'psycho-hygienic and prophylactic work both inside' and outside institutions, alongside preventive measures and medical interventions.[58] Narcology was established in order to ensure continuous surveillance of patients by the Ministry of Internal Affairs and the Ministry of Health, with the former having the last say in the case of any potential difference of opinion.[59]

The field of narcology was not only focused on alcohol – involving research, medical examinations and treatment – but was also based on coercion. Narcology seeped into the structures of everyday Soviet life as broad networks of narcological dispensaries in the work sphere were established alongside the organisation of independent workshops and departments at industrial factories, where alcoholics continued to work while receiving medical treatment.[60] One narcologist praised the 'possibilities in social-labour re-adaptation of alcoholic patients by helping them to stop hard drinking and return them to the normal social-productive life'.[61] Despite the comprehensive authority of narcology, a distinction (with regard to their respective functions) between LTPs and 'drunk-tanks', on the one hand, and research facilities, on the other, was officially upheld. According to this separation, the former were under the jurisdiction of the Ministry of Internal Affairs, while the latter remained under the control of the Ministry of Health.[62] As both ministries cooperated closely, narcologists were in fact provided with powers commonly reserved for the police. Narcologists thus held the authority to interfere in the private and work sphere alike in order to enforce ideas of normalcy. This panoptical approach relied on co-workers and relatives to discipline and report on the drinking behaviour of potential alcoholics.[63] Even healthcare professionals monitored each other's alcohol consumption.[64] Fear of coercion caused potential alcoholics to stop drinking in order to avoid forced contact with health institutions, counselling and doctors.[65] This development was encouraged by diagnostic categories that lacked clarity, as related in the popular Vyso□tskiĭ song mentioned above. Narcology fostered a precedence of the penal code. Difficulty in abstaining after a couple of drinks was considered a 'pathological drive towards alcohol' and therefore constituted an official reason for treatment, even against the patient's will.[66] Enforced treatment was usually the unavoidable endpoint of a heavy drinker's struggle with drinking, although narcology always provided alternative voluntary medical treatment options earlier on.

Medical treatment, stigma, labour and social control

Alcoholism was the most commonly diagnosed condition in regular psychiatric institutions. By the end of the Soviet era alcoholics made up roughly one half of the total number of patients in psychiatric hospitals, as well as in clinics attached to factories and dispensaries, where medicine and other treatment were administered.[67] The majority of patients with alcoholism in dedicated treatment centres were admitted involuntarily, though some did go voluntarily to sober up, obtaining free care and receiving sick pay at the same time.[68]

Narcology addressed those deemed to be substance abusers in a plethora of situations and at different stages. Potential alcoholics were initially confronted with psychiatrist-narcologists and police officers, not with social workers, since this profession did not exist in the Soviet Union.[69] The patient's fate was then determined not only by medical necessity, but also by the availability of particular treatments and on the basis of ideological preconditions. Some forms of treatment, like altitude chambers or specific medication, were not readily available on the medical map of the late Soviet Union and were therefore limited to patients in large urban institutions.[70]

The anthropologist Eugene Raikhel outlined three different avenues in the admittedly fairly heterogeneous treatment of Soviet alcoholics.[71] Those in one group, usually first-time patients, were treated locally as outpatients, in local clinics or in psychiatric hospitals. More serious cases were admitted to narcological clinics, where they participated in work therapy, providing a cheap work force, with 40 per cent of the earnings being kept by the institution.[72] The last group of patients, so-called chronic alcoholics 'who [were] considered dangerous to society', were sent to special colonies or LTPs.[73] The purpose of these institutions was to isolate patients from society in order to provide 'compulsory treatment and labour re-education', which could last from six months to up to two years. Alcoholics were sent to the LTPs by district courts without a chance to appeal the verdict.[74]

The first time many heavy drinkers came into contact with narcology was in one of the many drunk tanks in the Soviet Union at that time. These holding cells were maintained to supervise intoxicated people until they sobered up. Depending on the size of the facility, up to thirty beds might be available for patients who were picked up in a severely intoxicated state, usually during night-time. In the morning, patients were required to pay a fee to the nurse on site, and failing this they were transferred to hospitals for further treatment.[75] The public were aware of drunk tanks, not least because they entered popular consciousness in 1971 through Vladimir Vyso□tskiĭ's song 'Militseĭskiĭ protokol' (Police protocol), in which he describes two friends picked up by the designated police squad and brought to a drunk tank. The song goes on to recount how, as the morning dawns and they awaken, the narrator suggests to his friend that they continue drinking.[76] Each year, drunk tanks were frequented by up to 15 per cent of the adult population of the USSR.[77] These institutions were criticised for not providing sufficient medical care and for neglecting drunken inmates, frequently with fatal consequences. As Treml suggests, the high number of alcohol-related fatalities was therefore caused not solely by excessive drinking, but also by the 'deterioration of the quality and availability of health and medical services in the USSR'.[78] Treml, writing in 1982, suspected these institutions of 'benign neglect', for alcoholics were officially stigmatised and their lives were not held in high esteem.[79] Since the cells were overseen by local police, they also served punitive purposes. An involuntary overnight stay at a holding station usually also resulted in notification of the individual's employer.[80] This measure aggravated social pressure at work and triggered financial concerns, since employers were able to withhold as much as one third of monthly pay or to cancel or reduce vacation entitlements in a case of poor performance, especially if this was due to alcohol abuse.[81]

Outpatient detoxification at hospitals lasted from eight to ten days, during which time vitamins, tranquillisers and antidepressants were administered.[82] Some factories even had their own dispensaries, where on-site alcohol therapy was provided, including detoxification, medical and psychological evaluations and, eventually, prophylactic work therapy. These measures could be prolonged indefinitely, and, even after treatment was considered completed, patients remained on the passive register of the respective dispensary for a minimum of two years.[83] These registers primarily served purposes of social control, and policing not only helped state healthcare institutions to evaluate dispensaries' overall performance, but also allowed close supervision of former and active patients. They therefore contributed to the overall climate of control in the health sector. Once on the list, the patient was not allowed to hold occupations of responsibility or obtain a driving licence or a gun permit.[84] In 1984 2.7 million people were registered as alcoholics, amounting to about 2 per cent of the Soviet population.[85]

Not every alcoholic was treated on an outpatient basis, and personnel were aware of institutions' limitations, especially when it came to 'degraded alcoholics'.[86] Some of the more severe cases with little hope of recovery remained outpatients. This enabled them to live in their familiar surroundings, with family or work ties more or less functional. While this was sometimes justified as a means of upholding the patients' social setting, it also allowed the state to avoid costly periods of treatment.[87] Outpatient treatment, to some degree, mirrored Soviet ideas of collectivism and socially useful work, and was aimed at convincing patients of their irrational state, thus healing them as individuals and as social beings; Michel Foucault's analysis of psychiatric institutions during the European Enlightenment was based on a critique of a similar kind of thinking.[88] Although alcoholism was considered incurable, one case of complete convalescence is documented. The psychiatric Serbsky Institute in the centre of Moscow 'cured' the alcoholic Yuriĭ Brezhnev (1933–2013) after three weeks of treatment for alcoholism.[89] He was the son of the leader of the Soviet Union in 1964–82, Leonid Brezhnev. Prominent patients, it seems, could be freed of the branding 'alcoholic'.

Like other fields of psychiatry, narcology emphasised the curative function of work when it came to re-integrating people exhibiting deviant behaviour into society. In the Soviet Union the role of labour was of fundamental importance and was repeatedly mentioned in the Brezhnev Constitution of 1977.[90] Failure to work was considered parasitic and therefore pathological.[91] Not only did the vocabulary used by Soviet psychiatrists bear resemblance to National Socialist phraseology, but, as E. Follath and R. Oltmanns have pointed out, the psychiatrists also made use of German research that had originally supported the Nazi euthanasia programme during World War II.[92] Soviet psychiatry and narcology depicted useful work as a prime indicator of successful medical treatment.[93] Ideas of rehabilitation were thus closely connected to the patient's work performance, ultimately determining their social standing and political allegiance.[94] Accordingly, poor work performance due to alcohol consumption was a fast track to involuntary therapy. As Anderson noted, 'A 1967 decree permit[ted] compulsory treatment for alcoholics who "violate[d] labour discipline, public order, and the rules of the socialist community".'[95] Work therapy did not only serve medical and financial interests; it also combined curative and penal measures – a repeatedly surfacing theme throughout the history of work therapy in clinical settings.[96] The importance of the role of punishment is particularly apparent in the case of LTPs, where patients were mandated to work at factories without receiving any particular medical treatment.[97] It is important to consider that the concept of involuntary patient labour was not limited solely to the context of the psychiatric system, since in the Soviet Union 'work, society and psychiatry [were] intrinsically bound up', as recent comprehensive research has pointed out.[98]

Labour therapy was highly compatible with the Soviet understanding of psychiatry; psychoanalysis and other individual psychotherapeutic approaches, however, were readily dismissed.[99] Although the conflict between Pavlovians and psychoanalysts had ebbed away by the 1960s, psychoanalysis continued to be under attack by Soviet officials because it supposedly supported bourgeois and non-scientific positions. Group counselling, thanks to its collective approach, constituted an acceptable form of talking therapy. Likewise, charismatic psychiatrists, selected staff and recovering alcoholics were encouraged to influence patients by questioning their precarious lifestyle.[100] Whenever Soviet publications or professionals mentioned psychotherapy, they usually referred to lengthy, strictly hierarchical conversations between psychiatrist and patients. Such sessions were peppered with political recommendations and often accompanied by hypnosis. Therapeutic group sessions and work therapy complemented the programme, as social performance and work productivity held substantial ideological value.[101] Treatment also included clinically administered drugs. A combination of methods was used in aversion therapy, also known as conditioned reflex therapy, and in Disulfiram therapy.[102]

Aversion or conditioned reflex therapy attempted to create a link between alcohol and negative connotations, the aim being that the sight, smell and taste of alcohol would induce reactions like nausea and vomiting. This goal was achieved by injecting patients with the emetic apomorphine, after which they consumed an alcoholic drink, which they were not able to keep down. Narcologists also called this procedure active anti-alcohol therapy.[103] Because of the efficacy and immediate results witnessed by patients and physicians, the procedure was highly appraised and was even performed against a patient's will.[104] It is also an example of Pavlovian medical practice, which was highly compatible with the Soviet understanding of alcoholism.

Disulfiram therapy was the second most prominent form of medication-based therapy in narcology. Disulfiram, available in the Soviet Union under the brand name Antabuse, is a medication that inhibits the breakdown of acetaldehyde in the liver, causing discomfort and the symptoms of an immediate hangover when taken with alcohol. Depending on the amount of alcohol ingested, a life-threatening condition may arise. The medication was given orally, in a subcutaneous injection or as a suppository. Patients treated with Antabuse were informed of the potentially lethal consequences and were required to accept personal liability before treatment; after they were released, their spouses or employers were entrusted with monitoring their continuous sobriety.[105] Because this treatment was given only to selected patients, results were fairly positive. However, once people who were determined to drink removed their implants or were convinced they had received only a placebo, the deterrent effect of Antabuse vanished.[106]

The combination of detoxification, rational conversations with the narcologist, conditioned reflex therapy and disulfiram therapy was the ideal model for treatment proposed by Soviet narcology.

Other factors that were deemed important for recovery involved steady work, a stable social surrounding and the development of new interests, free of alcohol.[107] The success of this ideal approach strongly depended on the patient's cooperation. For unwilling or hesitant alcoholics, the Soviet Union created additional measures that did not require the patient's approval.

Legal and penal measures against alcoholics

Narcology consolidated the links between the medical and penal field, while affirming the moral condemnation of alcoholism. During the mid-1980s, clinically identified alcoholics had to comply with treatment; otherwise they were committing a punishable crime.[108] It is revealing that a substantial number of alcoholics, about 5–6 per cent of the registered alcoholics in the 1980s, underwent compulsory treatment, usually work therapy, in corrective labour colonies under supervision of the Ministry of Internal Affairs.[109] These developments were partly prompted by economic necessity.[110] The institutional association between treatment centre and prison also reflected the continuing Soviet conception of alcoholism as a moral shortcoming.[111]

Compulsory hospitalisation represents one of the most infamous chapters of Soviet psychiatry and received considerable attention in the Western world.[112] Human rights groups like Amnesty International called this practice 'spiritual murder' and a 'variation of gas chambers', while the dissident Andreĭ Amal'rik spoke of 'Stalinism without [open] violence'.[113] The legal provision for coerced treatment appears intentionally vague and vested the medical committees with excessive powers. In 1962 the Ministry of Health issued instruction no. 04–14/32, which listed the criteria required for involuntary hospitalisation. The criteria included aggressive tendencies against people or institutions, 'anomalous' behaviour and a variety of mental disorders – including dissimulation, where patients lack pathological symptoms altogether. In 1969 the instruction was extended by the Ministries of Health and Internal Affairs' joint order no. 345–209, extending the grounds for coerced treatment to 'potentially improper behaviour and socially dangerous tendencies'.[114] Instruction no. 06-14/43 of 26 August 1971, issued by the Ministry of Health, confirmed the practice of pre-emptive treatment whenever a psychiatrist was convinced of the necessity.[115] This development was followed by corresponding regulations for alcoholics and addicts. A Soviet textbook on the treatment of alcoholism demanded: 'When the behaviour of a person suffering from alcoholism or drug addiction is considered socially dangerous, this constitutes an absolute indication for immediate hospitalization.'[116] Because of the broad catalogue of pathological criteria, forensic psychiatrists essentially held universal powers to treat virtually everybody. The orders highlight the close connection between the Ministry of Health and the Ministry of Internal Affairs, even before the establishment of narcology in the mid-1970s. The human rights abuses associated with treating patients against their will have been the target of severe criticism in Western societies, as the anti-psychiatric movement in the late twentieth century has shown.[117]

Soviet authorities sometimes accused political dissidents of being alcoholics in order to incarcerate them in treatment centres. The underground publication *A Chronicle of Current Events* quoted Ida Nudel (born 1931), a Soviet Jewish woman who had repeatedly demanded permission to emigrate to Israel:

> I have waited quietly and obediently for my exit visa. No; rather, I have been a nuisance to the authorities. They put me in prison three times for short periods; in 1973 they fabricated a medical diagnosis that I was an alcoholic, intending to shut me up in a lunatic asylum.[118]

The legislation did not only provide opportunities for abuse and punishment. Some Soviet psychiatrists took advantage of the chance to remove alcoholics from their surroundings in order to protect those most affected by the consequences of excessive drinking. According to Soviet legal understanding, compulsory treatment of alcoholics was acceptable because it was determined by a people's court and therefore legitimised by Soviet society.[119] And despite the Helsinki Conference on Security and Co-operation in Europe in 1975, collective rights still dominated over individual rights in Soviet legal tradition.[120] Narcology was confronted with complaints by

> the great majority of patients in the treatment-and-labour preventoriums [who] do not consider themselves to have alcoholic illness. They thus look upon their stay in the treatment-and-labour preventorium and the compulsory treatment of alcoholism as a punishment.[121]

Any such complaint was considered a lack of insight into one's illness and was hence countered by re-education measures, which could last up to two years.[122]

Inpatients were subjected to the same treatment as outpatients. After detoxification, they underwent aversion or conditioned reflex therapy, and some were treated with disulfiram before being released. Labour therapy played a major role, as did re-education measures. After inpatient treatment, treatment on an outpatient basis was provided for three to four years, with the ultimate goal of 'helping the patients to cease hard drinking and bring them back to the full value of social-industrial activity'.[123] Strikingly, only 'hard drinking' was considered to be the root of all evils, not drinking in general.

Igor Sytinsky praised the important and positive role of the alcoholic's family and community in successful treatment.[124] However, this viewpoint disregards the fact that institutions also heavily relied on information obtained from relatives and co-workers in order to control the alcoholic probationer. Proceedings, eventually leading to repeated forced confinement, were frequently initiated by informers among colleagues, peers and family members, and once suspicious behaviour was reported, the medical process took over again. During the legal proceedings, the alcoholic's procedural rights were revoked. The recidivist was then left in the hands of a medical committee, a procedure which, as reported by Raikhel, was sometimes abused by relatives and even malicious neighbours, who denounced the alcoholic for selfish reasons.[125] This was true not only for substance abusers, but also in the case of potential candidates for a psychiatric institution. Presumption of sanity was not legally enshrined during the process of admission to a medical institution. Rather, the alleged alcoholic, schizophrenic or depressive was required to prove her or his sanity, without the support of legal procedures.[126]

Compulsory treatment for alcoholism provided the same loopholes that prevailed in regard to the potential for abuse in psychiatry, focusing on punitive measures rather than clear diagnostics. Criminals, alcoholics and the mentally ill could all be diagnosed and treated on the basis of similar assumptions and procedures. Significantly, labour therapy centres were overseen by the Ministry of Internal Affairs, which was in charge of the Soviet prison and labour colonies.[127] This moral and administrative proximity between the punitive and the curative was apparent in many elements of the regimes of medical institutions. Even psychiatrists wore uniforms, institutions were surrounded by barbed-wire fences, and escape attempts were treated as criminal offences.[128]

Involuntarily hospitalisation kept alcoholics under a prison-like regime. They could be medicated against their will and were required to perform forced labour. These procedures were officially sanctioned in the name of medical necessity, but in reality remained highly compatible with and hardly separable from the actual penal system. What is more, a steady exchange of prisoners and patients between medical institutions, penal colonies, the Gulag and regular prisons took place, encouraged by vague symptom classifications and ambiguous medical diagnoses. Michel Foucault considered this interchangeability a result of moral condemnation of medical conditions. In this sense, he characterised addiction and psychiatric illness in the Soviet context as 'crime's strange twin'.[129]

Despite the widespread acceptance of liquor in Soviet everyday life, the legal system relentlessly pursued criminal offences committed under the influence of alcohol. Article 39 no. 10 of the Penal Code of the RSFSR of 27 October 1960 called for harsher sentences for inebriated perpetrators.[130] The intention was to deter potential criminals from drinking. Arguably, legislators feared that an exculpating court ruling would increase the numbers of alcohol-related crimes, such as vandalism and assault. The criminalisation of heavy drinking was also consistent with the official government view on alcohol abuse and counted in the courts as an aggravating factor; for example, it could lead to an individual being tried for murder instead of manslaughter. According to Soviet legal scholars, excessive drinking was responsible for the creation of unsafe environments, and it was considered a constitutive precondition for certain crimes.

The penal code also provided the legal foundation for the compulsory medical treatment of alcoholic perpetrators. Potentially, not only did alcoholic criminals face harsher sentences for crimes committed in a state of inebriety, but Article 62 of the above-mentioned legislative text also allowed for additional sentences and coerced treatment for alcohol abuse. During the 1960s, the Supreme Court of the RSFSR proposed to the Supreme Soviet the expansion of legal jurisdiction to non-criminal alcoholics, in order to curb increasing rates of vandalism and street violence.[131] Although the proposal was not successful, the establishment of narcology in the following decade opened the path for the involuntary treatment of alcoholics, which was consistent with the proposal's main intention. Stricter measures against 'hooligans, parasites, and alcoholics' were eventually introduced under Andropov, and were intensified under his successor Konstantin Chernenko (1911–1985). Both of these officials believed alcoholism to be a severe threat to the Soviet people.[132]

Alcoholics kept under lock and key were not treated like non-alcoholic perpetrators. Even the official amnesty when the sixtieth anniversary of the USSR was celebrated in late 1982 excluded detainees who were incarcerated for alcohol-related crimes.[133] This decision was consistent with previous amnesties, like the pardon of 27 June 1980, which was extended to numerous groups of incarcerated patients 'serving sentences of up to five years'.[134] Among the exceptions to this act of grace were 'those serving a sentence, who have not yet completed their course of treatment for alcoholism, drug addiction or venereal disease'.[135] The actual end of a criminal sentence therefore depended upon the *completion* of treatment, which was to be determined by the institution.

Civil court claims and litigation against alcoholics could lead to their being deprived of their parental rights and being evicted from their homes; they were stripped of their legal capacity. If workers sustained injuries in a drunken state, they could be demoted; scientists could lose their university degrees if deemed to be inebriated, and families could be denied compensation if a relative died as a result of alcohol abuse.[136] In the Soviet Union, anti-alcohol legislation can be more accurately described as anti-alcoholism legislation, since alcohol remained a highly esteemed source of national income and social stability. Mikhail Gorbachëv (born 1931) was the only general secretary who tried to tackle the problem on a more comprehensive level.

The political campaign for sobriety under Mikhail Gorbachëv

Although Mikhail Gorbachëv is most commonly associated with the battle against Soviet alcohol abuse, his aspirations for a sober society were not new and merely intensified a political aim that had existed ever since the establishment of the USSR. All four of the general secretaries covered in this chapter attempted to eradicate the grave societal consequences of alcohol abuse, especially its impact on individuals' health and the negative consequences of alcohol abuse for workplace safety and production.[137] Gorbachëv's far-reaching approach began with the resolution 'O merakh po preodoleni□iu p'□ianstva i alkogolizma' (On measures to overcome drunkenness and alcoholism), which was adopted by the Soviet Communist Party on 7 May 1985.[138] The implementation of these measures was fast, as Gorbachëv's polity benefited from the more stringent administrational network that had been re-established during the Andropov era. But Gorbachëv's strategy also differed from that of his predecessors in one important aspect. He identified alcohol as the prime target in the battle against alcoholism and attempted to change societal views on the substance itself.[139] The motivation for this course of action was consistent with his comparatively liberal political position, soon to surface in his groundbreaking (and eventually Union-shattering) reforms. Gorbachëv encouraged people to openly address problems – including the extensive alcoholism prevalent in Soviet society. At the same time, his anti-alcohol campaign was the last project of attempted large-scale 'social engineering directed by the party state'.[140]

A broad catalogue of measures was imposed, including raising the drinking age, an increase in the price of alcohol, a ban on alcohol advertisements, restrictions on the production and availability of alcohol and intensification of anti-alcohol propaganda.[141]

The field of narcology was expanded and strengthened by means of extra funding. New sanctions on public and workplace intoxication were imposed, coerced treatment was made even easier, and new categories of alcohol-related offences were introduced.[142] In combination with the politics of *glasnost* (openness, transparency), the crackdown on alcohol triggered a sharp increase in alcohol-related trials and admissions to treatment centres. According to Biss, under Gorbachëv's administration the former secrecy that had surrounded the topic of alcohol abuse was gradually lifted.[143] In this sense, as in regard to the poor state of the Soviet economy, light was shed upon alcoholism, revealing it to be one of the most (de)pressing societal issues at that time.

The immediate results of these concerted actions were impressive, for heavy drinking in public and in the workplace came to be increasingly condemned among men, and subsequently decreased. While the average life expectancy for men had been only sixty-two years in 1984, it rose to sixty-five in 1987, when the campaign ended. (Life expectancy returned to its initial low level in 1991–92.)[144] Between 1984 and 1988, alcohol-related fatal accidents plummeted and the number of new inpatients for alcoholism treatment decreased by 25 per cent.[145] People who found it difficult to stop or restrict their alcohol consumption continued to drink in illegal bars, in dormitories and in private apartments. In these areas domestic alcohol-related criminal offences increased.[146]

During the Gorbachëv years alcoholics found themselves in an invidious situation, because alcohol ceased to be a readily available commodity. Vodka was substituted with 'shoe polish, cologne, glue, varnish, disinfectants, anti-freeze, insecticides and other toxic spirits', and the black market prospered.[147] This new custom led to a surge in poisonings: in the year 1987, 40,000 people became seriously unwell, and more than a quarter of that number died, as a result of drinking these toxic liquids.[148] Despite the positive impact of Gorbachëv's anti-alcohol measures overall, especially in the medical field, they were disobeyed by a staggering 85 per cent of the overall population.[149] As enthusiasm for Gorbachëv's reforms died away and other political and societal challenges, such as the national independence movements, surfaced, the anti-alcohol campaign soon lost its momentum. When it ended after just three years, alcohol-related death rates soared immediately, especially among Slavic men. The number of male fatalities in the age range from thirty-five to forty-four years rose by 75 per cent.[150] This development was made worse by social and political insecurity, unscrupulous producers of low-grade alcohol and the increasing availability of narcotics.[151] Gorbachëv's campaign therefore could be considered a success – but only while it lasted. After the imposed dry spell, alcoholism raged on.

Narcology ended with the Soviet system, as market economy principles entered the clinical field in post-Soviet Russia. Private and state-sponsored treatment initiatives began to work with patients, and the former exclusive official view on and the moral condemnation of alcoholics was complemented by 'imported methods and movements, ranging from Alcoholics Anonymous to Scientology'.[152] However, the problem of high alcohol consumption was unaltered and, as more recent evidence has shown, Russian alcohol consumption remains extremely high.[153]

Conclusion

This chapter has examined some of the particularities of Russian and Soviet alcohol abuse and the government responses to it. Because the state relied on fiscal revenues from the taxation of alcohol, widespread drinking was tolerated to a certain extent. Private and public alcohol consumption was part of particular regions' culture, and excessively heavy-handed interference by the authorities risked resistance or at least the proliferation of moonshining. At the same time, the pathologisation of heavy drinking, the criminalisation of drunkards and the conflation of punitive and medical treatments within forensic settings and penal work regimes became characteristic of the period preceding Gorbachëv.

It has been shown that Soviet state measures were inapt at changing the firmly entrenched heavy drinking culture. This was especially true for the Slavic and Baltic Soviet republics, where drinking traditions weighed more heavily than in the Muslim republics. The creation of narcology as a field of psychiatry by the Soviet state had established a firm link between health and security politics and provided narcologists with great powers. However, medical concerns were not the only motivation behind this development. It also offered a means of social control and a punitive approach founded on the civil and penal legal opportunities for compulsory medical treatment. Coherent political measures as introduced by Gorbachëv in 1985 alleviated the problems, but the political system collapsed before a change in popular attitudes to alcohol consumption could take hold. As the transition to the Commonwealth of Independent States took shape, political challenges outweighed ambitions to tackle post-Soviet alcoholism in the young republics. Private institutions and self-help groups like Alcoholics Anonymous soon replaced concerted state policies, which for the most part lacked the ambition and public support to successfully address the individual and societal harm of alcoholism.

Notes

1 For a detailed overview and a diverse range of case-studies, see Waltraud Ernst (ed.), *Work, Psychiatry, and Society, c. 1750–2015* (Manchester: Manchester University Press, 2016). Information on LTPs is scarce. For a brief overview on the emergence of the LTPs see F.B. Plotkin, 'Novye tendentsii v rossiĭskoĭ narkologii: vozvrat k starym silovym metodam prinuditel'nogo lecheni□ia' [New tendencies in Russian narcology: a return to the old methods of compulsory treatment], *Independent Psychiatric Journal* (ed. Independent Psychiatric Association of Russia), 4 (2015), 13–24, at 14–15.

2 See for example Mark Lawrence Schrad, *Vodka Politics: Alcohol, Autocracy, and the Secret History of the Russian State* (Oxford: Oxford University Press, 2014); Patricia Herlihy, *The Alcoholic Empire: Vodka and Politics in Late Imperial Russia* (New York: Oxford University Press, 2004).

3 J. Bhattacharya, C. Gathmann and G. Miller, 'The Gorbachev anti-alcohol campaign and Russia's mortality crisis' (NBER Working Paper Series, Working Paper 18589), 1–71, at 3. The non-peer-reviewed working papers from the National Bureau of Economic Research in Cambridge, Massachusetts, can be found online at https://www.nber.org/papers?page=1&perPage=50 (accessed 3 December 2020).

4 V. Treml, 'Death from alcohol poisoning in the USSR', *Soviet Studies*, 34, no. 4 (1982), 487–505, at 487.

5 Treml, 'Death from alcohol poisoning in the USSR', 487.
6 Treml, 'Death from alcohol poisoning in the USSR', 496.
7 S. C. Anderson, 'Alcoholism in the Soviet Union', *International Social Work*, 35, no. 4 (1992), 441–453, at 441.
8 Aleksandr Nemtsov, 'Russia: alcohol yesterday and today', *Addiction*, 100, no. 2 (2005), 146–9, at 146, https://onlinelibrary.wiley.com/doi/pdf/10.1111/j.1360-0443.2005.00971.x (accessed 23 February 2022).
9 D. Tarschys, 'The success of a failure: Gorbachev's alcohol policy, 1985–88', *Europe-Asia Studies*, 45, no. 1 (1993), 7–25, at 16.
10 Tarschys, 'The success of a failure', 16; Anderson, 'Alcoholism in the Soviet Union', 442.
11 Nemtsov, 'Russia: alcohol yesterday and today', 146–7.
12 Tarschys, 'The success of a failure', 16.
13 Bhattacharya, Gathmann and Miller, 'The Gorbachev anti-alcohol campaign', 4.
14 Quoted in Schrad, *Vodka Politics*, 261.
15 W.A. Pridemore, 'Heavy drinking and suicide in Russia', *Social Forces*, 85 no. 1 (2006), 413–30, at 425.
16 C. Biss, *Alkoholkonsum und Trunkenheitsdelikte in Russland mit vergleichenden Bezügen zu Deutschland* (Hamburg: LIT Verlag, 2006), 89.
17 Biss, *Alkoholkonsum und Trunkenheitsdelikte*, 91.
18 Biss, *Alkoholkonsum und Trunkenheitsdelikte*, 94.
19 Treml, 'Death from alcohol poisoning in the USSR', 491.
20 Biss, *Alkoholkonsum und Trunkenheitsdelikte*, 95.
21 V.S. Vysotskiĭ, *Sobranie cochineniĭ v chetyrekh tomakh* [Collected Works in Four Volumes], vol. 2: *Pesni 1971–1980* [Songs 1971–1980] (Moscow: Vremya, 2009).
22 W.D. Connor, 'Alcohol and Soviet society', *Slavic Review*, 30 no. 3 (1971), 570–88, at 574.
23 Connor, 'Alcohol and Soviet society', 581; B.P. Hinote and G.R. Webber, 'Drinking toward Manhood', *Men and Masculinities*, 15, no. 3 (2012), 292–310, at 301.
24 Hinote and Webber, 'Drinking toward manhood', 300, 304.
25 Connor, 'Alcohol and Soviet society', 582.
26 Hinote and Webber, 'Drinking toward manhood', 302, 304; E.A. Raikhel, *Governing Habits: Treating Alcoholism in the Post-Soviet Clinic* (Ithaca: Cornell University Press, 2016), 58.
27 J. Dutton, 'Changes in Soviet mortality patterns, 1959–77', *Population and Development Review*, 5, no. 2 (1979), 267–91, at 289.

28 Hinote and Webber, 'Drinking toward manhood', 304; Connor, 'Alcohol and Soviet society', 576. For gender-based drinking patterns, see S. Eriksen, 'Alcohol as a Gender Symbol', *Scandinavian Journal of History*, 24, no. 1 (2010), 45–73.
29 M. Foucault, *Psychologie und Geisteskrankheit* (Frankfurt am Main: Suhrkamp Verlag, 1968), 94.
30 Sergej V. Jargin, 'Letter to the editor: on the causes of alcoholism in the former Soviet Union', *Alcohol and Alcoholism*, 45 (2010), 104–5, at 104.
31 Connor, 'Alcohol and Soviet society', 580.
32 S.F. Wiseman, 'Communist ideology and the substance abuser: a peripatetic look at the use of the medical paradigm to oppress political deviants', *Journal of Drug Issues*, 15, no. 2 (1985), 247–61, at 248.
33 E.A. Babajan, *Textbook on Alcoholism and Drug Abuse in the Soviet Union* (New York: International Universities Press, 1985), 26.
34 Raikhel, *Governing Habits*, 65.
35 Adéla Gjuričová's contribution on Czechoslovakia in Chapter 11 of this volume illustrates the potential under state Communism for the emergence of alternative approaches that relied on individual initiatives. See also Mat Savelli's discussion of Yugoslavia in Chapter 10 of this volume.
36 Anderson, 'Alcoholism in the Soviet Union', 443.
37 Ivan Pavlov (1849–1936) was a Russian physiologist and Nobel Prize laureate, mostly known for his work on conditioning, according to which (obtained) reflexes determine one's behaviour.
38 Raikhel, *Governing Habits*, 61.
39 I.A. Sytinsky and Z.P. Gurevitch, 'Modern methods in treatment of chronic alcoholism: a review of the Soviet literature', *Addictive Behaviors*, 1, no. 4 (1976), 269–9, at 276.
40 I.A. Sytinsky, 'Alcohol control policy in the USSR', in P.M. Miller and T.D. Nirenberg (eds), *Prevention of Alcohol Abuse* (New York: Plenum Press, 1984), 245–51, at 247.
41 Sytinsky and Gurevitch, 'Modern methods in treatment of chronic alcoholism', 276.
42 Anderson, 'Alcoholism in the Soviet Union', 444.
43 Tarschys, 'The success of a failure', 18.
44 Wiseman, 'Communist ideology and the substance abuser', 256–7.
45 Tarschys, 'The success of a failure', 18.
46 Tarschys, 'The success of a failure', 18.
47 For more on late Soviet double-talk, see A. Yurchak, *Everything Was Forever, until It Was No More: The Last Soviet Generation* (Princeton: Princeton University Press, 2006).

48 Connor, 'Alcohol and Soviet society', 580, 588.
49 On socialist consumption, see Natalya Chernyshova, *Soviet Consumer Culture in the Brezhnev Era* (New York: Routledge, 2013).
50 In 1975 a governmental order separated the narcological system from the established psychiatric regime for pragmatic reasons, since most alcoholics had previously been treated in regular psychiatric hospitals. For a brief overview of Soviet narcology see Plotkin, 'Novye tendentsii v rossiĭskoĭ narkologii', 14–15. Eugene Raikhel devoted large sections of his excellent book to the tradition of narcology in today's Russia and traced it back to Soviet times; see introduction and chapter 2, 'Assembling narcology', in Raikhel, *Governing Habits*.
51 A. Prokopenko (ed.), *Bezumnaja psikhiatriya. Sekretnye materialy o primenenii v SSSR psikhiatrii v karatel'nykh tselyakh* [New Tendencies in Russian Narcology: A Return to the Old Coercive Methods of Compulsory Treatment] (Moscow: Sovershenno sekretno, 1997), 146.
52 Raikhel, *Governing Habits*, 66.
53 Raikhel, *Governing Habits*, 56, 67; Anderson, 'Alcoholism in the Soviet Union', 445.
54 Raikhel, *Governing Habits*, 64, 55.
55 See Gjuričová's discussion in Chapter 11 of this volume.
56 Boris Lewytzkyj (ed.), *Politische Opposition in der Sowjetunion, 1960–1972. Analyse und Dokumentation* (Munich: Deutscher Taschenbuchverlag, 1972), 202.
57 Raikhel, *Governing Habits*, 66.
58 Sytinsky, 'Alcohol control policy in the USSR', 248.
59 Raikhel, *Governing Habits*, 7.
60 Sytinsky, 'Alcohol control policy in the USSR', 249.
61 Sytinsky, 'Alcohol control policy in the USSR', 250. Note the emphasis on hard drinking. Even in the mid-1980s Soviet officials tried to change the drinking behaviour from wine to vodka. Wiseman, 'Communist Ideology and the substance abuser', 254.
62 Raikhel, *Governing Habits*, 66.
63 Raikhel, *Governing Habits*, 68.
64 E. Follath and R. Oltmanns, 'Das Mysterium der vierten Abteilung für Wladimir Bukowski', *Der Stern*, 14 (6 April 1978).
65 Raikhel, *Governing Habits*, 135.
66 Anon., *Sovetskoe ugolovnie pravo. Obshchoe chast'* [Soviet Criminal Law: General Part] (Moscow: □IUrisdicheska□ia Literatura, 1977), 466.
67 Anderson, 'Alcoholism in the Soviet Union', 441.

68 Raikhel, *Governing Habits*, 3; Connor, 'Alcohol and Soviet society', 585.
69 Anderson, 'Alcoholism in the Soviet Union', 444.
70 Sytinsky and Gurevitch, 'Modern methods in treatment of chronic alcoholism', 275; Raikhel, *Governing Habits*, 132.
71 Raikhel, *Governing Habits,* 33.
72 Anderson, 'Alcoholism in the Soviet Union', 441.
73 See Raikhel, *Governing Habits*, 68; quoted in Sytinsky and Gurevitch, 'Modern methods in treatment of chronic alcoholism', 270.
74 Sytinsky and Gurevitch, 'Modern methods in treatment of chronic alcoholism', 271, Plotkin, 'Novye tendentsii v rossiĭskoĭ narkologii', 14–15.
75 Anderson, 'Alcoholism in the Soviet Union', 445.
76 Many versions of the song are available on YouTube; the following clip features video material of drinking and drunk tanks from the late Soviet and early post-Soviet era: https://www.youtube.com/watch?v=F0CLqci2BGY (accessed 9 May 2022).
77 Anderson, 'Alcoholism in the Soviet Union', 445, Treml, 'Death from alcohol poisoning in the USSR', 497–8.
78 Treml, 'Death from alcohol poisoning in the USSR', 498.
79 Treml, 'Death from alcohol poisoning in the USSR', 499.
80 Raikhel, *Governing Habits*, 69.
81 Wiseman, 'Communist ideology and the substance abuser', 257.
82 Anderson, 'Alcoholism in the Soviet Union', 446. Some institutions also gave sulfazine, a chemical to trigger heavy sweating. Anderson, 'Alcoholism in the Soviet Union', 447.
83 Sytinsky, 'Alcohol control policy in the USSR', 248–9; Anderson, 'Alcoholism in the Soviet Union', 445.
84 Raikhel, *Governing Habits*, 70–1.
85 Nemtsov, 'Russia: alcohol yesterday and today'.
86 Sytinsky and Gurevitch, 'Modern methods in treatment of chronic alcoholism', 269.
87 Sytinsky and Gurevitch, 'Modern methods in treatment of chronic alcoholism', 270.
88 Anderson, 'Alcoholism in the Soviet Union', 445; Foucault, *Wahnsinn und Gesellschaft* (Berlin: Suhrkamp, 1973), 427; Amnesty International (ed.), *A Chronicle of Current Events*, nos 37–9 (London: Amnesty International Publications, 1978), 58, https://www.amnesty.org/en/documents/eur46/046/1978/en/ (accessed 30 September 2021).
89 E. Follath and R. Oltmanns, 'Wer verrückt ist, bestimmt die Partei', *Der Stern*, 13 (30 March 1978). Vladimir Serbsky (1858–1917)

dedicated his research largely to the establishment of links between social factors and forensic psychiatry. Although he died shortly after the February Revolution of 1917, his legacy remained untouched, and the Moscow-based State Scientific Centre for Social and Forensic Psychiatry carries his name to the present day. The institution was notorious especially in the second half of the twentieth century, when prominent dissidents were involuntarily admitted to and treated at the Serbsky Centre.

90 E. Schneider (ed.), *Breschnews neue Sowjetverfassung. Kommentar mit den Texten der UdSSR-Grundgesetze von Lenin über Stalin bis heute* (Stuttgart: Verlag Bonn Aktuell, 1978).

91 Amnesty International (ed.), *A Chronicle of Current Events*, nos 37–9, 58.

92 Follath and Oltmanns, 'Das Mysterium der vierten Abteilung für Wladimir Bukowski'.

93 Vasiliĭ IAkovlevich El'meev and Anatoliĭ Pavlovich Kazakov, *Kommunizm i sotsial'nyĭ progress* [Communism and Social Progress] (Leningrad: Izdatel'stvo Leningradskogo Universiteta, 1973), 198.

94 Akademiia Nauk SSSR, Institut gosudarstva i prava (ed.), *Kurs Sovetskogo ugolovnogo prava v shestikh tomakh* [Course of Soviet Criminal Law in Six Volumes], vol. 3: *Nakazanie* [Punishment] (Moscow: Nauka, 1970), 337.

95 Anderson, 'Alcoholism in the Soviet Union', 446.

96 For more information, especially on its origins, see Waltraud Ernst, 'Therapy and empowerment, coercion and punishment: historical and contemporary perspectives on work, psychiatry and society', in Ernst (ed.), *Work, Psychiatry, and Society*, 6.

97 Anderson, 'Alcoholism in the Soviet Union', 446.

98 Ernst, 'Therapy and empowerment, coercion and punishment', 10.

99 M. Thielen, *Sowjetische Psychologie und Marxismus. Geschichte und Kritik* (Frankfurt am Main: Campus Verlag, 1984), 275. Psychoanalysis had been under attack by Soviet officials, as it was thought to reify bourgeois and non-scientific positions. By the 1960s, the conflict between Pavlovians and psychoanalyts had ebbed away, see Alberto Angelini, 'History of the unconscious in Soviet Russia: from its origins to the fall of the Soviet Union', *International Journal of Psychoanalysis,* 89, no. 2 (2008), 369–88, at 376–8.

100 Anderson, 'Alcoholism in the Soviet Union', 447.

101 A striking example of the incompatibility of Western ideas of work therapy and Soviet idolisation of work was witnessed when political changes in Central Eastern European states occurred, such as the

Romanian example after World War II; see Valentin-Teron Toma, 'Work and occupation in Romanian psychiatry', c. 1883–1945', in Ernst (ed.), *Work, Psychiatry, and Society*, 194–219, at 212.

102 Sytinsky and Gurevitch, 'Modern methods in treatment of chronic alcoholism', 274.

103 Sytinsky and Gurevitch, 'Modern methods in treatment of chronic alcoholism', 272.

104 Raikhel, *Governing Habits*, 114–16.

105 Anderson, 'Alcoholism in the Soviet Union', 446–7.

106 Sytinsky and Gurevitch, 'Modern methods in treatment of chronic alcoholism', 273.

107 Anderson, 'Alcoholism in the Soviet Union', 447.

108 Wiseman, 'Communist ideology and the substance abuser', 256.

109 Nemtsov, 'Russia: alcohol yesterday and today'.

110 Connor, 'Alcohol and Soviet society', 585.

111 Raikhel, *Governing Habits*, 55.

112 One of the most comprehensive publications is S. Bloch and P. Reddaway, *Soviet Psychiatric Abuse: The Shadow over World Psychiatry* (Boulder, CO: Westview Press, 1984).

113 C. Mee, *Die Internierung sowjetischer Dissidenten in psychiatrischen Anstalten* (Hamburg: Amnesty International, Deutsche Sektion, 1971), 14; A. Amalrik, *Kann die Sowjetunion das Jahr 1984 erleben?* (Zurich: Diogenes Verlag, 1970), 32.

114 Boris Segal, 'Soviet approaches to involuntary hospitalisation', *International Journal of Social Psychiatry*, 23, no. 2 (1977), 94–102, at 95; Amnesty International (ed.), *A Chronicle of Current Events*, no. 50 (London: Amnesty International Publications, 1979), 99, https://www.amnesty.org/en/documents/eur46/008/1979/en/ (accessed 30 September 2021).

115 E. Nikolajew (ed.), *Gehirnwäsche in Moskau* (Munich: Schulz Verlag, 1983), 259.

116 Babajan, *Textbook on Alcoholism and Drug Abuse in the Soviet Union*, 210.

117 Besides the works of Michel Foucault, much has been published on the potential dangers of psychiatry, e.g. D. Blasius, *Der verwaltete Wahnsinn. Eine Sozialgeschichte des Irrenhauses* (Frankfurt am Main: Fischer Taschenbuchverlag, 1980): A. Monsorno, *Gesellschaft und Geisteskrankheit. Vom Versuch der 'Deinstitutionalisierung' der Psychiatrie in Italien* (Pfaffenweiler: Centaurus Verlag, 1997). The following authors have published comprehensive overviews on this topic; see Henry A. Nasrallah, 'The antipsychiatry movement:

who and why', *Current Psychiatry*, 12 (2011), 4, 6, 56; Mervat Nasser, 'The rise and fall of anti-psychiatry', *Psychiatric Bulletin*, 19 (1995), 743–6. For more current research see Peter Stastny et al. (eds), *Alternatives beyond Psychiatry* (Berlin: Peter Lehmann Publishing, 2007); Thomas Szasz, *Antipsychiatry: Quackery Squared* (Syracuse: Syracuse University Press, 2009).

118 Amnesty International (ed.), *A Chronicle of Current Events*, no. 50, p. 99.

119 Sytinsky, 'Alcohol control policy in the USSR', 250.

120 I. Hieblinger and R. Hieblinger, *Grundzüge des Staatsrechts sozialistischer Staaten. Leitfaden* (Halle an der Saale: Martin-Luther-Universität, 1987), 94; M.-E. Veya, *KSZE: Korb III. Rechtliche Aspekte der östlichen Menschenrechtspolitik* (Berlin: Monath Verlag, 1979), 8; M.G. Zhuravkov, *Sotsializm i moral'. Nekotorye cherty i osobennosti formirovani□ia morali sovetskogo obshchestvo* [Socialism and Morality: Some Features and Qualities of the Formation of the Morality of Soviet Society] (Moscow: Nauka, 1974), 211.

121 Sytinsky, 'Alcohol control policy in the USSR', 250.

122 Sytinsky, 'Alcohol control policy in the USSR', 250.

123 Sytinsky, 'Alcohol control policy in the USSR', 250.

124 Sytinsky, 'Alcohol control policy in the USSR', 249.

125 Raikhel, *Governing Habits*, 69, 74, 173.

126 Amnesty International, *Politische Gefangene in der UdSSR. Ihre Behandlung und ihre Haftbedingungen* (Frankfurt am Main: Fischer Taschenbuchverlag, 1980), 255.

127 Connor, 'Alcohol and Soviet society', 588; Raikhel, *Governing Habits*, 74.

128 Raikhel, *Governing Habits*, p. 74.

129 Foucault, *Wahnsinn und Gesellschaft*, 414–15; Amnesty International (ed.), *A Chronicle of Current Events*, no. 57 (London: Amnesty International Publications, 1981), 119, https://www.amnesty.org/en/documents/eur46/009/1981/en/ (accessed 9 May 2022).

130 Unless otherwise stated, the source for this paragraph is Biss, *Alkoholkonsum und Trunkenheitsdelikte*, 155, 145, 151.

131 Biss, *Alkoholkonsum und Trunkenheitsdelikte*, 144, 151.

132 Wiseman, 'Communist ideology and the substance abuser', 255.

133 Amnesty International (ed.), *A Chronicle of Current Events*, no. 57, p. 119. The legal text of the pardon specifically excludes, for example convicts who served sentences related to strong, poisonous and narcotic substances, malicious hooliganism and other typically alcohol-related crimes. Ukaz Prezidiuma Verkhovnogo Soveta SSSR

[Decree of the Presidium of the Supreme Soviet of the USSR], 'Ob amnistii v sv□iazi s 60-letiem Velikoĭ Okt□iabr'skoĭ sotsialisticheskoĭ revol□iutsii' [On amnesty in connection with the sixtieth anniversary of the Great October Socialist Revolution], http://docs.cntd.ru/document/901701190 (accessed 9 May 2022).

134 Amnesty International (ed.), *A Chronicle of Current Events*, no. 57, p. 119.

135 Amnesty International (ed.), *A Chronicle of Current Events*, no. 57, p. 119.

136 Anderson, 'Alcoholism in the Soviet Union', 448; Raikhel, *Governing Habits*, 68–9; V. Rich, 'Soviet alcoholism: drunk driver stripped of degree', *Nature*, 29 August 1985, 758.

137 Tarschys, 'The success of a failure', 15.

138 The resolution can be found at https://ru.wikisource.org/wiki-Постановление_Совета_Министров_СССР_от_7.05.1985 (accessed 9 May 2022).

139 Tarschys, 'The success of a failure', 7.

140 Raikhel, *Governing Habits*, 39.

141 Bhattacharya, Gathmann and Miller, 'The Gorbachev anti-alcohol campaign', 4; Anderson, 'Alcoholism in the Soviet Union', 450.

142 Bhattacharya, Gathmann and Miller, 'The Gorbachev anti-alcohol campaign', 4–5; Raikhel, *Governing Habits*, 67.

143 Biss, *Alkoholkonsum und Trunkenheitsdelikte*, 15; Raikhel, *Governing Gabits*, 74.

144 Nemtsov, 'Russia: alcohol yesterday and today', 147.

145 Tarschys, 'The success of a failure', 23.

146 Anderson, 'Alcoholism in the Soviet Union', 450.

147 Anderson, 'Alcoholism in the Soviet Union', 450.

148 Anderson, 'Alcoholism in the Soviet Union', 450.

149 Figures are quoted from Patricia Herlihy, *The Alcoholic Empire: Vodka and Politics in Late Imperial Russia* (New York: Oxford University Press, 2002), 157.

150 Bhattacharya, Gathmann and Miller, 'The Gorbachev anti-alcohol campaign', 2.

151 Bhattacharya, Gathmann and Miller, 'The Gorbachev anti-alcohol campaign', 12; Biss, *Alkoholkonsum und Trunkenheitsdelikte*, 16.

152 Raikhel, *Governing Habits*, 182.

153 World Health Organization, *Global Status Report on Alcohol and Health*, 2011, www.who.int/global-status-report-on-alcohol-and-health-2011 (accessed 9 May 2022).

Index

EU authorised representative for GPSR:
Easy Access System Europe, Mustamäe tee 50,
10621 Tallinn, Estonia
gpsr.requests@easproject.com

www.ingramcontent.com/pod-product-compliance
Ingram Content Group UK Ltd.
Pitfield, Milton Keynes, MK11 3LW, UK
UKHW021834100926
8556IPUK00004B/338
* 9 7 8 1 5 2 6 1 5 9 4 0 3 *